Neuroendocrine Neoplasms

Editor

RATHAN M. SUBRAMANIAM

PET CLINICS

www.pet.theclinics.com

Consulting Editor
ABASS ALAVI

April 2023 • Volume 18 • Number 2

ELSEVIER

1600 John F. Kennedy Boulevard • Suite 1800 • Philadelphia, Pennsylvania, 19103-2899

http://www.pet.theclinics.com

PET CLINICS Volume 18, Number 2
April 2023 ISSN 1556-8598, ISBN-13: 978-0-323-93843-3

Editor: John Vassallo (j.vassallo@elsevier.com)
Developmental Editor: Karen Justine S. Dino

PET Clinics (ISSN 1556-8598) is published quarterly by Elsevier Inc., 360 Park Avenue South, New York, NY 10010-1710. Months of issue are January, April, July, and October. Periodicals postage paid at New York, NY, and additional mailing offices. Subscription prices per year are $275.00 (US individuals), $500.00 (US institutions), $100.00 (US students), $304.00 (Canadian individuals), $563.00 (Canadian institutions), $100.00 (Canadian students), $297.00 (foreign individuals), $563.00 (foreign institutions), and $140.00 (foreign students). To receive student and resident rate, orders must be accompanied by name of affiliated institution, date of term, and the signature of program/residency coordinator on institution letterhead. Orders will be billed at individual rate until proof of status is received. Foreign air speed delivery is included in all Clinics subscription prices. All prices are subject to change without notice. POSTMASTER: Send address changes to PET Clinics, Elsevier Health Sciences Division, Subscription Customer Service, 3251 Riverport Lane, Maryland Heights, MO 63043. **Customer Service: 1-800-654-2452 (U.S. and Canada); 314-447-8871 (outside U.S. and Canada). Fax: 314-447-8029. E-mail: journalscustomerservice-usa@elsevier.com (for print support); journalsonlinesupport-usa@elsevier.com (for online support).**

Reprints. For copies of 100 or more of articles in this publication, please contact the Commercial Reprints Department, Elsevier Inc., 360 Park Avenue South, New York, NY 10010-1710. Tel.: 212-633-3874; Fax: 212-633-3820; E-mail: reprints@elsevier.com.

PET Clinics is covered in MEDLINE/PubMed (Index Medicus).

Contributors

CONSULTING EDITOR

ABASS ALAVI, MD, MD (Hon), PhD (Hon), DSc (Hon)
Professor of Radiology and Neurology, Director of Research Education, Division of Nuclear Medicine, Department of Radiology, Hospital of the University of Pennsylvania, Perelman School of Medicine, University of Pennsylvania, Philadelphia, Pennsylvania, USA

EDITOR

RATHAN M. SUBRAMANIAM, MBBS, MD, BMedSc, MClinEd, PhD, MPH, MBA, FRSN, FRANZCR, FACNM, FSNMMI, FAUR
Professor of Radiology and Nuclear Medicine, Department of Medicine, Otago Medical School, University of Otago, Dunedin, New Zealand; Department of Radiology, Duke University, Durham, North Carolina, USA

AUTHORS

CHANDRASEKHAR BAL, MD, DNB, DSc
Professor and Head, Department of Nuclear Medicine, All India Institute of Medical Sciences, New Delhi, India

EDWARD BARNETT, BSc(Hons)
Department of Pathology, Dunedin School of Medicine, University of Otago, Dunedin, New Zealand

LISA BODEI, MD, PhD
Attending, Director, Molecular Imaging and Therapy Service, Memorial Sloan Kettering Cancer Center, New York, New York, USA

KUNAL RAMESH CHANDEKAR, MD
Department of Nuclear Medicine, All India Institute of Medical Sciences, New Delhi, India

ANIRUDDHA CHATTERJEE, BSc, MSc, PhD
Department of Pathology, Dunedin School of Medicine, University of Otago, Dunedin, New Zealand

DILARA DENIZMEN, MD
Resident, Department of Nuclear Medicine, Istanbul Faculty of Medicine, Istanbul University, Istanbul, Turkey

HEYING DUAN, MD
Research Fellow, Department of Radiology, Division of Nuclear Medicine and Molecular Imaging, Stanford University, Stanford, California, USA

AMANDA HENDERSON, BS
Division of Nuclear Medicine and Molecular Imaging, The Russell H. Morgan Department of Radiology and Radiological Science, Johns Hopkins School of Medicine, Baltimore, Maryland, USA

ANDREI IAGARU, MD
Professor, Department of Radiology, Division of Nuclear Medicine and Molecular Imaging, Stanford University, Stanford, California, USA

VETRI SUDAR JAYAPRAKASAM, MBBS, FRCR, FEBNM
Assistant Attending, Molecular Imaging and Therapy Service, Memorial Sloan Kettering Cancer Center, New York, New York, USA

ASHA KANDATHIL, MBBS, DMRD, MD
Department of Radiology, The University of Texas Southwestern Medical Center, Dallas, Texas, USA

WAJAHAT KHATRI, MD
Division of Nuclear Medicine and Molecular Imaging, The Russell H. Morgan Department of Radiology and Radiological Science, Johns Hopkins School of Medicine, Baltimore, Maryland, USA

GUOBING LIU, MD, PhD
Department of Nuclear Medicine, Zhongshan Hospital, Institute of Nuclear Medicine, Shanghai Institute of Medical Imaging, Cancer Prevention and Treatment Center, Zhongshan Hospital, Fudan University, Shanghai, China

CHARLES MARCUS, MD
Assistant Professor, Division of Nuclear Medicine and Molecular Imaging, Department of Radiology and Radiological Sciences, Emory University School of Medicine, Atlanta, Georgia, USA

HYESUN PARK, MD
Department of Radiology, Lahey Hospital and Medical Center, Burlington, Massachusetts, USA

CHI QI, PhD
Department of Nuclear Medicine, Zhongshan Hospital, Institute of Nuclear Medicine, Fudan University, Shanghai Institute of Medical Imaging, Shanghai, China

AJITHA RAMESH, MBBS
Dunedin Hospital, Dunedin, New Zealand

EUAN J. RODGER, BSc, MSc, PhD
Department of Pathology, Dunedin School of Medicine, University of Otago, Dunedin, New Zealand

STEVEN P. ROWE, MD, PhD
Associate Professor, Division of Nuclear Medicine and Molecular Imaging, The Russell H. Morgan Department of Radiology and Radiological Science, Johns Hopkins School of Medicine, Baltimore, Maryland, USA

YASEMIN SANLI, MD
Professor, Department of Nuclear Medicine, Istanbul Faculty of Medicine, Istanbul University, Istanbul, Turkey

SWAYAMJEET SATAPATHY, MD
Department of Nuclear Medicine, All India Institute of Medical Sciences, New Delhi, India

HONGCHENG SHI, MD, PhD
Department of Nuclear Medicine, Zhongshan Hospital, Institute of Nuclear Medicine, Shanghai Institute of Medical Imaging, Cancer Prevention and Treatment Center, Zhongshan Hospital, Fudan University, Shanghai, China

JIM SMITH, MBChB, BMedSc(Hons)
Department of Pathology, Dunedin School of Medicine, University of Otago, Southern District Health Board, Dunedin Public Hospital, Dunedin, New Zealand

LILJA B. SOLNES, MD, MBA
Associate Professor, Division of Nuclear Medicine and Molecular Imaging, The Russell H. Morgan Department of Radiology and Radiological Science, Johns Hopkins School of Medicine, Baltimore, Maryland, USA

ERGI SPIRO, BS
Division of Nuclear Medicine and Molecular Imaging, The Russell H. Morgan Department of Radiology and Radiological Science, Johns Hopkins School of Medicine, Baltimore, Maryland, USA

RATHAN M. SUBRAMANIAM, MBBS, MD, BMedSc, MClinEd, PhD, MPH, MBA, FRSN, FRANZCR, FACNM, FSNMMI, FAUR
Professor of Radiology and Nuclear Medicine, Department of Medicine, Otago Medical School, University of Otago, Dunedin, New Zealand; Department of Radiology, Duke University, Durham, North Carolina, USA

Contents

Erratum xi

Preface: Neuroendocrine Neoplasms: Molecular Imaging and Therapy xiii

Rathan M. Subramaniam

Neuroendocrine Neoplasms: Epidemiology, Diagnosis, and Management 161

Ajitha Ramesh, Aniruddha Chatterjee, and Rathan M. Subramaniam

Neuroendocrine tumors have variety of biological and clinical characteristics. The classification of neuroendocrine neoplasm has evolved, and the newest 2019 World Health Organization classification outlines a well-differentiated high-grade G3 subtype, recognizing its differences from the poorly differentiated neuroendocrine carcinoma. ^{68}Ga-DOTAT PET has largely replaced somatostatin scintigraphy as the diagnostic workup choice for NENs. NETest, a multi-analyte liquid biopsy, is a promising recent development in the biochemical diagnosis. Management includes wait and watch approach, surgical resection, somatostatin analogs, ^{177}Lu DOTATATE therapy, chemotherapy, radiotherapy or immunotherapy combinations. Further clinical trials are necessary for determining the appropriate sequencing.

Neuroendocrine Neoplasms: Genetics and Epigenetics 169

Jim Smith, Edward Barnett, Euan J. Rodger, Aniruddha Chatterjee, and Rathan M. Subramaniam

Neuroendocrine neoplasms (NENs) are a group of rare, heterogeneous tumors of neuroendocrine cell origin, affecting a range of different organs. The clinical management of NENs poses significant challenges, as tumors are often diagnosed at an advanced stage where overall survival remains poor with current treatment regimens. In addition, a host of complex and often unique molecular changes underpin the pathobiology of each NEN subtype. Exploitation of the unique genetic and epigenetic signatures driving each NEN subtype provides an opportunity to enhance the diagnosis, treatment, and monitoring of NEN in an emerging era of individualized medicine.

Gastroenteropancreatic Neuroendocrine Tumor Diagnosis: DOTATATE PET/CT 189

Asha Kandathil and Rathan M. Subramaniam

Gastroenteropancreatic neuroendocrine tumors(NETs), which arise from the small intestine, rectum, colon, appendix, or pancreas, have variable malignant potential with clinical behavior determined by proliferative activity according to the Ki-67 index and tumor differentiation. Somatostatin receptor (SSTR) expression by NETs allows SSTR imaging using 68Ga-DOTATATE PET/computed tomography (CT) and treatment with octreotide or SSTR-targeted peptide receptor radionuclide therapy (PRRT). 68Ga-DOTATATE PET/CT is indicated for localization of the primary tumor in select cases, staging patients with known NET, and selecting patients for PRRT. NCCN guidelines consider imaging with 68Ga-DOTATATE PET/CT appropriate for staging and receptor status assessment.

Gastro-Enteric-Pancreatic Neuroendocrine Tumor Treatment: ^{177}Lu-DOTATATE 201

Yasemin Sanli, Dilara Denizmen, and Rathan M. Subramaniam

177Lu-DOTA-TATE therapy is a highly effective therapy in metastatic, well-differentiated, somatostatin receptor-positive GEP-neuroendocrine tumors (NETs) with mostly tolerable adverse effects. Guidelines generally refer to peptide receptor radionuclide therapy as a second-line therapy after SSA in gastroenteric and second- or third-line therapy in pancreatic NETs to improve survival rates and quality of life. Although we do not have sufficient data, 177Lu-DOTA-TATE therapy may also have a role in high-grade NET therapy, mostly in combination with other treatments such as chemotherapy.

Gastro-Enteric-Pancreatic Neuroendocrine Tumor Treatment: Actinium-225-DOTATATE and Combined Therapies 215

Swayamjeet Satapathy, Kunal Ramesh Chandekar, and Chandrasekhar Bal

The role of lutetium-177-DOTATATE in advanced well-differentiated gastro-entero-pancreatic neuroendocrine tumors is well established. However, there is a scope for improving treatment outcomes. Actinium-225-DOTATATE is a form of targeted alpha therapy (TAT) that results in more efficient tumor cell killing owing to the substantially higher linear energy transfer of alpha particles. Systemic TAT is also safe given that the shorter path length of the alpha particles spares the surrounding healthy tissue and results in relatively fewer adverse events. Combination therapies with radiosensitizing and other chemotherapeutic agents have also gained popularity, especially in the setting of higher grade and fluorodeoxyglucose-avid tumors.

Diagnosis and Treatment of Lung Neuroendocrine Neoplasms: Somatostatin Receptor PET Imaging and Peptide Receptor Radionuclide Therapy 223

Hyesun Park and Rathan M. Subramaniam

Recently, advancement of somatostatin receptor (SSTR) imaging and theragnostic approach using peptide receptor radionuclide therapy (PRRT) have changed the paradigm of diagnosis and management of neuroendocrine tumor. 68Ga-DOTA-TATE PET/CT can diagnose the lung carcinoids with high SSTR expression. With combination of 68Ga-DOTATATE PET/CT and 18F-FDG PET/CT, tumor heterogeneity of lung carcinoid can be identified, which may guide optimal patient selection for PRRT. PRRT may be an effective and safe treatment of advanced lung carcinoids during progression with first-line somatostatin analog therapy. This review provides updates on the diagnosis and management of lung carcinoids, focusing on SSTR imaging and PRRT.

Paragangliomas and Pheochromocytomas: Positron Emission Tomography/Computed Tomography Diagnosis and Therapy 233

Charles Marcus and Rathan M. Subramaniam

Molecular imaging evaluation of pheochromocytomas and paragangliomas depends on multiple factors, such as localized versus metastatic disease, the genetic, and biochemical profile of tumors. Positron emission tomography/computed tomography (PET/CT) imaging of these tumors outperforms Meta-Iodo-Benzyl-Guanidine (MIBG) scintigraphy in most cases. A few PET radiotracers have been studied in evaluating these patients with somatostatin receptor PET imaging and have shown superior performance compared with other agents in most of these patients. 18F-fluorodeoxyglucose PET/CT imaging is useful in select patients, such as those with succinate dehydrogenase complex subunit B–associated disease. Treatment strategy depends on multiple factors and necessitates a multidisciplinary approach.

Gastro-Entero-Pancreatic Tumors: FDG Positron Emission Tomography/Computed Tomography 243

Wajahat Khatri, Ergi Spiro, Amanda Henderson, Steven P. Rowe, and Lilja B. Solnes

Gastro-entero-pancreatic tumors comprise a group of heterogenous neoplasms, with medical imaging being paramount in the diagnosis, staging, and treatment planning of these tumors. Moreover, with the advent of newer radiopharmaceuticals, such as 68 Ga-labeled and 64 Cu-labeled somatostatin analogs (eg, 68 Ga-DOTATOC, 68 Ga-DOTATATE, 68 Ga-DOTANOC, and 64Cu-DOTATATE) that bind to the somatostatin receptor (SSTR), molecular imaging plays an increasing and critical role in the diagnosis, staging, and treatment planning of these neoplasms. Dual-tracer imaging with 18F-FDG PET/CT and SSTR agents may play a significant role in treatment planning and predicting patient outcomes in the setting of high-grade or poorly differentiated neuroendocrine tumors.

Neuroendocrine Neoplasms: Total-body PET/Computed Tomography 251

Guobing Liu, Chi Qi, and Hongcheng Shi

Total-body PET/computed tomography (CT) (uExplorer) static and dynamic scan using low-dose (48.1 to 73.6 MBq) gallium-68 (^{68}Ga) DOTATATE combined with low-dose (1.55 MBq/kg) or ultra-low-dose (0.37 MBq/kg) 18F-fluorodeoxyglucose (18F-FDG) were used as a routine in patients with neuroendocrine neoplasms (NENs). ^{68}Ga DOTATATE and 18F-FDG PET/CT static imaging play complementary roles in diagnosis, staging, and therapy-response evaluation in a patient with NENs. Kinetic parameters and time activity curve derived from the dynamic scan is helpful for understanding tumors biological characteristics and differential diagnosis of NENs.

Neuroendocrine Tumor Diagnosis: PET/MR Imaging 259

Heying Duan and Andrei Iagaru

Imaging plays a critical role in the diagnosis and management of neuroendocrine tumors (NETs). The initial workup of the primary tumor, including its characterization, local and distant staging, defines subsequent treatment decisions. Functional imaging using hybrid systems, such as PET combined with computed tomography, has become the gold standard. As NETs majorly arise from the gastrointestinal system and metastasize primarily to the liver, simultaneous PET and MR imaging with its high soft tissue contrast might be a valuable clinical one-stop-shop whole-body imaging tool. This review presents the current status and challenges of PET/MR imaging for diagnosis of NETs.

Neuroendocrine Tumor Therapy Response Assessment 267

Vetri Sudar Jayaprakasam and Lisa Bodei

Peptide receptor radionuclide therapy has become an integral part of management of neuroendocrine neoplasms. Gallium-68- and lutetium-177-labeled somatostatin receptor analogues have replaced yttrium-90- and 111-indium-based tracers. Several newer targeted therapies are also being used in clinical and research settings. It is imperative to accurately evaluate the response to these agents. The characteristics of NENs and the response patterns of the targeted therapies make response assessment in this group challenging. This article provides an overview of the strengths and weaknesses of the various biomarkers available for response assessment.

PET CLINICS

FORTHCOMING ISSUES

July 2023
Fibroblast Activation Protein Imaging
Frederik L. Giesel, Rodney J. Hicks, and Ken Herrmann, *Editors*

October 2023
Breast Cancer: Advances in Molecular Imaging
Gary A. Ulaner and Amy M. Fowler, *Editors*

January 2024
Advances in Organ-specific PET Instrumentation
Abass Alavi, Habib Zaidi, and Suleman Surti, *Editors*

RECENT ISSUES

January 2023
Critical Role of PET in Assessing Age Related Disorders
Abass Alavi, Babak Saboury, Ali Gholamrezanezhad, *Editors*

October 2022
Prostate Cancer
Harshad R. Kulkarni and Abass Alavi, *Editors*

July 2022
FDG vs. non-FDG Tracers in Less Explored Domains: An Appraisal
Sandip Basu, Rakesh Kumar, and Abass Alavi, *Editors*

PROGRAM OBJECTIVE

The goal of the *PET Clinics* is to keep practicing radiologists and radiology residents up to date with current clinical practice in positron emission tomography by providing timely articles reviewing the state of the art in patient care.

TARGET AUDIENCE

Practicing radiologists, radiology residents, and other health care professionals who provide patient care utilizing radiologic findings.

LEARNING OBJECTIVES

Upon completion of this activity, participants will be able to:

1. Review origins, classifications, and clinical behaviors of neuroendocrine neoplasms.
2. Discuss most common neuroendocrine neoplasms, such as gastro-enteric-pancreatic neuroendocrine tumors, and identify current treatment options.
3. Recognize diagnostic modalities used to confirm, stage, assist in treatment, and assess therapy responses with neuroendocrine neoplasms.

ACCREDITATION

The Elsevier Office of Continuing Medical Education (EOCME) is accredited by the Accreditation Council for Continuing Medical Education (ACCME) to provide continuing medical education for physicians.

The EOCME designates this journal-based CME activity for a maximum of 11 *AMA PRA Category 1 Credit*(s)™. Physicians should claim only the credit commensurate with the extent of their participation in the activity.

All other health care professionals requesting continuing education credit for this enduring material will be issued a certificate of participation.

DISCLOSURE OF CONFLICTS OF INTEREST

The EOCME assesses conflict of interest with its instructors, faculty, planners, and other individuals who are in a position to control the content of CME activities. All relevant conflicts of interest that are identified are thoroughly vetted by EOCME for fair balance, scientific objectivity, and patient care recommendations. EOCME is committed to providing its learners with CME activities that promote improvements or quality in healthcare and not a specific proprietary business or a commercial interest.

The planning committee, staff, authors, and editors listed below have identified no financial relationships or relationships to products or devices they or their spouse/life partner have with commercial interest related to the content of this CME activity:

Chandrasekhar Bal, MD, DNB, DSc; Edward Barnett, BSc(Hons); Lisa Bodei, MD, PhD; Kunal Ramesh Chandekar, MD; Aniruddha Chatterjee, BSc, MSc, PhD; Dilara Denizmen; Heying Duan, MD; Amanda Henderson, BS; Andrei Iagaru, MD; Vetri Sudar Jayaprakasam, MBBS, FRCR, FEBNM; Lynette Jones, MSN, RN-BC; Asha Kandathil, MBBS, DMRD, MD; Wajahat Khatri, MD; Mohana Manoj Krishnamoorthy, Guobing Liu, MD, PhD; Charles Marcus, MD; Hyesun Park, MD; Chi Qi, PhD; Ajitha Ramesh, MBBS; Euan J. Rodger, BSc, MSc, PhD; Yasemin Sanli, MD; Swayamjeet Satapathy, MD; HuHongcheng Shi, MD, PhD; Jim Smith, MBChB, BMedSc (Hons); Ergi Spiro, BS; Rathan M. Subramaniam, MD, MPH, PhD, MBA, FRSN, FRANZCR, FACNM, FSNMMI, FAUR

The planning committee, staff, authors, and editors listed below have identified financial relationships or relationships to products or devices they or their spouse/life partner have with commercial interest related to the content of this CME activity:

Steven P. Rowe, MD, PhD: Research funding and consulting: Progenics Pharmaceutical, Inc., Precision Molecular, Inc., PlenaryAI, Inc.; Ownership interest: Precision Molecular, Inc., PlenaryAI, Inc.

Lilja B. Solnes, MD, MBA: Research funding: Novartis AG Pharmaceutical Company, Cellectar, Inc., Precision Molecular, Inc.; Consultant: Progenics Pharmaceutical, Inc.

UNAPPROVED/OFF-LABEL USE DISCLOSURE

The EOCME requires CME faculty to disclose to the participants:

1. When products or procedures being discussed are off-label, unlabelled, experimental, and/or investigational (not US Food and Drug Administration [FDA] approved); and
2. Any limitations on the information presented, such as data that are preliminary or that represent ongoing research, interim analyses, and/or unsupported opinions. Faculty may discuss information about pharmaceutical agents that is outside of FDA-approved labelling. This information is intended solely for CME and is not intended to promote off-label use of these medications. If you have any questions, contact the medical affairs department of the manufacturer for the most recent prescribing information.

TO ENROLL

To enroll in the *PET Clinics* Continuing Medical Education program, call customer service at 1-800-654-2452 or sign up online at http://www.theclinics.com/home/cme. The CME program is available to subscribers for an additional annual fee of USD 254.00.

METHOD OF PARTICIPATION

In order to claim credit, participants must complete the following:

1. Complete enrolment as indicated above.
2. Read the activity.
3. Complete the CME Test and Evaluation. Participants must achieve a score of 70% on the test. All CME Tests and Evaluations must be completed online.

CME INQUIRIES/SPECIAL NEEDS

For all CME inquiries or special needs, please contact elsevierCME@elsevier.com.

Erratum

In the January 2023 *PET Clinics* (Volume 18, number 1) article, "Brain PET Imaging: Approach to Cognitive Impairment and Dementia," pages 103-113, an author's name was missing the initial. The author should be listed as "Ana M. Franceschi, MD, PhD."

PET Clin 18 (2023) xi
https://doi.org/10.1016/j.cpet.2023.01.002

Preface

Neuroendocrine Neoplasms: Molecular Imaging and Therapy

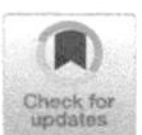

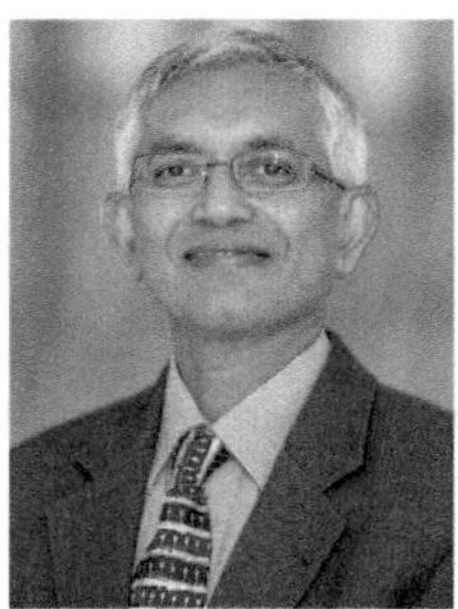

Rathan M. Subramaniam, MBBS, PhD, MPH, MBA, FRANZCR, FACNM, FSNMMI, FAUR
Editor

There have been transformative changes in molecular imaging diagnosis and radiopharmaceutical therapy for neuroendocrine neoplasms. This issue of *PET Clinic* "Neuroendocrine Neoplasms: Molecular Imaging and Therapy" updates critical basic and clinical practice aspects of PET imaging and therapy.

^{68}Ga-DOTATATE and ^{18}F-FDG-PET/CT are now used as the standard of care in the molecular imaging phenotyping of patients. As DOTATATE PET/CT is more sensitive for well-differentiated, and FDG-PET/CT is more sensitive for poorly differentiated, neuroendocrine neoplasms or neuroendocrine carcinomas, these two imaging tests provide complementary information that allows the most accurate phenotyping, illustrating the intralesion and interlesion heterogeneity of these tumors. Moderate to intense DOTATATE uptake (above liver uptake) indicates sufficient expression of somatostatin type-2 receptors, making patients eligible for ^{177}Lu DOTATATE therapy. However, FDG-PET/CT provides prognostic information, as patients with no FDG uptake have better survival outcomes, even among patients with well-differentiated neuroendocrine tumors (NETs). Therefore, patients who demonstrate intense FDG uptake and no DOTATATE uptake are deemed ineligible for ^{177}Lu DOTATATE therapy due to poor response and survival outcomes. This strategy of selecting patients based on the molecular expression of targets and patients who would benefit most from ^{177}Lu DOTATATE therapy prevents unnecessary comorbidities from ineffective treatment and would minimize inappropriate health system expenses. In addition, total body dynamic PET/CT could provide kinetic parameters and time activity curves, which may provide further biologic information for tumor heterogeneity and the potential for predicting therapy selection and response.

Increasingly, ^{177}Lu DOTATATE therapy is used as the standard of care to treat well-differentiated, locally advanced, inoperable NETs progressing on somatostatin analogues. Long-term follow-up data have confirmed the significant progression-free survival advantage and excellent tolerability. Ongoing further clinical trials are investigating the utility of ^{177}Lu DOTATATE against Everolimus (COMPETE; NCT03049189), ^{177}Lu DOTATATE versus standard of care for patients with aggressive grade 2 and 3 GEP NETs (COMPOSE; NCT04919226), and ^{177}Lu DOTATATE with long-acting octreotide versus high-dose (60 mg) long-acting octreotide as first-line therapy (NETTER-2; NCT03972488), which will further expand the indications in the future. In addition, other studies are investigating the use of ^{177}Lu DOTATATE for other somatostatin receptor–expressing tumors, such as small cell lung cancer (NCT05142696) and meningiomas (NCT03971461). Furthermore, real-world data are evolving from India for treating NET patients (PRRT naive and those refractory to ^{177}Lu DOTATATE) with ^{225}Ac DOTATATE.

PET Clin 18 (2023) xiii–xiv
https://doi.org/10.1016/j.cpet.2022.12.001
1556-8598/23/© 2022 Published by Elsevier Inc.

At the time of analysis, median progression-free survival was not achieved for the population in this study and was about 30 months for those who received ^{177}Lu DOTATATE. Ongoing clinical trials (NCT05153772, NCT05477576) in this space will shed more information on the success of alpha therapy in the future.

The therapy response assessment in neuroendocrine neoplasms is challenging due to tumor heterogeneity, their slow-growing nature, and longer time for response to manifest. Therefore, a combination of biologic, anatomic, and functional response parameters is necessary to estimate the accurate therapy response.

The scientific and clinical opportunities in diagnosing and treating neuroendocrine neoplasms are unlimited, and the future of the field is promising. This issue of *PET Clinic* outlines the current clinical practice and explores the scientific and clinical opportunities in the future.

Rathan M. Subramaniam, MBBS, PhD, MPH, MBA, FRANZCR, FACNM, FSNMMI, FAUR
Department of Medicine
Otago Medical School
University of Otago
201 Great King Street
Dunedin Hospital, First Floor
Dunedin 9016, New Zealand

E-mail address:
rathan.subramaniam@otago.ac.nz

Neuroendocrine Neoplasms

Epidemiology, Diagnosis, and Management

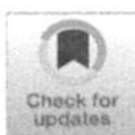

Ajitha Ramesh, MBBS[a], Aniruddha Chatterjee, BSc, MSc, PhD[b], Rathan M. Subramaniam, MD, MPH, PhD, MBA, FRSN, FAUR, FRANZCR, FSNMMI[c,d,*]

KEYWORDS

• Neuroendocrine neoplasms • Classification • Diagnosis • Management

KEY POINTS

- Neuroendocrine neoplasms (NENs) are a heterogeneous group of tumors arising from almost all organ systems, with unique biological and clinical behavior.
- The classification of NENs has been refined over the years to more accurately delineate the differences in grading and clinical progression of the different types. The newest World Health Organization Grading outlines a well-differentiated high-grade G3 subtype, recognizing its differences from the poorly differentiated neuroendocrine carcinoma.
- Anatomic and functional imaging modalities are used to confirm the diagnosis, localize the primary tumor, for staging, determine treatment and assess response to therapy. ^{68}Ga-DOTATE PET has largely replaced somatostatin scintigraphy as the diagnostic workup choice for NENs. In addition, NETest, a multi-analyte liquid biopsy, is a promising recent development in the biochemical testing of neuroendocrine tumors.
- The management of NENs is complex and involves different modalities, including surgical resection, somatostatin analogs, ^{177}Lu radiopharmaceutical therapy, chemotherapy, radiotherapy and immunotherapy. Recommendations based on disease burden and grade have been developed, but specific recommendations on the sequence of different treatment modalities have not been specified and require further clinical trials.

INTRODUCTION

Neuroendocrine neoplasms (NENs) are a heterogeneous group of tumors that arise from cells with a neuroendocrine phenotype. These cells secrete specific peptide hormones and biogenic amines stored within electron-dense membrane-bound granules.[1] NEN consists of a diverse range of tumors with varying locations, clinical syndromes, and biological activity associated with each type. NEN has characteristic immunostaining and is positive for general markers synaptophysin, chromogranin A, and neuron-specific enolase.[2,3]

NEN is generally divided into functional tumors, associated with a clinical syndrome due to excess secretion of hormones, and nonfunctional, which comprise most cases. These tumors can arise from a wide variety of neuroendocrine cells in the body. NENs occur most frequently in the gastrointestinal tract (62% to 67%), followed by the lungs (22% to 27%).[4] Poorly-differentiated neuroendocrine carcinomas (NECs) represent 10% to 20% of all NENs.[5] Of the gastropancreatic tumors, the most common are those arising from the small intestine (30.8%), rectum (26.3%), colon (17.6%), pancreas (12.1%), and appendix (5.7%).[6]

[a] Dunedin Hospital, 201 Great King Street, Dunedin 9016, New Zealand; [b] Department of Pathology, Dunedin School of Medicine, University of Otago, PO Box 56, Dunedin 9054, New Zealand; [c] Department of Medicine, Otago Medical School, University of Otago, 201 Great King Street, Dunedin, New Zealand; [d] Department of Radiology, Duke University, Durham, NC, USA

* Corresponding author. 201 Great King Street, Dunedin, New Zealand.
E-mail address: rathan.subramaniam@otago.ac.nz

PET Clin 18 (2023) 161–168
https://doi.org/10.1016/j.cpet.2022.10.002
1556-8598/23/

Neuroendocrine tumors (NETs) also form almost 20% of primary lung tumors, with small cell carcinoma being the most common at around 15%.[7] Medullary carcinomas of the thyroid and tumors arising from the parathyroid and pituitary glands may be classified under NENs. Rare NETs of the breast, vulva, and vagina have also been reported.[8,9]

The management of NENs requires a multimodal approach under a team including an endocrinologist, radiologist, nuclear medicine physician, oncologist, surgeon, and pathologist. A wait-and-watch approach can manage[9] asymptomatic low-grade tumors. However, surgery is the curative option in any local, regional disease with a possibility of >90% tumor reduction. Surgery can also be considered for advanced diseases with obstructive symptoms.[10] The somatostatin analogs, octreotide (SSA) and lanreotide, have been the backbone of medical therapy of NEN and are used to control symptoms of hormone excess in patients with functional NENs and to inhibit tumor growth.[11] Peptide receptor radionuclide therapy (PRRT) is a novel form of second-line treatment for patients who are nonresponsive to SSA and is a targeted therapy with radiolabeled somatostatin analogs.[12] For well-differentiated advanced tumors, Cepacitabine in combination with Temozolomide (CAPTEM) has proven to be an effective second-line and salvage therapy following treatment with somatostatin analogs and first-line chemotherapy, which includes fluorouracil, doxorubicin, and streptozocin.[13–15] First-line therapy for poorly differentiated NECs includes etoposide and platinum-based regimens. Newer studies have shown the efficacy of second-line treatment with folinic acid, 5-fluorouracil, and irinotecan (FOLFIRI) and FOLFIRI with Oxaliplatin (FOLFIRINOX).[16]

Epidemiology

The United States Cancer Statistics (USCS) Registry reports an overall incidence of 2.89 per 100,000 people per year from 2001 to 2015, with a reported male preponderance of three times more than females.[17] The Surveillance, Epidemiology, and End Results (SEER) Program of the National Cancer Institute reported a 6.4-fold increase in age-adjusted incidence from 1.09 per 100,000 in 1973 to 6.98 per 100,000 in 2012. This increase in incidence has been more pronounced among early-stage NENs and the older-age group of patients >65 years.[18] Comparing worldwide, there has been a similar increasing trend in the incidence of NETs as found in studies conducted in Europe and Asia, in which all sites average incidence increase in cases per 100,000 per year has varied from 0.05 (In Switzerland) to 0.23 (In Canada), compared with 0.16 in the United States.[19,20] Regional distribution of GEP-NENs has also been shown, with rectal NENs being the most common in Asia, followed by pancreatic and gastric NENs. In contrast, small intestinal and appendiceal NENs are more prevalent in Europe.[21] Several studies have also reported racial differences in the United States, with a greater incidence among African- American people, followed by Caucasians and Asians.[22] This difference is also reflected in overall survival and treatment outcomes, with African-Americans and Hispanics with SI and pancreatic NETs less likely to receive surgery.[23,24]

The median overall survival for all NENs from a recent US-based population study was 9.3 years, with localized NETs (>30 years) having a better median overall survival compared with regional NETs (10.2 years) and distant NETs (12 months).[18] NECs, which are poorly differentiated, have a much poorer prognosis; lung NECs with a median survival of 7.6 months, small intestinal NEC was more than 25.1 months, and pancreatic NEC at 5.7 months. The overall survival for patients with unknown NEC was 2.5 months.[25] However, overall survival rates have improved over the years from 2000, and this improvement is more prominent in the distant well-differentiated GI NET group.[18]

Classification

The classification of NENs has been challenging due to the heterogeneity of these tumors, and different classification systems have been proposed and modified over the years. The term "carcinoid" was first coined by Oberndorf in 1907, and the term was used to refer to "carcinoma-like," or the benign behavior of small bowel tumors that secreted bioactive amines.[26] In 2000, World Health Organization (WHO) introduced the term NET for Gastroenteropancreatic tumors and differentiated them into three histologic categories based on tumor differentiation. In 2004, the WHO divided the neoplasms of the lung and thymus into three grades based on mitotic index and necrosis.[4] The first TNM Classification was proposed by Rindi and colleagues,[6] adopted by the European Neuroendocrine Tumor Society (ENETS) in 2006[27] and by the American Joint Committee on Cancer (AJCC) in 2010. This was further refined by the WHO in 2010, introducing the term NENs to refer to all tumors of neuroendocrine origin irrespective of grade and anatomic location. These were further classified into well-differentiated NET, which could be of Grades G1, and G2 based on the mitotic count, and poorly differentiated NEC, which was G3 by definition.

In 2019, further refining the classification introduced the well-differentiated NET G3 subtype among GEP-NET, recognizing its differences from the poorly differentiated NEC. These tumors have a high mitotic count and Ki 67 index and a better prognosis than NECs. Further, NECs are classified as either large-cell neuroendocrine carcinoma (LCNEC) or small-cell neuroendocrine carcinoma (SCNEC).[28] The dichotomy between well-differentiated NETs, in particular, well-differentiated G3 tumors and poorly-differentiated NECs, differ in genetic markers, response to treatment, and prognostic markers. Mixed adenoneuroendocrine carcinomas were renamed mixed neuroendocrine neoplasm (MiNEN), which refers to tumors with >30% of cells of non-neuroendocrine origin adenocarcinoma or squamous cell carcinoma.[29] The current WHO classification scheme is outlined in **Table 1**.

There has been a recent proposal for the molecular classification of lung NENs into three distinct types with unique molecular signatures and clinical behavior- primary high-grade NENs, secondary high-grade NENs, and indolent low-grade NENs. This distinction is based on morphology, proliferation index, involvement of different molecular pathways, and clinical progression.[30] Similar morpho molecular classification systems have been proposed among thymic NENs, based on molecular features and proliferation rate. However, it was found that morphology and proliferation rate alone was insufficient to classify individual cases for clinical treatment correctly.[31] Further studies may lead to a more concise classification system incorporating molecular features, should it become more practically feasible to include molecular testing of samples.

Diagnosis and Staging

Endoscopy with biopsy is generally the first line in the workup of gastrointestinal NETs. For pancreatic NENs, the most sensitive examination is endoscopic ultrasound, with a mean sensitivity of 86% (range 82% to 93%) and a mean specificity of 92% (ranges from 74% to 96%), which additionally allows for biopsy.[32] A magnetic resonance cholangiopancreatographic scan (MRCP) can delineate the regional anatomy and the relation of the tumor to the pancreatic duct and the main bile duct. In addition, suspected NETs of the lung may present as a lung mass, and biopsy is obtained via transbronchial or a transthoracic method.

Depending on the disease site, biochemical evaluation may include gastrin levels, 24- hour plasma, urinary HIAA (5- hydroxy indole acetic acid), or ACTH (adrenocorticotropic hormone). Testing of chromogranin-A, which was sometimes used as a biochemical marker in nonfunctional tumors, is no longer included in the latest NCCN diagnostic algorithm due to its low specificity and the fact that it can be high in a range of other conditions such as hepatic and renal impairment and PPI (proton-pump inhibitor) use, leading to false-positive results.[33–36] NETest, a multi-analyte liquid biopsy, is a promising recent development in the biochemical testing of NETs, with a sensitivity of >95% and specificity of >90%. However, phase 2 data are still lacking and has limited clinical application.[37–39] For PPGL, Biochemical testing includes plasma-free or 24-h urine fractionated metanephrines, and in cervical paragangliomas, serum and urine testing of catecholamines or methoxytyramine can be considered.

Adequate biopsy specimens and interpretation by an expert pathologist are crucial in the workup of NENs. Pathologic assessment includes conventional hematoxylin and eosin (H&E) stained slides to confirm the morphology of neuroendocrine cells and assess differentiation. Mitotic activity is determined by examining ten fields at 40x magnification and counting the active cells in these areas. Immunohistochemical studies using MIB-1 antibody to label Ki67 are used to establish tumor grade with Ki-67 proliferation index by counting the number of mitotic cells per 10 high power fields or 2 mm^2 on H&E stained slides.[40] It is recommended that both the mitotic index and Ki-67 index be measured, and the higher parameter should be selected if there is a discrepancy between them.[41] Biopsy of a metastatic lesion may be preferred to guide therapy options as the tumor grade may increase between primary and metastatic lesions.[42]

Anatomic (computed tomography [CT], MR, and ultrasonography [US]) and functional (Gallium 68 (^{68}Ga) 1,4,7,10-tetraazacyclododecane-1,4,7,10-tetraacetic acid (DOTA)–octreotate [^{68}Ga-DOTATATE] PET, Octreoscan, ^{18}F FDG-PET) imaging modalities are used to confirm the diagnosis, localization of the primary tumor, determination of staging, determine treatment, and assess response to therapy.[43] Cross-sectional imaging should be done to include the primary site of disease using either CT or MRI and ^{68}Ga-DOTATATE PET/CT. According to NCCN Guidelines (Version 4.2021),[33] imaging of the chest is optional for GI NET unless there is clinical suspicion or a known tumor in the chest. Similarly, imaging of the brain is generally not required for well-differentiated NETs. As small intestinal NETs frequently present with mesenteric metastases, these tumors can cause an intense desmoplastic reaction reflected in CT as an irregular soft tissue mass, typically with one or more areas of calcifications surrounded by radiating

Table 1
Neuroendocrine tumor/carcinoma classification

Neuroendocrine Neoplasm WHO classification 2017/2019				
Family	Differentiation	Grade	Mitotic Count/10 HPFs	Ki 67 Index
Neuroendocrine tumors	Well differentiated	G1	<2	<3%
	Well differentiated	G2	2–20	3% to 20%
	Well differentiated	G3	>20	>20%
Neuroendocrine carcinoma	Poorly differentiated	Small cell	>20	>20%
	Poorly differentiated	Large cell	>20	>20%
MiNENs (Mixed neuroendocrine/ non-neuroendocrine tumors)	Variable	Variable	Variable	Variable

Abbreviation: HPF, high-power field.

streaks in mesenteric fat. There is consensus that CT or MRI should be used with functional imaging. ^{68}Ga-DOTA-PET/CT is now the preferred method compared with the previously used ^{111}In-pentetreotide scintigraphy.[44]

In the recent past, functional imaging with somatostatin receptor scintigraphy has emerged as the diagnostic workup of choice for NENs, as well as for evaluating receptor status before administration of somatostatin analogs or peptide-receptor-targeted radionuclide therapy. However, this modality has largely been replaced by ^{68}Ga-DOTA PET/CT. The drawbacks of scintigraphy are limited spatial resolution and lower tumor-to-background ratio. In addition, NENs that have a different subset of SSR (other than SSR2 or SSR4) may not be picked up by this method.[45] A systematic review and meta-analysis of 22 studies found that ^{68}Ga-DOTATATE PET had a pooled sensitivity and specificity of 91% and 94%, respectively.[46] For liver metastases, metabolic imaging with ^{68}Ga- DOTA PET/CT should be performed to detect extra-hepatic disease in the first place.[47] If hepatic metastases are present and the patient is considered for hepatic resection, a liver MRI should be performed, as MRI provides high-resolution anatomic information before surgery.

For PPGL, ^{68}Ga- DOTA PET/CT, MIBG scan, and CT or MRI can be considered in staging the disease. However, multiple studies have shown greater sensitivity of ^{68}Ga-DOTATATE and 68Ga-DOTANOC over MIBG scanning and octrescan. Therefore, it is recommended as the first line investigation for diagnosis and follow-up of PPGL, replacing previously used MIBG scanning.[48–50]

Management

a. Well-differentiated Grade 1 or 2 NETs

For gastrointestinal NETs, small tumors less than 2 cm are amenable to wait and watch approach. Bowel resection with regional lymphadenectomy is recommended if there is a spread to surrounding tissues (locoregional disease). If there is an advanced locoregional disease with or without distant metastases, several options are available depending on several clinical parameters. If the patient is asymptomatic with a low tumor burden, observation may be sufficient, or treatment with octreotide/lanreotide[11] can be considered. If the patient is locally symptomatic from the primary tumor, consideration of resection of the primary tumor followed by observation is indicated with CT or MRI every 12 weeks - 12 months, as appropriate. If complete resection is possible, resecting the primary tumor with metastases is recommended. If there is a clinically significant tumor burden, treatment can be started with octreotide or lanreotide.[51] Other options in case of significant disease are PRRT with ^{177}Lu-DOTATATE,[52] liver-directed therapy for a liver predominant disease, or everolimus.[53,54] Palliative radiotherapy for bone metastases can be considered. Cytotoxic chemotherapy is regarded as the last option.

Nonfunctioning pancreatic tumors are treated with surgical resection if they are well-differentiated. In locoregional disease, tumors less than or equal to 2 cm can be removed with enucleation and regional lymphadenectomy. The approach for tumors greater than 2 cm invasive or node-positive is pancreatoduodenectomy with regional lymphadenectomy (if the tumor is in the pancreatic head) or distal pancreatectomy, splenectomy, and regional lymphadenectomy.[55] If complete resection is possible in metastatic disease, it should be attempted. In the case of asymptomatic metastatic disease with low tumor burden, treatment with somatostatin analogs and surveillance with abdominal/pelvic/chest CT/MRI/ DOTATATE PET/CT for disease progression is usually done. If there is evidence of disease progression, or if there is a symptomatic metastatic disease with clinically significant tumor burden, enrollment in clinical trials with front-line therapy with sunitinib[56] or Everolimus (category 1)[57,58] is suitable. Other options are chemotherapy with temozolomide and cepacitabine,[59] PRRT, or palliative radiotherapy. Belzutifan can be considered in the population of patients with germline VHL mutations with progressive pNETs.

In localized disease of lung NETs, the tumor should be resected. Complete resection should be aimed at locoregional disease (stage IIA/B). However, in case of incomplete resection or positive margins, typical carcinoids can be treated with observation with consideration for radiotherapy.[60] Additional cytotoxic chemotherapy can be considered for atypical carcinoids, with appropriate follow-up. In the case of locally advanced unresectable disease, typical carcinoids can be managed by observation if asymptomatic, somatostatin analogs, everolimus, temozolomide, and cepcitabine[61–63] or radiotherapy are used if symptomatic. Concurrent radiotherapy and cytotoxic chemotherapy can be considered for locally advanced unresectable atypical carcinoids.

Metastatic disease of lung NETs can be treated with observation if asymptomatic with low tumor grade. If Somatostatin receptor-positive or hormonal symptoms are present, somatostatin analogs can be used. For clinically significant tumor burden with low grade or intermediate grade, or if there is evidence of disease progression, referral to a clinical trial is indicated, along with treatment with Everolimus (category 1), PRRT with ^{177}Lu-Dotatate (if SSR-positive),[55] or with chemotherapy options. Liver disease can be treated with liver-directed therapy. However, a palliative approach with somatostatin analogs is appropriate if multiple lung nodules exist.

b. Well-differentiated Grade 3 NETs

Depending on the biology, locoregional disease with a possibility of resection can be approached. Favorable tumor biology, that is, low Ki-67 counts, SSR-positive on PET imaging, and slow growing, can allow complete tumor resection with regional lymphadenectomy followed by aggressive follow-up every 12 to 24 weeks for 2 years, then every 6 to 12 months for up to 10 years.[64] Follow-up can be done with histopathology and or appropriate imaging, as clinically indicated. If the tumor burden is unresectable, but there is a clinically significant tumor burden with evidence of disease progression, enrollment in a clinical trial is recommended. There is also a role for starting treatment with somatostatin analogs, Everolimus, sunitinib (for pancreas only),[56] PRRT,[65] pembrolizumab, or chemotherapy. Follow-up, in this case, is as above, but routine functional imaging (using SSR-PET/CT or SSR PET/MRI) and biochemical markers as clinically indicated. If tumor burden proves to be unresectable, but is low and asymptomatic, observation with short interval follow-up scans can be considered, with or without treatment with octreotide or lanreotide, if SSR positive. Resection with regional lymphadenectomy can still be considered with unfavorable tumor biology, but enrollment in a clinical trial is warranted if not feasible.

c. Poorly differentiated Grade 3 tumors

If the disease is considered resectable, depending on the site of the disease, therapy options include resection with adjuvant or neoadjuvant chemotherapy and radiotherapy.[66,67] chemotherapy or radiotherapy can be used alone, or definitive chemoradiation with cisplatin and etoposide or carboplatin and etoposide can be considered.[68,69] If there is locoregional spread without the option of resection, concurrent or sequential chemotherapy with radiotherapy can be considered, or just chemotherapy.

The main option is chemotherapy if there is a metastatic disease that is not amenable to resection. If there is still progression of the disease, Nivolumab or ipilimumab can be considered.[70,71]

SUMMARY

NETs are a group of heterogeneous tumors that can arise from almost any organ system and have a variety of biological and clinical characteristics. The classification of NEN has evolved over many decades, and the newest is the 2019 WHO Classification of these tumors. The newest WHO Grading outlines a well-differentiated high-grade G3 subtype, recognizing its differences from the poorly differentiated NEC. ^{68}Ga-DOTATE PET has largely replaced somatostatin scintigraphy as the diagnostic workup choice for NENs. NETest, a multi-analyte liquid biopsy, is a promising recent development in the biochemical diagnosis of NETs. Management includes wait and watch approach, surgical resection, somatostatin analogs, ^{177}Lu radiopharmaceutical therapy, chemotherapy, and radiotherapy. Further clinical trials are necessary for determining the appropriate sequencing of different treatment modalities.[30,72]

CLINICS CARE POINTS

- Imaging of Neuroendocrine Neoplasm is undertaken with a combination of 68Ga DOTATATE PET/CT, MRI and CT, as appropriate.
- NEN patients are best managed by a multidisciplinary team consisting of surgeons, endocrinologists, oncologists, nuclear medicine physicians, radiologists and palliative care specialists.

DISCLOSURE

The authors have nothing to disclose.

REFERENCES

1. Klöppel G. Neuroendocrine neoplasms: dichotomy, origin and classifications. Visc Med 2017;33(5):324.
2. Ma ZY, Gong YF, Zhuang HK, et al. Pancreatic neuroendocrine tumors: a review of serum biomarkers, staging, and management. World J Gastroenterol 2020;26(19):2305–22. Available at: http://www.wjgnet.com/.
3. Wiedenmann B, Franke WW, Kuhn C, et al. Synaptophysin: a marker protein for neuroendocrine cells and neoplasms. Proc Natl Acad Sci U S A 1986; 83(10):3500–4.
4. Oronsky B, Ma PC, Morgensztern D, et al. Nothing but NET: a review of neuroendocrine tumors and carcinomas. Neoplasia (United States) 2017;19(12): 991–1002.
5. Pavel M, Öberg K, Falconi M, et al. Gastroenteropancreatic neuroendocrine neoplasms: ESMO Clinical Practice Guidelines for diagnosis, treatment and follow-up. Ann Oncol 2020;31(7):844–60.
6. Cives M, Strosberg JR. Gastroenteropancreatic neuroendocrine tumors. CA Cancer J Clin 2018; 689(6):471–87.
7. Rekhtman N. Lung neuroendocrine neoplasms: recent progress and persistent challenges. Mod Pathol 2022;35(Suppl 1):36.
8. Georgescu TA, Bohiltea RE, Munteanu O, et al. Emerging therapeutic concepts and latest diagnostic advancements regarding neuroendocrine tumors of the gynecologic tract. Medicina (Kaunas) 2021;57(12).
9. Rosen LE, Gattuso P. Neuroendocrine tumors of the breast. Arch Pathol Lab Med 2017;141(11):1577–81.
10. Kunz PL, Reidy-Lagunes D, Anthony LB, et al. Consensus guidelines for the management and treatment of neuroendocrine tumors. Pancreas 2013;42(4):557.
11. Rinke A, Müller HH, Schade-Brittinger C, et al. Placebo-controlled, double-blind, prospective, randomized study on the effect of octreotide LAR in the control of tumor growth in patients with metastatic neuroendocrine midgut tumors: a report from the PROMID Study Group. J Clin Oncol 2009; 27(28):4656–63.
12. Starr JS, Sonbol MB, Hobday TJ, et al. Peptide receptor radionuclide therapy for the treatment of pancreatic neuroendocrine tumors: recent insights. Onco Targets Ther 2020;13:3545.
13. Chatzellis E, Angelousi A, Daskalakis K, et al. Activity and safety of standard and prolonged capecitabine/temozolomide administration in patients with advanced neuroendocrine neoplasms. Neuroendocrinology 2019. https://doi.org/10.1159/000500135.
14. Lu Y, Zhao Z, Wang J, et al. Safety and efficacy of combining capecitabine and temozolomide (CAPTEM) to treat advanced neuroendocrine neoplasms: a meta-analysis. Medicine (Baltimore) 2018;97(41). https://doi.org/10.1097/MD.0000000000012784.
15. Kouvaraki MA, Ajani JA, Hoff P, et al. Fluorouracil, doxorubicin, and streptozocin in the treatment of patients with locally advanced and metastatic pancreatic endocrine carcinomas. J Clin Oncol 2004;22(23):4710–9.
16. Hentic O, Hammel P, Couvelard A, et al. FOLFIRI regimen: an effective second-line chemotherapy after failure of etoposide–platinum combination in patients with neuroendocrine carcinomas grade 3. Endocr Relat Cancer 2012;19(6):751–7.
17. Patel N, Benipal B. Incidence of neuroendocrine tumors in the United States from 2001-2015: a United States cancer statistics analysis of 50 states. Cureus 2019;11(3). https://doi.org/10.7759/CUREUS.4322.
18. Dasari A, Shen C, Halperin D, et al. Trends in the incidence, prevalence, and survival outcomes in patients with neuroendocrine tumors in the United States. JAMA Oncol 2017;3(10):1335.
19. Leoncini E, Boffetta P, Shafir M, et al. Increased incidence trend of low-grade and high-grade neuroendocrine neoplasms. Endocrine 2017;58(2):368.
20. Das S, Dasari A. Epidemiology, incidence, and prevalence of neuroendocrine neoplasms: are there global differences? Curr Oncol Rep 2021;23(4). https://doi.org/10.1007/S11912-021-01029-7.
21. Takayanagi D, Cho H, Machida E, et al. Update on epidemiology, diagnosis, and biomarkers in gastroenteropancreatic neuroendocrine neoplasms. Cancers (Basel) 2022;14(5):1119.
22. Shen C, Gu D, Zhou S, et al. Racial differences in the incidence and survival of patients with neuroendocrine tumors. Pancreas 2019;48(10):1373–9.
23. Kessel E, Naparst M, Alpert N, et al. Racial differences in gastroenteropancreatic neuroendocrine tumor treatment and survival in the United States. Pancreas 2021;50(1):29–36.
24. Zhou H, Zhang Y, Wei X, et al. Racial disparities in pancreatic neuroendocrine tumors survival: a SEER study. Cancer Med 2017;6(11):2745–56.

25. Dasari A, Mehta K, Byers LA, et al. Comparative study of lung and extrapulmonary poorly differentiated neuroendocrine carcinomas: a SEER database analysis of 162,983 cases. Cancer 2018;124(4):807–15.
26. Modlin IM, Shapiro MD, Kidd M. Siegfried Oberndorfer: origins and perspectives of carcinoid tumors. Hum Pathol 2004;35(12):1440–51.
27. Rindi G, Klöppel G, Alhman H, et al. TNM staging of foregut (neuro)endocrine tumors: a consensus proposal including a grading system. Virchows Arch 2006;449(4):395–401.
28. Popa O, Taban SM, Pantea S, et al. The new WHO classification of gastrointestinal neuroendocrine tumors and immunohistochemical expression of somatostatin receptor 2 and 5. Exp Ther Med 2021; 22(4). https://doi.org/10.3892/ETM.2021.10613.
29. Assarzadegan N, Montgomery E. What is new in the 2019 World Health Organization (who) classification of tumors of the digestive system: review of selected updates on neuroendocrine neoplasms, appendiceal tumors, and molecular testing. Arch Pathol Lab Med 2021;145(6):664–77.
30. La Rosa S, Uccella S. Classification of neuroendocrine neoplasms: lights and shadows. Rev Endocr Metab Disord 2021;22(3):527–38.
31. Dinter H, Bohnenberger H, Beck J, et al. Molecular classification of neuroendocrine tumors of the thymus. J Thorac Oncol 2019;14(8):1472–83.
32. Sundin A, Arnold R, Baudin E, et al. ENETS consensus guidelines for the standards of care in neuroendocrine tumors: radiological, nuclear medicine and hybrid imaging. Neuroendocrinology 2017;105(3):212–44.
33. Guidelines detail. Available at: https://www.nccn.org/guidelines/guidelines-detail?category=1&id=1448. Accessed April 18, 2022.
34. Marotta V, Zatelli MC, Sciammarella C, et al. Chromogranin A as circulating marker for diagnosis and management of neuroendocrine neoplasms: more flaws than fame. Endocr Relat Cancer 2018; 25(1):R11–29.
35. Kidd M, Bodei L, Modlin IM. Chromogranin A: any relevance in neuroendocrine tumors? Curr Opin Endocrinol Diabetes Obes 2016;23(1):28–37.
36. Malczewska A, Kidd M, Matar S, et al. An assessment of circulating chromogranin a as a biomarker of bronchopulmonary neuroendocrine neoplasia: a systematic review and meta-analysis. Neuroendocrinology 2020;110(3–4):198–216.
37. Modlin IM, Kidd M, Malczewska A, et al. The NETest: the clinical utility of multigene blood analysis in the diagnosis and management of neuroendocrine tumors. Endocrinol Metab Clin North Am 2018;47(3): 485–504.
38. Liu E, Paulson S, Gulati A, et al. Assessment of NETest clinical utility in a U.S. Registry-Based Study. Oncologist 2019;24(6):783–90.
39. Puliani G, Di Vito V, Feola T, et al. NETest: a systematic review focusing on the prognostic and predictive role. Neuroendocrinology 2021. https://doi.org/10.1159/000518873. Published online August 5.
40. Dillon JS. Work up of gastroenteropancreatic neuroendocrine tumors. Surg Oncol Clin N Am 2020; 29(2):165.
41. Köseoğlu H, Duzenli T, Sezikli M. Gastric neuroendocrine neoplasms: a review. World J Clin Cases 2021; 9(27):7973.
42. Keck KJ, Choi A, Maxwell JE, et al. Increased grade in neuroendocrine tumor metastases negatively impacts survival. Ann Surg Oncol 2017; 24(8):2206–12.
43. Sanli Y, Garg I, Kandathil A, et al. Neuroendocrine tumor diagnosis and management: 68 Ga-DOTATATE PET/CT. AJR Am J Roentgenol 2018; 211(2):267–77.
44. Oberg K, Krenning E, Sundin A, et al. A delphic consensus assessment: imaging and biomarkers in gastroenteropancreatic neuroendocrine tumor disease management. Endocr Connect 2016;5(5):174.
45. Orlefors H, Sundin A, Garske U, et al. Whole-body 11C-5-hydroxytryptophan positron emission tomography as a universal imaging technique for neuroendocrine tumors: comparison with somatostatin receptor scintigraphy and computed tomography. J Clin Endocrinol Metab 2005;90(6):3392–400.
46. Singh S, Poon R, Wong R, et al. 68Ga PET imaging in patients with neuroendocrine tumors: a systematic review and meta-analysis. Clin Nucl Med 2018; 43(11):802–10.
47. Ronot M, Clift AK, Baum RP, et al. Morphological and functional imaging for detecting and assessing the resectability of neuroendocrine liver metastases. Neuroendocrinology 2018;106(1):74–88.
48. Mojtahedi A, Thamake S, Tworowska I, et al. The value of 68Ga-DOTATATE PET/CT in diagnosis and management of neuroendocrine tumors compared with current FDA approved imaging modalities: a review of literature. Am J Nucl Med Mol Imaging 2014; 4(5):426.
49. Singh D, Shukla J, Walia R, et al. Role of [68Ga]DOTANOC PET/computed tomography and [131I]MIBG scintigraphy in the management of patients with pheochromocytoma and paraganglioma: a prospective study. Nucl Med Commun 2020;41(10): 1047–59.
50. Jaiswal SK, Sarathi V, Malhotra G, et al. The utility of 68 Ga-DOTATATE PET/CT in localizing primary/metastatic pheochromocytoma and paraganglioma in children and adolescents - a single-center experience. J Pediatr Endocrinol Metab 2020;34(1): 109–19.
51. Caplin ME, Pavel M, Ćwikła JB, et al. Lanreotide in metastatic enteropancreatic neuroendocrine tumors. N Engl J Med 2014;371(3):224–33.

52. Strosberg J, El-Haddad G, Wolin E, et al. Phase 3 trial of 177 Lu-Dotatate for midgut neuroendocrine tumors. N Engl J Med 2017;376(2):125–35.
53. Pavel ME, Baudin E, Öberg KE, et al. Efficacy of everolimus plus octreotide LAR in patients with advanced neuroendocrine tumor and carcinoid syndrome: final overall survival from the randomized, placebo-controlled phase 3 RADIANT-2 study. Ann Oncol 2017;28(7):1569.
54. Pavel ME, Singh S, Strosberg JR, et al. Health-related quality of life for everolimus versus placebo in patients with advanced, non-functional, well-differentiated gastrointestinal or lung neuroendocrine tumours (RADIANT-4): a multicentre, randomised, double-blind, placebo-controlled, phase 3 trial. Lancet Oncol 2017;18(10):1411–22.
55. Souche R, Hobeika C, Hain E, et al. Surgical management of neuroendocrine tumours of the pancreas. J Clin Med 2020;9(9):1–18.
56. Raymond E, Dahan L, Raoul J-L, et al. Sunitinib malate for the treatment of pancreatic neuroendocrine tumors. N Engl J Med 2011;364(6):501–13.
57. Yao JC, Pavel M, Lombard-Bohas C, et al. Everolimus for the treatment of advanced pancreatic neuroendocrine tumors: overall survival and circulating biomarkers from the randomized, Phase III RADIANT-3 study. J Clin Oncol 2016;34(32): 3906–13.
58. Yao JC, Shah MH, Ito T, et al. Everolimus for advanced pancreatic neuroendocrine tumors. N Engl J Med 2011;364(6):514–23.
59. Fine RL, Gulati AP, Krantz BA, et al. Capecitabine and temozolomide (CAPTEM) for metastatic, well-differentiated neuroendocrine cancers: the Pancreas Center at Columbia University experience. Cancer Chemother Pharmacol 2013;71(3):663–70.
60. Bilski M, Mertowska P, Mertowski S, et al. The role of conventionally fractionated radiotherapy and stereotactic radiotherapy in the treatment of carcinoid tumors and large-cell neuroendocrine cancer of the lung. Cancers (Basel) 2022;14(1):177.
61. Al-Toubah T, Morse B, Strosberg J. Capecitabine and temozolomide in advanced lung neuroendocrine neoplasms. Oncologist 2020;25(1):e48–52.
62. Papaxoinis G, Kordatou Z, McCallum L, et al. Capecitabine and temozolomide in patients with advanced pulmonary carcinoid tumours. Neuroendocrinology 2020;110(5):413–21.
63. Mirvis E, Toumpanakis C, Mandair D, et al. Efficacy and tolerability of peptide receptor radionuclide therapy (PRRT) in advanced metastatic bronchial neuroendocrine tumours (NETs). Lung Cancer 2020;150:70–5.
64. Coriat R, Walter T, Terris B, et al. Gastroenteropancreatic well-differentiated grade 3 neuroendocrine tumors: review and position statement. Oncologist 2016;21(10):1191.
65. Sharma N, Naraev BG, Engelman EG, et al. Peptide receptor radionuclide therapy outcomes in a north american cohort with metastatic well-differentiated neuroendocrine tumors. Pancreas 2017;46(2): 151–6.
66. Petrella F, Bardoni C, Casiraghi M, et al. The role of surgery in high-grade neuroendocrine cancer: indications for clinical practice. Front Med 2022;9: 869320.
67. Pellat A, Cottereau AS, Terris B, et al. Neuroendocrine carcinomas of the digestive tract: what is new? Cancers (Basel) 2021;13(15).
68. Frizziero M, Spada F, Lamarca A, et al. Carboplatin in combination with oral or intravenous etoposide for extra-pulmonary, poorly-differentiated neuroendocrine carcinomas. Neuroendocrinology 2019; 109(2):100–12.
69. Strosberg JR, Halfdanarson TR, Bellizzi AM, et al. The north american neuroendocrine society (NANETS) consensus guidelines for surveillance and medical management of midgut neuroendocrine tumors. Pancreas 2017;46(6):707.
70. Patel SP, Othus M, Chae YK, et al. A phase II basket trial of dual anti-CTLA-4 and Anti-PD-1 blockade in rare tumors (DART SWOG 1609) in patients with nonpancreatic neuroendocrine tumors. Clin Cancer Res 2020;26(10):2290–6.
71. Patel SP, Mayerson E, Chae YK, et al. A phase II basket trial of dual anti-CTLA-4 and anti-PD-1 blockade in rare tumors (DART) SWOG S1609: high-grade neuroendocrine neoplasm cohort. Cancer 2021;127(17):3194–201.
72. Rindi G, Klimstra DS, Abedi-Ardekani B, et al. A common classification framework for neuroendocrine neoplasms: an International Agency for Research on Cancer (IARC) and World Health Organization (WHO) expert consensus proposal. Mod Pathol 2018;31(12):1770.

Neuroendocrine Neoplasms
Genetics and Epigenetics

Jim Smith, MBChB, BMedSc(Hons)[a,b,*], Edward Barnett, BSc(Hons)[a], Euan J. Rodger, BSc, MSc, PhD[a], Aniruddha Chatterjee, BSc, MSc, PhD[a], Rathan M. Subramaniam, MBBS, BMedSc, MClinEd, MPH, PhD, MBA, FRANZCR, FSNMMI, FAUR[c,d]

KEYWORDS

• Neuroendocrine neoplasms • Genetics • Epigenetics • Molecular landscape

KEY POINTS

- Neuroendocrine neoplasms (NENs) are a group of rare and clinically heterogeneous tumors affecting a range of different organs, for which early diagnosis and effective management are often significant challenges.
- Each NEN subtype is driven via a complex host of genetic and epigenetic changes, which may be subtype-specific and promote neoplastic progression through the dysregulation of critical cellular pathways.
- Investigation of these unique genetic and epigenetic changes continues to elucidate the molecular landscape, which underpins NEN tumorigenesis with greater detail.
- Recent and ongoing clinical trials have focused on exploiting these molecular aberrations to provide improved diagnostic and management approaches.
- Ongoing exploitation of the molecular landscape of individual tumors and tumor subtypes forms the basis of future NEN management through more personalized diagnosis, treatment, and disease monitoring.

INTRODUCTION

Neuroendocrine neoplasms (NENs) comprise a heterogeneous group of rare tumors from various anatomical sites.[1] NENs are defined by histological evidence of neuroendocrine differentiation and the corresponding expression of immunohistochemical markers of neuroendocrine differentiation, including chromogranin A (CgA) and synaptophysin. Neuroendocrine histological features are well-conserved irrespective of the organ of origin and neoplasms range from well to very poorly differentiated.[2] Most of the NENs originate de novo from neuroendocrine cell lineages, although there is increasing recognition of NEN development via lineage plasticity in response to targeted treatment approaches.[1,2] NENs display a broad spectrum of clinical aggressiveness based on the level of differentiation and proliferative index; these tumors may also secrete bioactive substances in a tumor-specific manner, leading to the development of clinical syndromes with high intertumoral variability.[1,3] Clinical diagnosis and staging of NENs is based on a combination of tissue

Funded by: No funding was used in the production of this article.

[a] Department of Pathology, Dunedin School of Medicine, University of Otago, PO Box 56, Dunedin 9054, New Zealand; [b] Te Whatu Ora - Southern, Dunedin Public Hospital, 270 Great King Street, PO Box 913, Dunedin, New Zealand; [c] Department of Medicine, Otago Medical School, University of Otago, PO Box 56, Dunedin 9054, New Zealand; [d] Department of Radiology, Duke University, 2301 Erwin Rd, BOX 3808, Durham, NC 27705, USA

* Corresponding author. Te Whatu Ora - Southern, Dunedin Public Hospital, 270 Great King Street, PO Box 913, Dunedin, New Zealand

E-mail address: jim.smith2@southerndhb.govt.nz

PET Clin 18 (2023) 169–187
https://doi.org/10.1016/j.cpet.2022.11.003

biopsy, tumor- or syndrome-specific testing for secreted substances and radiological imaging approaches, including computed tomography (CT), MR, and PET-based investigation.[3] Given the heterogeneous nature of NENs and limitations of current screening approaches, the importance of understanding the molecular pathways that drive NEN tumorigenesis is becoming increasingly clear. Well-differentiated, low-grade neuroendocrine tumors (NETs) are molecularly distinct from higher grade neuroendocrine carcinomas (NECs), which are aggressive, poorly differentiated, and highly proliferative.[1,2] The development of both de novo and treatment-induced NENs is driven by the acquisition of characteristic genetic and epigenetic alterations. As our understanding of these molecular alterations in the clinical context advances, so too does our ability to exploit these signatures for improving diagnosis, prognostication, and targeted treatment modalities. Here, we define the molecular landscape of three major NEN subtypes: gastroenteropancreatic NENs (GEP-NENs); lung NENs (L-NENs); and paraganglioma and phaeochromocytoma (PGPCs) and highlight the current and prospective applications of these molecular signatures for clinical applications.

DEFINING THE GENOMIC AND EPIGENOMIC LANDSCAPE OF NEUROENDOCRINE NEOPLASMS

Biologically, the landscape of NENs is heterogeneous and often mixed, though several common alterations have been characterized. Genomic instability, including chromothripsis and localized hypermutation and tumor mutational burden (TMB), typically increases in proportion to NEN aggressiveness, with NECs displaying average TMB rates around five times higher than NETs.[4] Indeed, several major drivers of NEC carcinogenesis have now been documented; disruption of *TP53* or *RB1* is observed in up to 80% of NECs, whereas other commonly affected genes include *KRAS*, *CSMD3*, *APC*, *CSMD1*, *LRATD2*, *TRRAP*, and *MYC*.[4,5] Overall, NENs display a much lower TMB than other solid malignancies and higher grade NECs comprise only 10% to 20% of all NENs.[6]

As for many malignancies, genome-wide losses of DNA methylation are documented in NENs, which results in the inappropriate activation of DNA repetitive elements and increased genomic instability. Methylation changes in regulatory elements such as gene promoters and enhancers also occur in a subtype-specific manner, altering the expression of tumor suppressor and oncogenes. Posttranslational histone modifications are similarly altered at the genome-wide and individual gene level; these mechanisms regulate chromatin conformation and subsequently, transcriptomic profiles to drive tumor development via aberrant cellular pathway activation or repression alongside genetic influences. The corresponding dysregulation of epigenetic machinery is also observed, with DNA methylation- and histone-modifying enzymes demonstrating altered expression in NENs. Another class of major epigenetic regulators, noncoding RNAs (ncRNA), is nonprotein-coding genomic elements that display numerous multilevel interactions with RNA, DNA, proteins, and epigenetic marks, thereby contributing to the complex coregulation of biological networks in conjunction with other genomic and epigenomic mechanisms. The role of ncRNAs in NEN has been comprehensively reviewed in the literature, and detailed discussion of these molecules is beyond the scope of this review.[7,8]

Gastroenteropancreatic Neuroendocrine Neoplasms

GEP-NENs comprise all NENs arising from the gastrointestinal system and are the second most common malignancy of the gastrointestinal tract; GEP-NENs vary substantially by anatomical site, from both a clinical and biological perspective.[9] Pancreatic NEN (P-NEN) and small intestinal NEN (SI-NEN) are the most widely studied GEP-NEN subtypes and demonstrate a number of distinct molecular features (**Fig. 1**); evidence is continuing to emerge for additional subtypes, including colonic and rectal NENs.[4,9,10]

Broadly, the molecular landscape of GEP-NEN is dominated by the inactivation of crucial tumor suppressor genes, whereas the activation of oncogenic drivers is comparatively rare in these tumors.[11] Chromosomal instability (CIN) is a noted feature of almost all GEP-NEN, with numerous chromosomal deletions documented in a high proportion of both P-NEN and SI-NEN, respectively.[12–18] Microsatellite instability (MSI), contrastingly, is implicated in around 10% of P-NEN and is enriched in colonic NEN but is rarely observed in SI-NEN. Concordant with findings in colorectal adenocarcinoma, MSI is observed in tumors displaying concomitant *BRAF* mutation.[10,19,20] Conserved genetic events across subtypes of GEP-NEN are in line with the aberrations described across all NETs. Similarly, mutational load and genomic instability are typically increased in GEP-NECs and in the context of more aggressive disease.[4] Several epigenetic features are also common to multiple

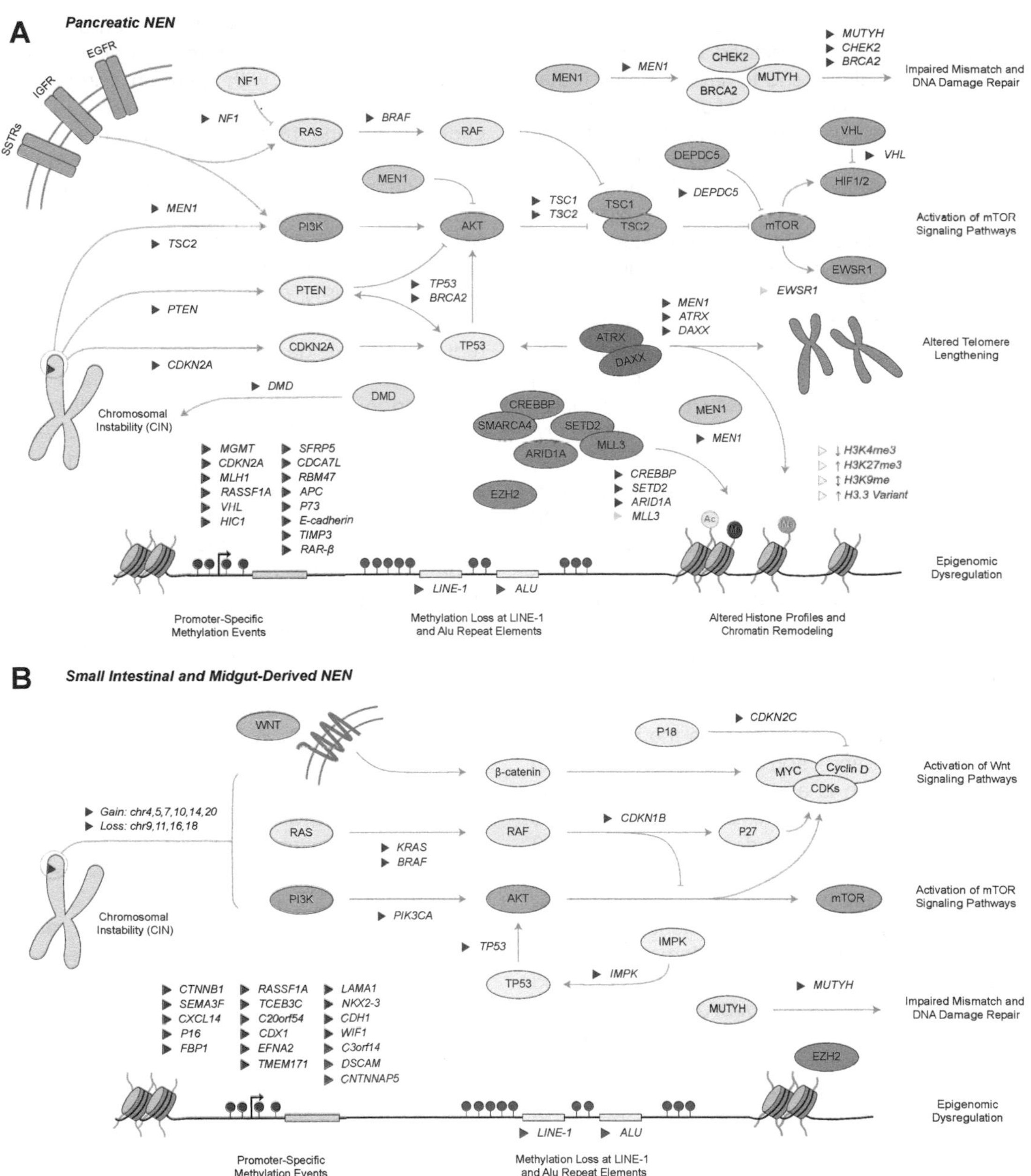

Fig. 1. Major molecular pathways involved in the tumorigenesis of pancreatic and small intestinal neuroendocrine neoplasms. (*A*) Pancreatic NEN display aberrations in a number of key molecular pathways, including DNA damage and mismatch repair, mTOR signaling, alternative telomere lengthening, and epigenetic pathways. *MEN1* loss is heavily implicated in the vast majority of these pathways. (*B*) Midgut-derived or small intestinal NENs are genetically stable tumors with a handful of aberrations documented in the TGF-β/Wnt, mTOR, and DNA repair pathways. Epigenomic alterations in SI-NEN are largely related to altered genome-wide and promoter-specific DNA methylation profiles. Chromosomal instability plays a significant role in the pathobiology of both pancreatic and small intestinal NEN.

GEP-NEN subtypes; for example, the histone methyltransferase *EZH2* is overexpressed in both P-NEN and SI-NEN, emerging as a novel prospective therapeutic target.[21–23] Further, unique mutational and methylomic signatures are being identified, which allow for cell-of-origin determination for NENs, including tumors of small versus large-cell lineage. However, further validation of these signatures is required for use in a clinically relevant manner.[24–26]

Pancreatic neuroendocrine neoplasm

Perhaps the most well defined from a molecular perspective, P-NENs tend to have a higher mutational burden than GEP-NENs of other sites of origin and are more genetically unstable. CIN in P-NEN results in characteristic losses of tumor suppressor genes, for example, *CDKN2A*, *TSC2*, and *PTEN*, with subsequent impacts on downstream pathways. A variety of germline and somatic mutations or gene fusions have been observed in P-NEN, which contribute to the dysregulation of several main cellular pathways, including DNA damage repair (*MUTYH*, *CHEK2*, *BRCA2*); telomere maintenance (*ATRX*, *DAXX*) and chromatin remodeling (*SETD2*, *ARID1A*, *MLL3*); and RAS/RAF (neurofibromatosis type 1 [*NF1*]) and PI3K/AKT/mTOR (*PTEN, TSC1, TSC2, DEPDC5, EWSR1, YY1, FOXO3*) signaling pathways.[27–32] Germline Von-Hippel Lindau (*VHL*) mutations, which result in a deregulated hypoxic response, have also been implicated in P-NEN tumorigenesis.[28,31] The loss of *DMD* has been identified in advanced P-NEN, which predisposes to DNA damage and genomic instability.[4,33,34] *MEN1*, which encodes menin, is a key genomic driver in P-NEN that impacts these aforementioned pathways, alongside TGF-β and GLI/hedgehog signaling; *MEN1* loss is the most common germline and somatic genetic event in P-NEN.[27,31] Menin is a central component of the MLL2 histone methyltransferase complex, the loss of which results in global depletion of H3K4me3 and corresponding enrichment of H3K27me3.[35] Histone profiles are further altered in P-NEN via the loss of SWI/SNF complex components *ATRX* and *DAXX*, which results in impaired telomeric and pericentric incorporation of histone variant H3.3 and altered H3K9me levels; ATRX/DAXX and menin act in concert to induce context-specific deposition or removal of the repressive histone modification H3K9me3.[36] Loss of the CREBBP histone H3K27 acetyltransferase, an aberration also common to SCLC, is a feature of advanced P-NEN.[4,37] From a DNA methylation standpoint, P-NEN is characterized by both global and promoter-specific methylation changes. Concordant with other GEP-NEN subtypes, P-NENs display DNA hypomethylation of DNA repeat elements, including *LINE-1* and *Alu*.[38] Promoter hypermethylation-induced gene repression is also common in P-NEN, affecting numerous genes with significant overlap to the aforementioned genomically altered cellular pathways.[19,39–43]

Small intestinal and midgut-derived neuroendocrine neoplasm

SI-NENs, comparatively, are genetically stable tumors with very few characterized mutational events.[17,44,45] Instead, CIN and chromosomal rearrangements hold a more central role in SI-NEN tumorigenesis, with gains in chromosome (chr)4, 5, 7, 10, 14, and 20, as well as loss of chr9, 11, 16, and 18 documented across various tumors; loss of chr18 occurs in 66% to 88% of tumors and is proposed to drive tumorigenesis via the TGF-β/Wnt and PI3K/mTOR signaling pathways.[4,12,17,46,47] Of note, *CDKN1B* is mutated in approximately 8% of SI-NEN and up to 23% of advanced SI-NEN; *CDKN1B* encodes p27, which acts as a tumor suppressor in SI-NEN via cell cycle regulation.[4,44] Aside from aberrations of *CDKN1B*, low rates of sporadic mutation have been observed in a handful of genes, including *APC*, *CDKN2C*, *BRAF*, *KRAS*, *PIK3CA*, and *TP53*.[47] Two germline variants have also been identified, implicating *IMPK*, the regulator of p53 activation, and *MUTYH*, a gene involved in DNA damage repair.[48,49] Epigenomic changes are, thus far, understudied in the context of SI-NEN, although they seem to be highly relevant. High rates of promoter-specific and gene body DNA methylation changes have been documented in SI-NEN with subsequent transcriptional impacts; over 30 affected genes have now been characterized, including *RASSF1A*, *WIF1*, *TCEB3C*, *CDX1*, and *SEMA3F*.[38,45,50–52] These alterations largely converge on the PI3K/mTOR and TGF-β/Wnt signaling pathways. Further, global methylation losses and hypomethylation of genomic repeat elements *LINE-1* and *Alu* are more extensive in SI-NEN than GEP-NEN of other sites of origin, potentially via passive methylation loss, as decreases of 5-hydroxymethylcytosine with the concordant loss of TET1 and nuclear exclusion of TET2 have also been observed.[53,54]

Other gastroenteropancreatic-neuroendocrine neoplasm subtypes

Limited evidence currently exists in the published literature concerning other subtypes of GEP-NEN, although a small number of aberrations have been characterized for colonic and rectal NEN. Recent high-throughput analyses have identified an overrepresentation of *BRAF* mutation in colonic NEN and *FBXW7* in rectal NEN.[10,55,56] A subset of rectal and anal NEN were identified to have an absence of *TP53* and *RB1* mutation but were positive for high-risk human papillomavirus.[57] Further investigation of these, and other GEP-NEN subtypes, is required to elucidate the unique molecular networks underpinning their development and progression.

Lung Neuroendocrine Neoplasms

NENs of the lung (**Fig. 2**) encompass typical carcinoid (TC) and atypical carcinoid (AC), large cell

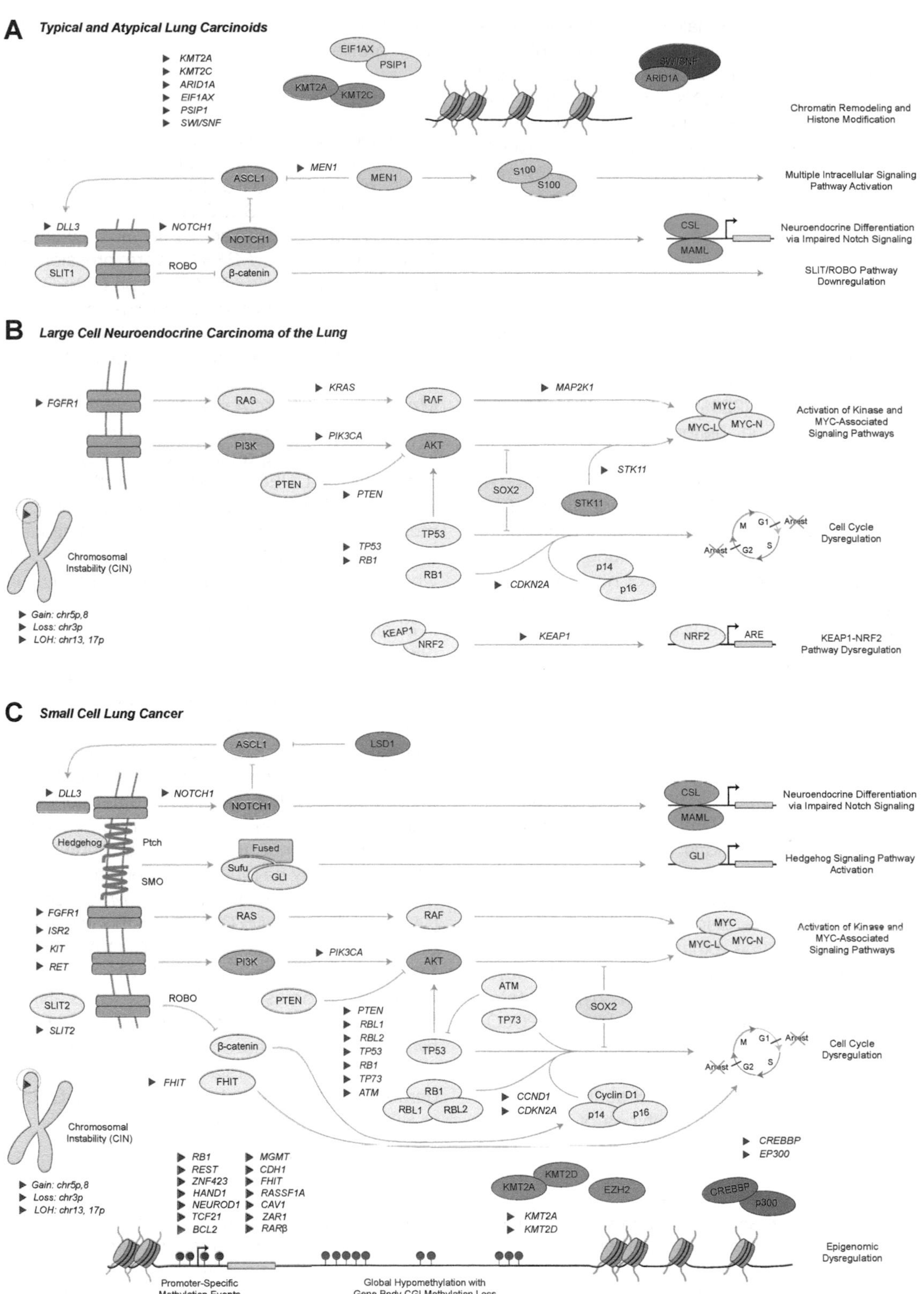

Fig. 2. Key molecular pathways underpinning the major clinical subtypes of lung neuroendocrine neoplasms. (*A*) Molecular features in typical and atypical lung carcinoid tumors are largely limited to dysregulated histone and chromatin remodeling pathways, with a handful of aberrations documented in the SLIT/ROBO, Notch, and MEN-mediated cellular signaling pathways. (*B*) Large cell neuroendocrine carcinomas display variable phenotypes with

NEC (LCNEC), and small cell lung carcinoma (SCLC) separated by discrete histomorphological criteria.[58] TC and AC define low- and intermediate-grade NENs, respectively, and generally carry a favorable clinical prognosis. Comparatively, SCLC and LCNEC are strongly associated with cigarette smoking, display very high TMB, and almost invariably have a poor prognosis.[59–62]

Lung carcinoid neoplasms

TC and AC are molecularly similar and commonly possess mutations in histone modification pathways, with 45% displaying mutations in chromatin remodeling genes, including components of the SWI/SNF complex (22%); a further 40% demonstrate mutations in histone methyltransferases and demethylases, concomitant with reduced histone methylation.[60,62] Loss of *PSIP1, ARID1A, EIF1AX, KMT2A, KMT2C*, and especially *MEN1* is particularly prevalent.[60,63,64] Distinct molecular clusters have been identified in lung carcinoids: one displaying overexpression of neuroendocrine transcription factors *ASCL1* and *DLL3*, similar to SCLC and LCNEC type I; another with recurrent *EIF1AX* mutations and *SLIT1/ROBO1* pathway downregulation; and a third with a loss of *MEN1* alongside monocyte invasion and dendritic cell depletion suggesting immune evasion.[65] Loss of *MEN1* is a poor prognostic factor in carcinoids and correlates with increased *S100* expression alongside decreased *ASCL1* expression.[63,66] Inactivation of *TP53/RB1* is rare in pulmonary carcinoids, as are mutations associated with non-small cell lung cancers (NSCLC; *BRAF, KRAS, SMAD4*, and *PIK3CA*).[62,63,67,68] Chromosomal rearrangements are also comparatively uncommon, although some exhibit chr11q deletions or chromothripsis, generally associated with *MEN1* loss.[60,62,69,70] In rare cases, a hypermutated phenotype has been demonstrated in *POLQ*-mutant carcinoids.[62] The DNA methylation landscape of pulmonary carcinoids remains largely understudied, although small-scale analyses have proposed molecular subtypes of carcinoids based on combined transcriptomic and methylation profiles.[63]

Lung neuroendocrine carcinoma

Multiomic analyses have demonstrated two major LCNEC subtypes, with molecular similarities to SCLC and non-small cell lung tumors (NSCLC), respectively.[62,71,72] SCLC-like LCNEC is defined by *RB1* and *TP53* co-inactivation, alongside *MYC, SOX2*, and *FGFR1* overexpression and *PTEN* inactivation.[71,73] NSCLC-type LCNEC often exhibits *TP53* inactivation with wild-type *RB1* and *STK11* or *KEAP1* inactivation; *KRAS* mutation, reminiscent of lung adenocarcinoma, is also common, with occasional losses of *CDKN2A, MAP2K1*, and *PI3KCA*.[72] *RB1* mutation is associated with distinct chemotherapeutic response in LCNEC, suggesting an important therapeutic role in stratifying LCNEC based on *RB1* status.[62,74,75] Both LCNEC and SCLC commonly display chromosomal rearrangement, including deletions of chr3p, loss of heterozygosity (eg, chr13, 17p, where *RB1* and *TP53* are located), and copy number gains at chr5p and 8.[62,76]

Bi-allelic inactivation of *RB1* (90%) and *TP53* (98%) hallmarks SCLC; in rare tumors with wild-type *RB1*, alternative pathways of deregulation, such as downstream *CCND1* overexpression, commonly occur.[67] *RBL1* and *RBL2*, closely related to *RB1*, are also commonly inactivated, and *CDKN2A*, which activates *RB1* and *TP53*, is often lost.[67,77] *ATM* mutation is often concurrent with *TP53* mutation.[67,78] SCLC is characterized by several distinct transcriptional subtypes, of which there may be multiple present in a single tumor. Amplification of different *MYC* isoforms (*MYC, MYCL*, and *MYCN*) drives the progression of various subtypes.[67,79,80] SCLC-A (70% of SCLC) highly expresses *ASCL1*, whereas smaller numbers express *NEUROD1* (SCLC-N) or *POU2F3* (SCLC-P); the existence of a *YAP1*-positive SCLC subtype associated with wild-type *RB1* (SCLC-Y) is controversial.[79–82] In vitro work has demonstrated temporal evolution from SCLC-A to SCLC-N and then SCLC-Y.[79]

similarities to either small cell or non-small cell lung cancers, including aberrations in the RAS/RAF, PI3K/AKT, and MYC-signaling pathways, among other common changes in cell cycle regulation such as *TP53/RB1* inactivation. The KEAP1/NRF2 axis is also often dysregulated, with subsequent impacts on androgen response element (ARE) signaling. (*C*) Small cell lung cancer is the best defined from a molecular perspective, with pathognomonic *TP53/RB1* loss and aberrations in associated pathways driving cell cycle dysregulation. Impaired Notch signaling is also prevalent, alongside hyperactivation of Hedgehog, kinase, and other MYC-associated pathways. Epigenomic changes are common, with alterations to histone and chromatin remodeling machinery widely observed. Promoter DNA methylation changes facilitate the transcriptional regulation of tumor suppressors, oncogenes, and factors involved in neuroendocrine differentiation, whereas losses of gene body methylation occur globally.

Disrupted Notch signaling occurs in 25% of lung NEN patients. Inactivating *NOTCH* mutations drive SCLC via *ASCL1* expression, negatively regulating Notch signaling via *DLL3* expression.[67,83] *DLL3* is expressed in 75% of stage IV LCNEC, associated with concomitant *ASCL1* expression.[84] A subset of SCLC also displays increased Notch signaling, which may be indirectly tumorigenic via growth signaling of adjacent neuroendocrine cells and provides chemoresistance.[85] PD-L1 expression is usually low in SCLC, although a small proportion of SCLC and 16% of stage IV LCNEC tumors display PD-L1 overamplification, which is associated with better prognosis.[75,86] *PI3KCA* mutations, which impact the PI3K/AKT signaling pathway, occur in SCLC and LCNEC with greater frequency than in carcinoids.[62,87] Sporadic *KRAS* mutations may also occur.[62] Around 25% of lung NENs also show copy number gains in *TERT, SDHA,* and *RICTOR*.[62]

Posttranslational histone modifications occur with even greater frequency in lung NEC, with 55% demonstrating mutations in chromatin remodeling pathways.[62] Increased expression of LSD1, an H3K4 and H3K27 demethylase, is associated with SCLC progression both in vitro and in vivo.[88] Similarly, overexpression of *EZH2* occurs in a small proportion of SCLC via *RB1* inactivation, promoting tumor progression by suppressing the TGF-β-Smad-ASCL1 pathway.[89,90] A range of genes involved in cellular regulatory pathways and neuroendocrine differentiation display altered promoter methylation profiles in SCLC, including *ZAR1*, *RASSF1A*, *CDH1*, and *RARβ*, which are hypermethylated in SCLC compared with carcinoids.[91–94] Globally, SCLC displays predominant hypomethylation within gene bodies and intergenic regions, consistent with other tumor types.

Contrary to findings in other NEN subtypes, cluster analyses suggest that pulmonary carcinoids may represent a precursor lesion to NEC. Overlapping transcriptional states have been identified in AC and LCNEC, which suggest a possible continuum of progression from AC to LCNEC,[95] further supported by observations of tumors with carcinoid morphology but genetic features of NEC. Progression from carcinoids to NEC is proposed via *RB1/TP53* inactivation and the subsequent accumulation of NEC-associated mutations; however, this concept remains the focus of ongoing debate.[59,64,96]

Paraganglioma and Pheochromocytoma

PGPCs define two catecholamine-hypersecreting NEN subtypes, which originate from the chromaffin cells of the adrenal medulla or the extra-adrenal sympathetic ganglia, respectively. The two are histologically indistinguishable, and both commonly manifest with nonspecific features of catecholamine excess.[97] At least 20 germline genetic mutations are associated with PGPC susceptibility, many of which define known autosomal dominant syndromes that affect multiple organ systems, including multiple endocrine neoplasia type 2B (MEN-2B; *RET*), *VHL*, and *NF1*.[98–100] Around 30% of patients presenting with PGPCs carry germline mutations, whereas a further 30%–40% of PGPCs display identifiable somatic mutations, highlighting the high level of genetic determinism in PGPC tumorigenesis.[101,102] Clinical manifestations of heritable PGPCs are typically unique to each syndrome, and heritable tumors tend to present around 15 years earlier in life than sporadic tumors.[97] Several major metabolic and cell regulatory pathways are uniquely impacted in the tumorigenesis of PGPC, defining three distinct genomic and epigenomic clusters (**Fig. 3**).[101,102] Complex interplay between these molecular pathways facilitates multilevel deregulation to promote tumor development irrespective of the initial driver event.

Pseudohypoxia

Aberrations are often observed in regulators of metabolic function, thereby promoting pseudohypoxia via metabolic reprogramming. Mutations in the genes encoding subunits of succinate dehydrogenase (*SDHA, SDHB, SDHC, SDHD, SDHAF2*)—an essential catalyst of the tricarboxylic acid (TCA) cycle and component of the electron transfer chain—are particularly prevalent.[101,102] Impaired succinate dehydrogenase (SDH) activity in chromaffin cells results in truncation of the TCA cycle and subsequent succinate and fumarate accumulation. Broadly, metabolite excess drives the widespread inhibition of α-ketoglutarate (2-oxoglutarate)-dependent dioxygenases, which are critical regulators of metabolic sensing, hypoxic response, and epigenetic function; DNA and histone demethylases are particularly impacted, resulting in characteristic patterns of epigenetic silencing.[102] Alongside mitochondrial dysfunction, mutations affecting a range of proteins involved in the downstream hypoxia signaling pathway have also been identified, for example, alterations to hypoxia-inducible factors (HIFs; *EPAS1*, *ARNT*), prolyl hydroxylases that mediate HIF stability (*PHD1, PHD2*), or the VHL-mediated (*VHL*) HIF degradation process.[101] Fundamentally, these changes drive oxygen-independent activation of HIFs in PGPC tumorigenesis, contributing to metabolic switching, tumor cell

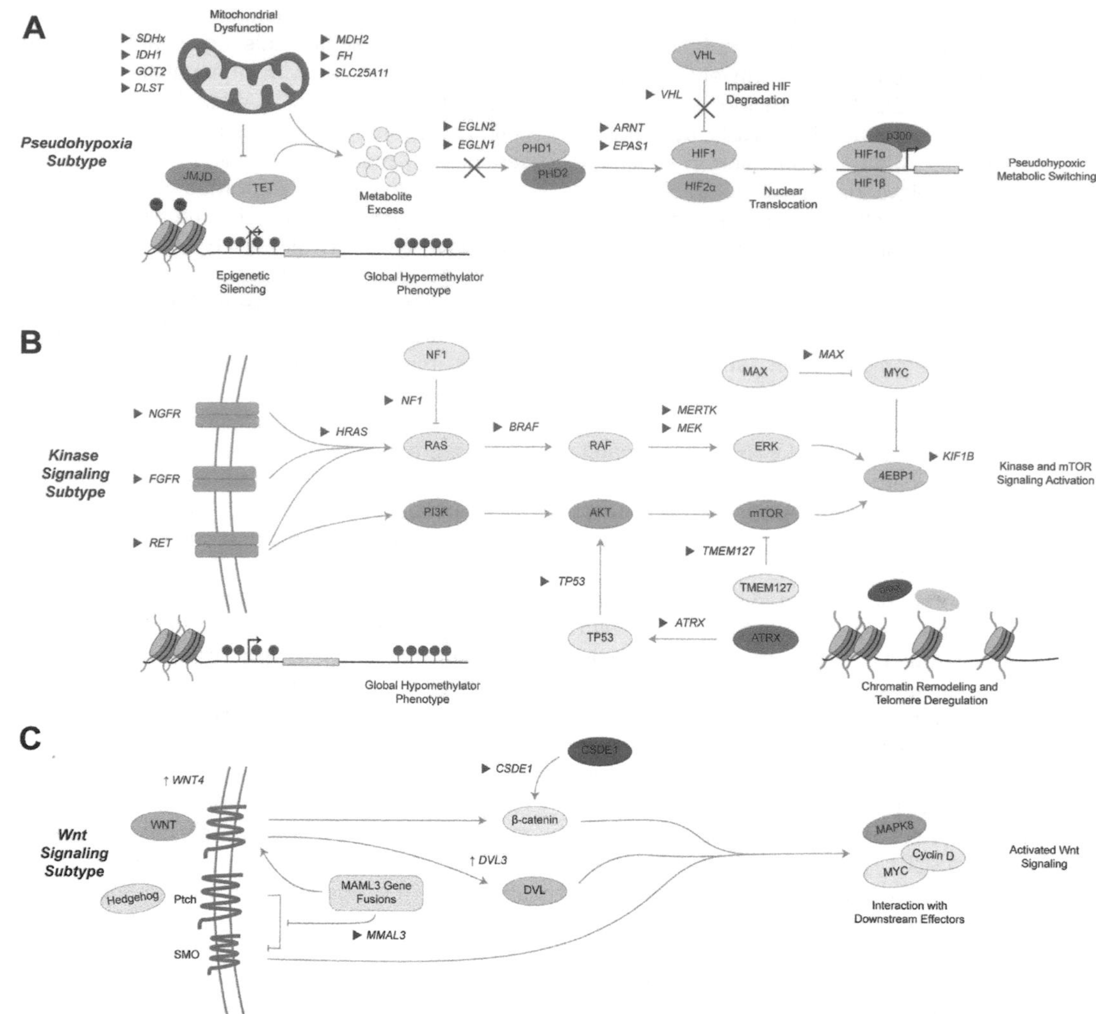

Fig. 3. Three major molecular clusters involved in paraganglioma and pheochromocytoma tumorigenesis. (*A*) Pseudohypoxia subtype tumors are characterized by disrupted mitochondrial function and inappropriate downstream activation of hypoxic response pathways. (*B*) Kinase signaling subtype tumors display hyperactivation of the RAS/RAF/MEK and PI3K/AKT/mTOR pathways, as well as altered telomere lengthening and chromatin remodeling. (*C*) Least well-defined of the PGPC subtypes, the Wnt signaling cluster of tumors, are associated with MMAL3 gene fusions, CSDE1 aberrations, and hyperactivation of the Wnt and Hedgehog signaling pathways to drive tumorigenesis.

proliferation, angiogenesis, and the development of metastasis.[103]

Abnormal kinase signaling and mTOR activation

The kinase signaling subtype of PGPCs is commonly characterized by germline or somatic mutations in the *RET*, *NF1*, or *HRAS*.[98,100,101,104] Further, alterations in *MAX, TMEM127, KIF1Bβ, BRAF, FGFR, NGFR, MERTK, MET,* and subunits of protein kinase A have been documented.[101,105–107] Wider contributors to this cluster include somatic aberrations of *TP53*, a key mediator of apoptosis, and *ATRX*, a SWI/SNF component that functions in chromatin remodeling and normal restraint of telomere length.[101,108] Aberrations in these kinase signaling pathways ultimately drive apoptotic evasion and enhanced cell growth, proliferation, and survival.[101,109]

Wnt-signaling activation

Alongside the two aforementioned subtypes, a third cluster of genes has been implicated in PGPC tumorigenesis via the activation of abnormal Wnt and Hedgehog signaling.[101] Gain-of-function *MAML3* fusion genes and loss-of-function *CSDE1* mutations have been implicated as driver events in Wnt-subtype PGPCs.[101]

Tumors of this subtype exhibit increased expression of Wnt pathway components, including *WNT4* and *DVL3*, alongside *CHGA*, which encodes the neuroendocrine-associated marker CgA.[101] Wnt and Hedgehog are developmental pathways involved in embryonic patterning and growth; constitutive activation of these pathways in tumorigenesis results in unrestrained proliferation, invasion, and metastasis.[110,111]

Emerging epigenetic contributors to paraganglioma and phaeochromocytoma tumorigenesis

Epigenetic contributors to PGPC tumorigenesis, similar to other NEN, remain comparatively understudied; however, roles for several epigenetic regulators are now emerging. On a global scale, different PGPC subtypes display contrasting patterns of DNA methylation, wherein pseudohypoxia subtype tumors are broadly characterized by genome-wide hypermethylation, whereas the kinase signaling subtype is associated with global methylation loss.[112,113] Gain-of-function mutations in *DNMT3A* have been described in a small number of PGPCs, associated with promoter hypermethylation, particularly homeobox-containing genes.[114] Promoter-specific methylation changes are documented in *PNMT*, *RDBP*, and *CDKN2A*, among other genes, correlated with differing phenotypic features.[115–118] Alongside DNA methylation changes, somatic and germline aberrations are seen in histone-related regulators, including histone subunit variant 3.3 (*H3F3A*) and a range of histone demethylases (*JMJD1C*, *KDM2B*) and methyltransferases (*KMT2B*, *EZH2*, *SETD2*); interestingly, these mutations were commonly observed in tumors that lacked a distinct germline mutation and had minimal overlap with kinase signaling-type PGPCs.[107] Together, this host of epigenomic changes comprises an ever-increasing component of the complex molecular landscape governing PGPC.

Clinical Application of Molecular Signatures in Neuroendocrine Neoplasms

Biomarkers for diagnosis and treatment monitoring

NENs are often detected at later disease stages due to their slow progression and vague symptomatology, although advances in diagnostic techniques have led to improved rates of timely diagnosis. The ongoing discovery and application of molecular biomarkers will further enhance disease detection for NENs, with greater subtype specificity.

Somatostatin receptors (SSTRs) are commonly expressed in NENs and are involved in complex antiproliferative signaling via regulation of the PI3K and MAPK pathways.[119] NEN-specific SSTR expression is commonly exploited for both tumor detection and management. Indeed, functional radiological imaging using radiolabeled somatostatin analogues (SSAs) is a mainstay for disease staging for the majority of NEN, most commonly using ^{68}Ga/^{64}Cu-DOTA-SSA PET/CT; 2-deoxy-2-[fluorine-18]fluoro-D-glucose PET/CT remains more appropriate in the characterization of higher grade lesions, and CXCR4-targeted imaging provides another emerging option for tumors with high Ki-67.[120–122] Further, SSTR-2 or SSTR-5 are markers which may be detected immunohistochemically where functional imaging is unavailable. Immunohistochemical staining can similarly be performed for other prognostic biomarkers, including DAXX/ATRX and p53/pRb, which aid in classifying G3 NETs versus NEC, particularly in the context of P-NEN.[6]

Traditional serum-based markers of NEN, such as CgA, have poor accuracy in the context of diagnosis; however, there has been increasing focus on identifying blood-based signatures with clinical utility over recent years. NETest, an mRNA-based signature comprising 51 NEN-specific transcripts, has emerged as a serum-based tool with high prospective utility. Now validated across GEP-NEN, L-NEN, and tumors of unknown primary, NETest displays 95% accuracy for diagnosing new NEN. Furthermore, NETest also shows efficacy for disease monitoring, offering 84.5% to 85.5% accuracy in differentiating between stable versus progressive disease and 94% accuracy for detecting disease recurrence postoperatively.[123–125] This seems to be a promising serum-based test for diagnosis and monitoring disease progression.

Current targeted treatment approaches

Given the rarity and clinical heterogeneity of NENs, management can often be challenging. A range of surgical, chemotherapeutic, radionuclide, and biological treatment options are now available for NEN, although the response to these therapies is highly variable between different tumors and disease contexts. Symptomatic management, particularly functioning neoplasms, is another central facet of NEN treatment. Surgical resection remains the cornerstone of definitive management for localized disease and offers the only opportunity for cure. Further, surgical cytoreduction of tumor burden may offer symptomatic relief and prolonged survival as a palliative treatment measure in more advanced disease.[6,126] Indeed, many NENs are diagnosed at an advanced stage with unresectable, metastatic disease, where the use of medical therapies is required.[127] Systemic chemotherapy remains a first-line treatment option in selected tumors, for example, the use of platinum-based agents in SCLC, capecitabine, and temozolomide for advanced P-NEN, or cyclophosphamide, vincristine, and dacarbazine in PGPCs; the efficacy of alternative systemic agents continues to be explored, with mixed results.[126,128–131] There is an increasing focus on exploiting the unique molecular features of individualized tumors to maximize clinical outcomes with targeted therapies (**Fig. 4**).

SSAs, which target commonly expressed SSTRs, are now widely used as antisecretory and antiproliferative agents in SSTR-positive NENs.[126,132–134] Octreotide- and lanreotide-based formulations displayed initial success in GEP-NEN, including the PROMID and CLARINET trials, with substantial survival benefits shown in patients with unresectable disease.[132,135] The advent of second-generation SSAs, including pasireotide, has led to further improvements in tumor control and progression-free survival rates, with trials now supporting the first-line use of SSAs for lung NETs alongside other NENs.[126,133] Peptide receptor radionuclide therapy (PRRT), most commonly using ^{99}Y- or ^{177}Lu-based-SSAs, similarly exploits SSTR expression to deliver targeted radionuclides (eg, DOTATATE or DOTATOC) to tumor cells. PRRT has shown efficacy in L-NEN, GEP-NEN, and PGPCs, including conferring superior progression-free survival than SSA treatment alone in the NETTER-1 trial.[136–139] PRRT agents are under continued investigation to determine their optimal role in adjunct and comparison to the other targeted therapies.[140] Intriguingly, epigenetic agents, including histone deacetylase and DNA methyltransferase inhibitors, have been shown in preclinical models to enhance PRRT

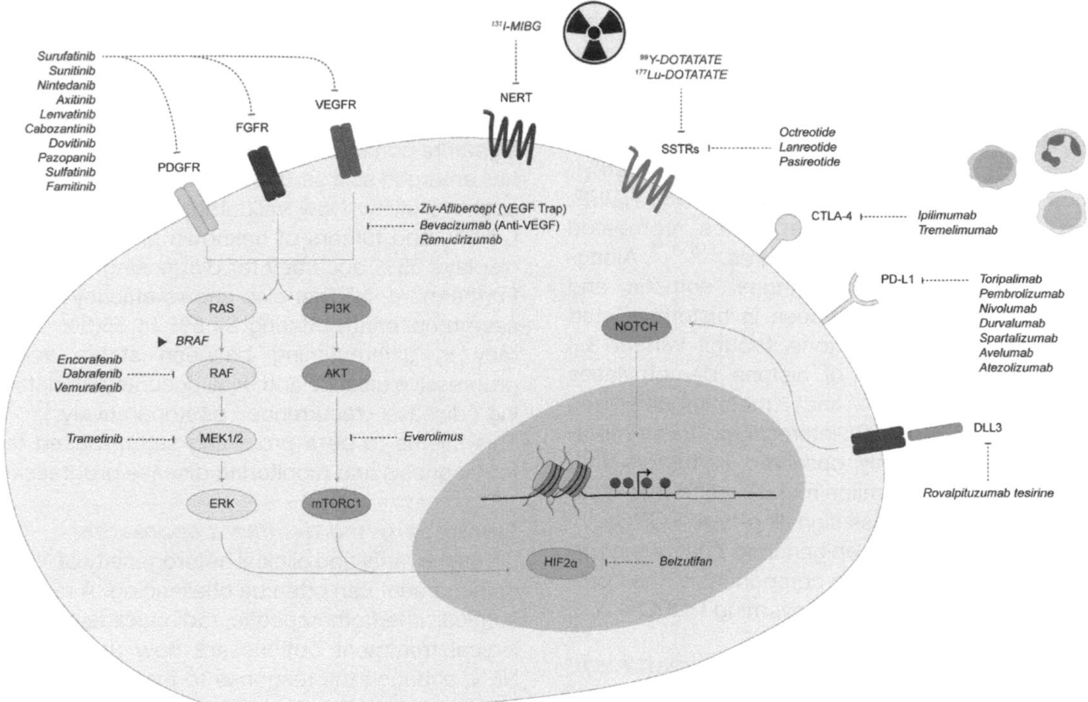

Fig. 4. Current targeted treatment modalities for neuroendocrine neoplasms. Numerous agents are currently used or under trial for use in the management of unresectable neuroendocrine tumors. Multi-target tyrosine kinase inhibitors and antiangiogenic agents (anti-VEGF agents and traps) disrupt often overactive kinase signaling pathways to prevent tumor proliferation and vascularization; targeted mTOR, *BRAF* V600 E, and MEK inhibitors act downstream within the PI3K/AKT/mTOR or RAS/RAF/MEK signaling pathways to disrupt tumorigenesis. Theranostic radionuclides exploit the expression of tumor-specific receptors (norepinephrine reuptake transporter, NERT; somatostatin receptor, SSTR) to deliver targeted radiation; somatostatin analogues similarly act on SSTRs to prevent tumor secretion and growth. Anti-CTLA-4 and anti-PD-L1 monoclonal antibodies enhance the native immune response to reactivate anti-tumorigenic pathways. Novel anti-hypoxia inducible factor agents (belzutifan) achieve symptomatic and tumor stabilization through abolishing inappropriate pseudohypoxic signaling pathways. Anti-DLL3 agents such as the antibody-drug conjugate rovalpituzumab tesirine modulate Notch pathway signaling and have direct cytotoxic effects. Only agents that have been trialed in a clinical setting are shown irrespective of efficacy.

efficacy through the upregulation of SSTRs.[141,142] Unique to PGPC management, the use of iodine-131 metaiodobenzylguanidine (^{131}I-MIBG) is a similar method of delivering targeted radiation, where MIBG is a substrate for norepinephrine re-uptake transporters expressed on the cell surface of PGPCs.[143]

Given the vascular nature of NENs and their propensity to display aberrant kinase signaling, numerous agents targeting these pathways have been evaluated. Multi-target tyrosine kinase inhibitors (TKIs) and other antiangiogenic agents, including anti-vascular endothelial growth factor (VEGF) monoclonal antibodies (bevacizumab) and immunoglobulin-based VEGF traps (ziv-aflibercept), continue to be trialed in NEN management.[144,145] Several of these agents have shown promise, including the vascular endothelial growth factor receptor inhibitor, sunitinib, approved for the treatment of advanced metastatic P-NETs.[6,146] Clinical trials for a range of TKIs are ongoing across multiple NEN contexts.[6] Targeting the overactivation of mTOR signaling pathways, everolimus is an mTOR inhibitor that has demonstrated significant benefits with respect to progression-free survival in the RADIANT trials and is now used in the management of P-NEN (G1/2), lung carcinoids, and nonfunctioning GEP-NETs, as well as showing promise in advanced PGPCs.[147–152] Combined therapy with everolimus and other agents, as well as the optimal order of treatment sequence to maximize efficacy, is the focus of ongoing research.[6,140,153] Specific to neoplasms with *BRAF* V600 E mutation, BRAF inhibitors (BRAFi; encorafenib, dabrafenib, vemurafenib) have been trialed in *BRAF*-mutant colonic and rectal NEN.[56,154] Encorafenib abolishes tumor growth in vitro in patient-derived xenografts of colonic NEN which display *EGFR* promoter hypermethylation—a known marker of BRAFi responsiveness.[56] In trials involving patients with Stage IV, G3 NEN, rectal, but not colonic, NEN were responsive to treatment with vemurafenib or dabrafenib, in combination with the MEK inhibitor (MEKi), trametinib.[154]

Targeted immunotherapies are currently being explored across numerous clinical trials for different NEN subtypes. Immune evasion remains a hallmark of malignant tumors and immunomodulators display noted benefits for several other cancer types. Common agents which disrupt the PD-1 or CTLA-4 axes have been trialed, specifically anti-PD-1 monoclonal antibodies (nivolumab, pembrolizumab, durvalumab, toripalimab, spartalizumab, avelumab, atezolizumab) alone, or in combination with anti-CTLA-4 agents (ipilimumab, tremelimumab). Efficacy of these medications has been variable, with ORRs ranging from 0% to 36% dependent on NEN subtype and grade, the specific agent used, and combinatorial approaches as an adjunct to treatment with TKIs, anti-VEGF antibodies, or chemotherapeutic regimens; despite these initial results, meaningful comparisons to standard management are yet to be made.[155–161] Interferon-alpha was previously recognized as an immunomodulatory treatment option; however, its use is now limited to refractory functional midgut NEN and selected patients due to a poor adverse reaction profile and limited clinical response.[3]

Specifically explored in SCLC, rovalpituzumab tesirine (Rova-T) is an antibody-drug conjugate that targets DLL3 to inhibit tumorigenesis via Notch signaling pathway modulation and direct cytotoxic effects. Although phase 1 trials were encouraging, subsequent phase 2 and 3 trials demonstrated limited efficacy of Rova-T alongside significant toxicity, both alone and in combination with immunomodulators. Alternative anti-DLL3 agents are now in ongoing trials.[162–165]

Prospective therapeutic targets and disease monitoring

A wide range of agents are now being used in the ever improving management of inoperable NENs, but several key molecular pathways are yet to be exploited. Future strategies may target alternative tumorigenic mechanisms, including epigenetic regulatory pathways such as dynamic DNA methylation changes, histone modifications, and chromatin remodeling, which remain thus far understudied in NEN. Few epigenetic treatments have been meaningfully trialed in NEN thus far, with only small phase two trials reported for histone deacetylase inhibitors (HDACi), including belinostat and panobinostat.[166,167] Further investigation of such epigenetic agents is warranted, with work in preclinical models demonstrating efficacy for HDACi and EZH2 inhibitors in reducing tumor burden and progression.[21,22,168,169]

Experimental in vitro and in vivo studies have identified several additional prospective molecular targets. In models of SCLC, for example, targeted inhibition of PTPN3 enhanced antitumor immune responses and prevented invasion, migration, and proliferation.[170] In PGPCs, hypoxic cluster and SDHx-deficient tumors have shown response to SUCNR1, COX-2, and PARP inhibitors in vitro, each modulating the activation of pseudohypoxic signaling pathways.[171–173] Further, the HIF2A inhibitor, belzutifan, has demonstrated a rapid and sustained tumor response and symptomatic control in a single case of *EPAS1*-mutant Pacak—Zhuang syndrome.[174] HIF2A antagonists are efficacious in the management of renal cell carcinoma.[175] Combinations of immunomodulators, including mannanBAM, TLR ligands, and anti-CD40 agents, are shown to substantially decrease liver metastases and tumor bulk in mouse xenografts of PGPC.[176] These represent several examples of areas for therapeutic exploitation in the future.

Many molecular markers have been identified with relevance for monitoring treatment response, including both chemotherapy and targeted treatment modalities. For example, *MGMT* promoter methylation as a predictor of response to temozolomide, *BRAF* V600 E levels in urine circulating tumor DNA for BRAFi, and MEKi response monitoring in colorectal NEN, and serum *SLFN11* as a predictor of response to platinum-based chemotherapy in lung LCNEC. Methylation-based biomarkers are an emerging field, with groups using in vitro disease models to identify them. Further, CgA levels, while not useful in NEN diagnosis, are widely used as a general marker of disease response and progression in all subtypes of NEN.[6,154,177,178] Serum-based detection of accurate markers to guide treatment selection is an attractive prospect and ongoing field of active research, offering the possibility of personalized management regimens without the need for more intensive molecular profiling or primary culturing of sampled patient tissue.

SUMMARY

As a rare and widely heterogeneous group of neoplasms, NENs pose ongoing challenges for timely detection and management, often diagnosed at advanced stages where curative surgical intervention is unachievable. A host of complex and often unique molecular changes underpin the pathobiology of each NEN subtype, our understanding of which continues to improve with ongoing research. The exploitation of these unique molecular signatures from a clinical perspective is not without challenges; however, the use of targeted treatment regimens and disease monitoring tailored to individual patients and tumor biology is undoubtedly the future of medical management in NEN. We have explored the genomic and epigenomic landscape of several major NEN subtypes based on current understanding. Further, we have detailed the current diagnostic, treatment, and monitoring approaches which exploit these unique molecular signatures to enhance clinical management of NEN; continued exploration of novel biomarkers and therapeutic targets will form a key component of improved NEN management in the future.

CLINICS CARE POINTS

- Advances in the genomic and epigenomic profiling of NENs continues to enhance our understanding of the pathways which drive tumourigenesis in different NEN subtypes – proffering new molecular targets for improving diagnosis, treatment, and disease monitoring.
- Whilst curative surgical management is often unachievable in advanced NEN, there is a growing range of available targeted treatment approaches that exploit these key molecular pathways.
- Evidence for the use of more targeted diagnostic, treatment, and monitoring approaches continues to build, with a number of clinical trials ongoing.
- Molecular profiling of individual tumours represents a future ideal to maximise patient outcomes through precision oncology.

DISCLOSURE

The authors have nothing to disclose.

ACKNOWLEDGMENTS

The authors would like to also thank TD Scott Chair in Urology Trust, Department of Surgical Sciences, and Department of Pathology at the Dunedin School of Medicine, University of Otago for supporting our work.

REFERENCES

1. Rickman DS, Beltran H, Demichelis F, et al. Biology and evolution of poorly differentiated neuroendocrine tumors. Nat Med 2017;23(6):664–73.
2. Rindi G, Inzani F. Neuroendocrine neoplasm update: toward universal nomenclature. Endocr Relat Cancer 2020;27(6):R211–8.
3. Hofland J, Kaltsas G, de Herder WW. Advances in the diagnosis and management of well-differentiated neuroendocrine neoplasms. Endocr Rev 2020;41(2):371–403.
4. van Riet J, van de Werken HJG, Cuppen E, et al. The genomic landscape of 85 advanced neuroendocrine neoplasms reveals subtype-heterogeneity and potential therapeutic targets. Nat Commun 2021;12(1):4612.
5. Kawasaki K, Toshimitsu K, Matano M, et al. An organoid biobank of neuroendocrine neoplasms

enables genotype-phenotype mapping. Cell 2020; 183(5):1420–35.
6. Pavel M, Öberg K, Falconi M, et al. Gastroenteropancreatic neuroendocrine neoplasms: ESMO Clinical Practice Guidelines for diagnosis, treatment and follow-up. Ann Oncol 2020;31(7):844–60.
7. Malczewska A, Kidd M, Matar S, et al. A comprehensive assessment of the role of miRNAs as biomarkers in gastroenteropancreatic neuroendocrine tumors. Neuroendocrinology 2018;107:73–90.
8. Turai PI, Nyírő G, Butz H, et al. MicroRNAs, long non-coding RNAs, and circular RNAs: potential biomarkers and therapeutic targets in pheochromocytoma/paraganglioma. Cancers (Basel) 2021; 13(7):1522.
9. Kidd M, Modlin I, Öberg K. Towards a new classification of gastroenteropancreatic neuroendocrine neoplasms. Nat Rev Clin Oncol 2016;13(11):691–705.
10. Venizelos A, Elvebakken H, Perren A, et al. The molecular characteristics of high-grade gastroenteropancreatic neuroendocrine neoplasms. Endocr Relat Cancer 2022;29(1):1–14.
11. Kidd M, Modlin IM, Bodei L, et al. Decoding the molecular and mutational ambiguities of gastroenteropancreatic neuroendocrine neoplasm pathobiology. Cell Mol Gastroenterol Hepatol 2015;1(2): 131–53.
12. Zikusoka MN, Kidd M, Eick G, et al. The molecular genetics of gastroenteropancreatic neuroendocrine tumors. Cancer Interdiscip Int J Am Cancer Soc 2005;104(11):2292–309.
13. Perren A, Komminoth P, Saremaslani P, et al. Mutation and expression analyses reveal differential subcellular compartmentalization of PTEN in endocrine pancreatic tumors compared to normal islet cells. Am J Pathol 2000;157(4):1097–103.
14. Hu W, Feng Z, Modica I, et al. Gene amplifications in well-differentiated pancreatic neuroendocrine tumors inactivate the p53 pathway. Genes Cancer 2010;1(4):360–8.
15. Kytölä S, Höög A, Nord B, et al. Comparative genomic hybridization identifies loss of 18q22-qter as an early and specific event in tumorigenesis of midgut carcinoids. Am J Pathol 2001;158(5):1803–8.
16. Kytölä S, Nord B, Edström Elder E, et al. Alterations of the SDHD gene locus in midgut carcinoids, Merkel cell carcinomas, pheochromocytomas, and abdominal paragangliomas. Genes Chromosomes Cancer 2002;34(3):325–32.
17. Banck MS, Kanwar R, Kulkarni AA, et al. The genomic landscape of small intestine neuroendocrine tumors. J Clin Invest 2013;123(6):2502–8.
18. Pipinikas CP, Berner AM, Sposito T, et al. The evolving (epi) genetic landscape of pancreatic neuroendocrine tumours. Endocr Relat Cancer 2019;26(9):R519–44.
19. House MG, Herman JG, Guo MZ, et al. Aberrant hypermethylation of tumor suppressor genes in pancreatic endocrine neoplasms. Ann Surg 2003; 238(3):423.
20. Kidd M, Eick G, Shapiro MD, et al. Microsatellite instability and gene mutations in transforming growth factor-beta type II receptor are absent in small bowel carcinoid tumors. Cancer 2005; 103(2):229–36.
21. April-Monn SL, Andreasi V, Schiavo Lena M, et al. EZH2 inhibition as new epigenetic treatment option for pancreatic neuroendocrine neoplasms (PanNENs). Cancers (Basel) 2021;13(19):5014.
22. Barazeghi E, Hellman P, Norlén O, et al. EZH2 presents a therapeutic target for neuroendocrine tumors of the small intestine. Sci Rep 2021;11(1): 22733.
23. Rahman MM, Qian ZR, Wang EL, et al. DNA methyltransferases 1, 3a, and 3b overexpression and clinical significance in gastroenteropancreatic neuroendocrine tumors. Hum Pathol 2010;41(8): 1069–78.
24. How-Kit A, Dejeux E, Dousset B, et al. DNA methylation profiles distinguish different subtypes of gastroenteropancreatic neuroendocrine tumors. Epigenomics 2015;7(8):1245–58.
25. Simon T, Riemer P, Jarosch A, et al. DNA methylation reveals distinct cells of origin for pancreatic neuroendocrine carcinomas and pancreatic neuroendocrine tumors. Genome Med 2022;14(1):1–14.
26. Hackeng WM, Dreijerink KMA, de Leng WWJ, et al. Genome methylation accurately predicts neuroendocrine tumor origin: an online tool. Clin Cancer Res 2021;27(5):1341–50.
27. Larsson C, Skogseid B, Öberg K, et al. Multiple endocrine neoplasia type 1 gene maps to chromosome 11 and is lost in insulinoma. Nature 1988; 332(6159):85–7.
28. Richard S, Giraud S, Beroud C, et al. Von Hippel-Lindau disease: recent genetic progress and patient management. Francophone Study Group of von Hippel-Lindau Disease (GEFVH). Ann Endocrinol (Paris) 1998;59(6):452–8.
29. Jiao Y, Shi C, Edil BH, et al. DAXX/ATRX, MEN1, and mTOR pathway genes are frequently altered in pancreatic neuroendocrine tumors. Science 2011;331(6021):1199–203.
30. Marinoni I, Kurrer AS, Vassella E, et al. Loss of DAXX and ATRX are associated with chromosome instability and reduced survival of patients with pancreatic neuroendocrine tumors. Gastroenterology 2014;146(2):453–60.
31. Scarpa A, Chang DK, Nones K, et al. Whole-genome landscape of pancreatic neuroendocrine tumours. Nature 2017;543(7643):65–71.
32. Puccini A, Poorman K, Salem ME, et al. Comprehensive genomic profiling of gastroenteropancreatic

neuroendocrine neoplasms (GEP-NENs). Clin Cancer Res 2020;26(22):5943–51.
33. Mitsui J, Takahashi Y, Goto J, et al. Mechanisms of genomic instabilities underlying two common fragile-site-associated loci, PARK2 and DMD, in germ cell and cancer cell lines. Am J Hum Genet 2010;87(1):75–89.
34. Jelinkova S, Fojtik P, Kohutova A, et al. Dystrophin deficiency leads to genomic instability in human pluripotent stem cells via NO synthase-induced oxidative stress. Cells 2019;8(1):53.
35. Lin W, Watanabe H, Peng S, et al. Dynamic epigenetic regulation by menin during pancreatic islet tumor formation. Mol Cancer Res 2015;13(4):689–98.
36. Di Domenico A, Wiedmer T, Marinoni I, et al. Genetic and epigenetic drivers of neuroendocrine tumours (NET). Endocr Relat Cancer 2017;24(9): R315–34.
37. Jia D, Augert A, Kim D-W, et al. Crebbp loss drives small cell lung cancer and increases sensitivity to HDAC inhibition. Cancer Discov 2018;8(11): 1422–37.
38. Fotouhi O, Adel Fahmideh M, Kjellman M, et al. Global hypomethylation and promoter methylation in small intestinal neuroendocrine tumors: an in vivo and in vitro study. Epigenetics 2014;9(7): 987–97.
39. Lakis V, Lawlor RT, Newell F, et al. DNA methylation patterns identify subgroups of pancreatic neuroendocrine tumors with clinical association. Commun Biol 2021;4(1):1–11.
40. Chan AO-O, Kim SG, Bedeir A, et al. CpG island methylation in carcinoid and pancreatic endocrine tumors. Oncogene 2003;22(6):924–34.
41. Walter T, Van Brakel B, Vercherat C, et al. O6-Methylguanine-DNA methyltransferase status in neuroendocrine tumours: prognostic relevance and association with response to alkylating agents. Br J Cancer 2015;112(3):523–31.
42. Schmitt AM, Schmid S, Rudolph T, et al. VHL inactivation is an important pathway for the development of malignant sporadic pancreatic endocrine tumors. Endocr Relat Cancer 2009;16(4):1219–27.
43. Tirosh A, Mukherjee S, Lack J, et al. Distinct genome-wide methylation patterns in sporadic and hereditary nonfunctioning pancreatic neuroendocrine tumors. Cancer 2019;125(8):1247–57.
44. Francis JM, Kiezun A, Ramos AH, et al. Somatic mutation of CDKN1B in small intestine neuroendocrine tumors. Nat Genet 2013;45(12):1483–6.
45. Karpathakis A, Dibra H, Pipinikas C, et al. Prognostic impact of novel molecular subtypes of small intestinal neuroendocrine tumor. Clin Cancer Res 2016;22(1):250–8.
46. Andersson E, Arvidsson Y, Swärd C, et al. Expression profiling of small intestinal neuroendocrine tumors identifies subgroups with clinical relevance, prognostic markers and therapeutic targets. Mod Pathol 2016;29(6):616–29.
47. Simbolo M, Vicentini C, Mafficini A, et al. Mutational and copy number asset of primary sporadic neuroendocrine tumors of the small intestine. Virchows Arch 2018;473(6):709–17.
48. Sei Y, Zhao X, Forbes J, et al. A hereditary form of small intestinal carcinoid associated with a germline mutation in inositol polyphosphate multikinase. Gastroenterology 2015;149(1):67–78.
49. Dumanski JP, Rasi C, Björklund P, et al. A MUTYH germline mutation is associated with small intestinal neuroendocrine tumors. Endocr Relat Cancer 2017;24(8):427–43.
50. Zhang H-Y, Rumilla KM, Jin L, et al. Association of DNA methylation and epigenetic inactivation of RASSF1A and beta-catenin with metastasis in small bowel carcinoid tumors. Endocrine 2006; 30(3):299–306.
51. Edfeldt K, Ahmad T, Åkerström G, et al. TCEB3C a putative tumor suppressor gene of small intestinal neuroendocrine tumors. Endocr Relat Cancer 2014;21(2):275–84.
52. Verdugo AD, Crona J, Starker L, et al. Global DNA methylation patterns through an array-based approach in small intestinal neuroendocrine tumors. Endocr Relat Cancer 2014;21(1):L5–7.
53. Choi I-S, Estecio MR, Nagano Y, et al. Hypomethylation of LINE-1 and Alu in well-differentiated neuroendocrine tumors (pancreatic endocrine tumors and carcinoid tumors). Mod Pathol 2007;20(7): 802–10.
54. Barazeghi E, Prabhawa S, Norlén O, et al. Decrease of 5-hydroxymethylcytosine and TET1 with nuclear exclusion of TET2 in small intestinal neuroendocrine tumors. BMC Cancer 2018;18(1):764.
55. Chen L, Liu M, Zhang Y, et al. Genetic characteristics of colorectal neuroendocrine carcinoma: more similar to colorectal adenocarcinoma. Clin Colorectal Cancer 2021;20(2):177–85.e113.
56. Capdevila J, Arqués O, Hernández Mora JR, et al. Epigenetic EGFR gene repression confers sensitivity to therapeutic BRAFV600E blockade in colon neuroendocrine carcinomas. Clin Cancer Res 2020;26(4):902–9.
57. Shamir ER, Devine WP, Pekmezci M, et al. Identification of high-risk human papillomavirus and Rb/E2F pathway genomic alterations in mutually exclusive subsets of colorectal neuroendocrine carcinoma. Mod Pathol 2019;32(2):290–305.
58. Pelosi G, Sonzogni A, Harari S, et al. Classification of pulmonary neuroendocrine tumors: new insights. Translational Lung Cancer Res 2017;6(5): 513.
59. Pelosi G, Bianchi F, Dama E, et al. Most high-grade neuroendocrine tumours of the lung are likely to secondarily develop from pre-existing carcinoids:

innovative findings skipping the current pathogenesis paradigm. Virchows Arch 2018;472(4):567–77.
60. Fernandez-Cuesta L, Peifer M, Lu X, et al. Frequent mutations in chromatin-remodelling genes in pulmonary carcinoids. Nat Commun 2014;5(1):1–7.
61. Rea F, Rizzardi G, Zuin A, et al. Outcome and surgical strategy in bronchial carcinoid tumors: single institution experience with 252 patients. Eur J Cardiothorac Surg 2007;31(2):186–91.
62. Simbolo M, Mafficini A, Sikora KO, et al. Lung neuroendocrine tumours: deep sequencing of the four World Health Organization histotypes reveals chromatin-remodelling genes as major players and a prognostic role for TERT, RB1, MEN1 and KMT2D. J Pathol 2017;241(4):488–500.
63. Laddha SV, Da Silva EM, Robzyk K, et al. Integrative genomic characterization identifies molecular subtypes of lung carcinoids. Cancer Res 2019; 79(17):4339–47.
64. Cros J, Théou-Anton N, Gounant V, et al. Specific genomic alterations in high-grade pulmonary neuroendocrine tumours with carcinoid morphology. Neuroendocrinology 2021;111(1–2):158–69.
65. Alcala N, Leblay N, Gabriel AAG, et al. Integrative and comparative genomic analyses identify clinically relevant pulmonary carcinoid groups and unveil the supra-carcinoids. Nat Commun 2019;10(1): 1–21.
66. Swarts DRA, Scarpa A, Corbo V, et al. MEN1 gene mutation and reduced expression are associated with poor prognosis in pulmonary carcinoids. J Clin Endocrinol Metab 2014;99(2):E374–8.
67. George J, Lim JS, Jang SJ, et al. Comprehensive genomic profiles of small cell lung cancer. Nature 2015;524(7563):47–53.
68. Armengol G, Sarhadi VK, Rönty M, et al. Driver gene mutations of non-small-cell lung cancer are rare in primary carcinoids of the lung: NGS study by ion Torrent. Lung 2015;193(2):303–8.
69. Walch AK, Zitzelsberger HF, Aubele MM, et al. Typical and atypical carcinoid tumors of the lung are characterized by 11q deletions as detected by comparative genomic hybridization. Am J Pathol 1998;153(4):1089–98.
70. Swarts DRA, Ramaekers FCS, Speel E-JM. Molecular and cellular biology of neuroendocrine lung tumors: evidence for separate biological entities. Biochim Biophys Acta (BBA)-Reviews Cancer 2012;1826(2):255–71.
71. Rekhtman N, Pietanza MC, Hellmann MD, et al. Next-generation sequencing of pulmonary large cell neuroendocrine carcinoma reveals small cell carcinoma–like and non–small cell carcinoma–like subsets. Clin Cancer Res 2016;22(14):3618–29.
72. George J, Walter V, Peifer M, et al. Integrative genomic profiling of large-cell neuroendocrine carcinomas reveals distinct subtypes of high-grade neuroendocrine lung tumors. Nat Commun 2018; 9(1):1–13.
73. Rudin CM, Durinck S, Stawiski EW, et al. Comprehensive genomic analysis identifies SOX2 as a frequently amplified gene in small-cell lung cancer. Nat Genet 2012;44(10):1111–6.
74. Derks JL, Leblay N, Thunnissen E, et al. Molecular subtypes of pulmonary large-cell neuroendocrine carcinoma predict chemotherapy treatment outcome. Clin Cancer Res 2018;24(1):33–42.
75. Hermans BCM, Derks JL, Thunnissen E, et al. Prevalence and prognostic value of PD-L1 expression in molecular subtypes of metastatic large cell neuroendocrine carcinoma (LCNEC). Lung Cancer 2019;130:179–86.
76. Wistuba II, Behrens C, Virmani AK, et al. High resolution chromosome 3p allelotyping of human lung cancer and preneoplastic/preinvasive bronchial epithelium reveals multiple, discontinuous sites of 3p allele loss and three regions of frequent breakpoints. Cancer Res 2000;60(7):1949–60.
77. Kim K-B, Kim Y, Rivard CJ, et al. FGFR1 is critical for RBL2 loss-driven tumor development and requires PLCG1 activation for continued growth of small cell lung cancer. Cancer Res 2020;80(22): 5051–62.
78. Vollbrecht C, Werner R, Walter RFH, et al. Mutational analysis of pulmonary tumours with neuroendocrine features using targeted massive parallel sequencing: a comparison of a neglected tumour group. Br J Cancer 2015;113(12): 1704–11.
79. Ireland AS, Micinski AM, Kastner DW, et al. MYC drives temporal evolution of small cell lung cancer subtypes by reprogramming neuroendocrine fate. Cancer Cell 2020;38(1):60–78.
80. Rudin CM, Poirier JT, Byers LA, et al. Molecular subtypes of small cell lung cancer: a synthesis of human and mouse model data. Nat Rev Cancer 2019;19(5):289–97.
81. Sutherland KD, Ireland AS, Oliver TG. Killing SCLC: insights into how to target a shapeshifting tumor. Genes Dev 2022;36(5–6):241–58.
82. Sonkin D, Thomas A, Teicher BA. Are neuroendocrine negative small cell lung cancer and large cell neuroendocrine carcinoma with WT RB1 two faces of the same entity? Lung Cancer Manag 2019;8(2):LMT13.
83. Meder L, König K, Ozretić L, et al. NOTCH, ASCL1, p53 and RB alterations define an alternative pathway driving neuroendocrine and small cell lung carcinomas. Int J Cancer 2016;138(4):927–38.
84. Hermans BCM, Derks JL, Thunnissen E, et al. DLL3 expression in large cell neuroendocrine carcinoma (LCNEC) and association with molecular subtypes and neuroendocrine profile. Lung Cancer 2019; 138:102–8.

85. Lim JS, Ibaseta A, Fischer MM, et al. Intratumoural heterogeneity generated by Notch signalling promotes small-cell lung cancer. Nature 2017;545(7654):360–4.
86. George J, Saito M, Tsuta K, et al. Genomic amplification of CD274 (PD-L1) in small-cell lung cancer. Clin Cancer Res 2017;23(5):1220–6.
87. Capodanno A, Boldrini L, Alì G, et al. Phosphatidylinositol-3-kinase α catalytic subunit gene somatic mutations in bronchopulmonary neuroendocrine tumours. Oncol Rep 2012;28(5):1559–66.
88. Mohammad HP, Smitheman KN, Kamat CD, et al. A DNA hypomethylation signature predicts antitumor activity of LSD1 inhibitors in SCLC. Cancer Cell 2015;28(1):57–69.
89. Sabari JK, Lok BH, Laird JH, et al. Unravelling the biology of SCLC: implications for therapy. Nat Rev Clin Oncol 2017;14(9):549–61.
90. Murai F, Koinuma D, Shinozaki-Ushiku A, et al. EZH2 promotes progression of small cell lung cancer by suppressing the TGF-β-Smad-ASCL1 pathway. Cell Discov 2015;1(1):1–17.
91. Toyooka S, Toyooka KO, Maruyama R, et al. DNA methylation profiles of lung tumors1. Mol Cancer Ther 2001;1(1):61–7.
92. Richter AM, Kiehl S, Köger N, et al. ZAR1 is a novel epigenetically inactivated tumour suppressor in lung cancer. Clin Epigenetics 2017;9(1):1–12.
93. Kalari S, Jung M, Kernstine KH, et al. The DNA methylation landscape of small cell lung cancer suggests a differentiation defect of neuroendocrine cells. Oncogene 2013;32(30):3559–68.
94. Sunaga N, Miyajima K, Suzuki M, et al. Different roles for caveolin-1 in the development of non-small cell lung cancer versus small cell lung cancer. Cancer Res 2004;64(12):4277–85.
95. Simbolo M, Barbi S, Fassan M, et al. Gene expression profiling of lung atypical carcinoids and large cell neuroendocrine carcinomas identifies three transcriptomic subtypes with specific genomic alterations. J Thorac Oncol 2019;14(9):1651–61.
96. Qiu H, Jin B-M, Wang Z-F, et al. MEN1 deficiency leads to neuroendocrine differentiation of lung cancer and disrupts the DNA damage response. Nat Commun 2020;11(1):1–12.
97. Neumann HPH, Young WF Jr, Eng C. Pheochromocytoma and paraganglioma. N Engl J Med 2019;381(6):552–65.
98. Mulligan LM, Kwok JBJ, Healey CS, et al. Germline mutations of the RET proto-oncogene in multiple endocrine neoplasia type 2A. Nature 1993;363(6428):458–60.
99. Latif F, Tory K, Gnarra J, et al. Identification of the von Hippel-Lindau disease tumor suppressor gene. Science 1993;260(5112):1317–20.
100. Bausch B, Borozdin W, Neumann HP, European-American pheochromocytoma study G. Clinical and genetic characteristics of patients with neurofibromatosis type 1. N Engl J Med 2006;1:2729–31.
101. Fishbein L, Leshchiner I, Walter V, et al. Comprehensive molecular characterization of pheochromocytoma and paraganglioma. Cancer Cell 2017;31(2):181–93.
102. Moog S, Lussey-Lepoutre C, Favier J. Epigenetic and metabolic reprogramming of SDH-deficient paragangliomas. Endocr Relat Cancer 2020;27(12):R451–63.
103. Favier J, Gimenez-Roqueplo A-P. Pheochromocytomas: the (pseudo)-hypoxia hypothesis. Best Pract Res Clin Endocrinol Metab 2010;24(6):957–68.
104. Crona J, Delgado Verdugo A, Maharjan R, et al. Somatic mutations in H-RAS in sporadic pheochromocytoma and paraganglioma identified by exome sequencing. J Clin Endocrinol Metab 2013;98(7):E1266–71.
105. Yeh IT, Lenci RE, Qin Y, et al. A germline mutation of the KIF1Bβ gene on 1p36 in a family with neural and nonneural tumors. Hum Genet 2008;124(3):279–85.
106. Qin Y, Yao L, King EE, et al. Germline mutations in TMEM127 confer susceptibility to pheochromocytoma. Nat Genet 2010;42(3):229–33.
107. Toledo RA, Qin Y, Cheng ZM, et al. Recurrent mutations of chromatin-remodeling genes and kinase receptors in pheochromocytomas and paragangliomas. Clin Cancer Res 2016;22(9):2301–10.
108. Fishbein L, Khare S, Wubbenhorst B, et al. Whole-exome sequencing identifies somatic ATRX mutations in pheochromocytomas and paragangliomas. Nat Commun 2015;6(1):6140.
109. Jochmanova I, Pacak K. Genomic landscape of pheochromocytoma and paraganglioma. Trends Cancer 2018;4(1):6–9.
110. Taipale J, Beachy PA. The Hedgehog and Wnt signalling pathways in cancer. Nature 2001;411(6835):349–54.
111. Pelullo M, Zema S, Nardozza F, et al. Wnt, Notch, and TGF-β pathways impinge on hedgehog signaling complexity: an open window on cancer. Front Genet 2019;10:711.
112. Letouzé E, Martinelli C, Loriot C, et al. SDH mutations establish a hypermethylator phenotype in paraganglioma. Cancer Cell 2013;23(6):739–52.
113. Backman S, Maharjan R, Falk-Delgado A, et al. Global DNA methylation analysis identifies two discrete clusters of pheochromocytoma with distinct genomic and genetic alterations. Sci Rep 2017;7(1):44943.
114. Remacha L, Currás-Freixes M, Torres-Ruiz R, et al. Gain-of-function mutations in DNMT3A in patients with paraganglioma. Genet Med 2018;20(12):1644–51.
115. Eisenhofer G, Klink B, Richter S, et al. Metabologenomics of phaeochromocytoma and paraganglioma: an

integrated approach for personalised biochemical and genetic testing. Clin Biochemist Rev 2017;38(2):69.

116. De Cubas AA, Korpershoek E, Inglada-Pérez L, et al. DNA methylation profiling in pheochromocytoma and paraganglioma reveals diagnostic and prognostic markers. Clin Cancer Res 2015; 21(13):3020–30.
117. Kiss NB, Geli J, Lundberg F, et al. Methylation of the p16INK4A promoter is associated with malignant behavior in abdominal extra-adrenal paragangliomas but not pheochromocytomas. Endocr Relat Cancer 2008;15(2):609.
118. Kiss NB, Muth A, Andreasson A, et al. Acquired hypermethylation of the P16INK4A promoter in abdominal paraganglioma: relation to adverse tumor phenotype and predisposing mutation. Endocr Relat Cancer 2013;20(1):65–78.
119. Briest F, Grabowski P. PI3K-AKT-mTOR-signaling and beyond: the complex network in gastroenteropancreatic neuroendocrine neoplasms. Theranostics 2014;4(4):336–65.
120. Sundin A, Arnold R, Baudin E, et al. ENETS consensus guidelines for the standards of care in neuroendocrine tumors: radiological, nuclear medicine and hybrid imaging. Neuroendocrinology 2017;105(3):212–44.
121. Werner RA, Weich A, Higuchi T, et al. Imaging of chemokine receptor 4 expression in neuroendocrine tumors-a triple tracer comparative approach. Theranostics 2017;7(6):1489.
122. Kaemmerer D, Träger T, Hoffmeister M, et al. Inverse expression of somatostatin and CXCR4 chemokine receptors in gastroenteropancreatic neuroendocrine neoplasms of different malignancy. Oncotarget 2015;6(29):27566.
123. Kidd M, Modlin IM, Drozdov I, et al. A liquid biopsy for bronchopulmonary/lung carcinoid diagnosis. Oncotarget 2018;9(6):7182.
124. Öberg K, Califano A, Strosberg JR, et al. A meta-analysis of the accuracy of a neuroendocrine tumor mRNA genomic biomarker (NETest) in blood. Ann Oncol 2020;31(2):202–12.
125. Modlin IM, Kidd M, Frilling A, et al. Molecular genomic assessment using a blood-based mRNA signature (NETest) is cost-effective and predicts neuroendocrine tumor recurrence with 94% accuracy. Ann Surg 2021;274(3):481–90.
126. Singh S, Bergsland EK, Card CM, et al. Commonwealth neuroendocrine tumour research collaboration and the north American neuroendocrine tumor society guidelines for the diagnosis and management of patients with lung neuroendocrine tumors: an international collaborative endorsement and update of the 2015 European neuroendocrine tumor society expert consensus guidelines. J Thorac Oncol 2020;15(10):1577–98.
127. Öberg K, Castellano D. Current knowledge on diagnosis and staging of neuroendocrine tumors. Cancer Metastasis Rev 2011;30(1):3–7.
128. Grogan RH, Mitmaker EJ, Duh Q-Y. Changing paradigms in the treatment of malignant pheochromocytoma. Cancer Control 2011;18(2):104–12.
129. Zandee WT, de Herder WW. The evolution of neuroendocrine tumor treatment reflected by ENETS guidelines. Neuroendocrinology 2018;106(4):357–65.
130. Lin JP, Zhao YJ, He QL, et al. Adjuvant chemotherapy for patients with gastric neuroendocrine carcinomas or mixed adenoneuroendocrine carcinomas. Br J Surg 2020;107(9):1163–70.
131. Schmitz R, Mao R, Moris D, et al. Impact of Postoperative chemotherapy on the survival of patients with high-grade gastroenteropancreatic neuroendocrine carcinoma. Ann Surg Oncol 2021;28(1): 114–20.
132. Rinke A, Müller HH, Schade-Brittinger C, et al. PROMID Study Group, Placebo-controlled, double-blind, prospective, randomized study on the effect of octreotide LAR in the control of tumor growth in patients with metastatic neuroendocrine midgut tumors: a report from the PROMID Study Group. J Clin Oncol 2009;27:4656–63.
133. Ferolla P, Brizzi MP, Meyer T, et al. Efficacy and safety of long-acting pasireotide or everolimus alone or in combination in patients with advanced carcinoids of the lung and thymus (LUNA): an open-label, multicentre, randomised, phase 2 trial. Lancet Oncol 2017;18(12):1652–64.
134. Caplin ME, Pavel M, Phan AT, et al. Lanreotide autogel/depot in advanced enteropancreatic neuroendocrine tumours: final results of the CLARINET open-label extension study. Endocrine 2021; 71(2):502–13.
135. Caplin ME, Pavel M, Ćwikła JB, et al. Lanreotide in metastatic enteropancreatic neuroendocrine tumors. N Engl J Med 2014;371(3):224–33.
136. Brabander T, Van der Zwan WA, Teunissen JJM, et al. Long-term efficacy, survival, and safety of [177Lu-DOTA0, Tyr3] octreotate in patients with gastroenteropancreatic and bronchial neuroendocrine tumors. Clin Cancer Res 2017;23(16): 4617–24.
137. Strosberg J, El-Haddad G, Wolin E, et al. Phase 3 trial of 177Lu-Dotatate for midgut neuroendocrine tumors. N Engl J Med 2017;376(2):125–35.
138. Satapathy S, Mittal BR, Bhansali A. Peptide receptor radionuclide therapy in the management of advanced pheochromocytoma and paraganglioma: a systematic review and meta-analysis. Clin Endocrinol (Oxf) 2019;91(6):718–27.
139. Taïeb D, Jha A, Treglia G, et al. Molecular imaging and radionuclide therapy of pheochromocytoma and paraganglioma in the era of genomic

characterization of disease subgroups. Endocr Relat Cancer 2019;26(11):R627–52.
140. Spyroglou A, Bramis K, Alexandraki KI. Neuroendocrine neoplasms: evolving and future treatments. Curr Opin Endocr Metab Res 2021;19:15–21.
141. Guenter RE, Aweda T, Carmona Matos DM, et al. Pulmonary carcinoid surface receptor modulation using histone deacetylase inhibitors. Cancers (Basel) 2019;11(6):767.
142. Jin X-F, Auernhammer CJ, Ilhan H, et al. Combination of 5-fluorouracil with epigenetic modifiers induces radiosensitization, somatostatin receptor 2 expression, and radioligand binding in neuroendocrine tumor cells in vitro. J Nucl Med 2019;60(9):1240–6.
143. Pryma DA, Chin BB, Noto RB, et al. Efficacy and safety of high-specific-activity 131I-MIBG therapy in patients with advanced pheochromocytoma or paraganglioma. J Nucl Med 2019;60(5):623–30.
144. Zhu M, Costello BA, Yin J, et al. Phase II trial of bevacizumab monotherapy in pancreatic neuroendocrine tumors. Pancreas 2021;50(10):1435–9.
145. Halperin DM, Lee JJ, Ng CS, et al. A phase II trial of ziv-aflibercept in patients with advanced pancreatic neuroendocrine tumors. Pancreas 2019;48(3):381–6.
146. Raymond E, Dahan L, Raoul J-L, et al. Sunitinib malate for the treatment of pancreatic neuroendocrine tumors. N Engl J Med 2011;364(6):501–13.
147. Yao JC, Lombard-Bohas C, Baudin E, et al. Daily oral everolimus activity in patients with metastatic pancreatic neuroendocrine tumors after failure of cytotoxic chemotherapy: a phase II trial. J Clin Oncol 2010;28(1):69.
148. Yao JC, Shah MH, Ito T, et al. Everolimus for advanced pancreatic neuroendocrine tumors. N Engl J Med 2011;364(6):514–23.
149. Yao JC, Fazio N, Singh S, et al. Everolimus for the treatment of advanced, non-functional neuroendocrine tumours of the lung or gastrointestinal tract (RADIANT-4): a randomised, placebo-controlled, phase 3 study. The Lancet 2016;387(10022):968–77.
150. Fazio N, Kulke M, Rosbrook B, et al. Updated efficacy and safety outcomes for patients with well-differentiated pancreatic neuroendocrine tumors treated with sunitinib. Target Oncol 2021;16(1):27–35.
151. Druce MR, Kaltsas GA, Fraenkel M, et al. Novel and evolving therapies in the treatment of malignant phaeochromocytoma: experience with the mTOR inhibitor everolimus (RAD001). Horm Metab Res 2009;41(09):697–702.
152. Oh DY, Kim TW, Park YS, et al. Phase 2 study of everolimus monotherapy in patients with nonfunctioning neuroendocrine tumors or pheochromocytomas/paragangliomas. Cancer 2012;118(24):6162–70.
153. Daskalakis K, Tsoli M, Angelousi A, et al. Antitumour activity of everolimus and sunitinib in neuroendocrine neoplasms. Endocr Connections 2019;8(6):641–53.
154. Klempner SJ, Gershenhorn B, Tran P, et al. BRAFV600E mutations in high-grade colorectal neuroendocrine tumors may predict responsiveness to BRAF–MEK combination therapy. Cancer Discov 2016;6(6):594–600.
155. Cao Y, Ma Y, Yu J, et al. Favorable response to immunotherapy in a pancreatic neuroendocrine tumor with temozolomide-induced high tumor mutational burden. Cancer Commun 2020;40(12):746–51.
156. Shen L, Yu X, Lu M, et al. Surufatinib in combination with toripalimab in patients with advanced neuroendocrine carcinoma: results from a multicenter, open-label, single-arm, phase II trial. J Clin Oncol 2021;39(15_suppl):e16199.
157. Halperin DM, Liu S, Dasari A, et al. A phase II trial of atezolizumab and bevacizumab in patients with advanced, progressive neuroendocrine tumors (NETs). Am Soc Clin Oncol 2020;38(4_suppl):619.
158. Klein O, Kee D, Markman B, et al. Immunotherapy of ipilimumab and nivolumab in patients with advanced neuroendocrine tumors: a subgroup analysis of the CA209-538 clinical trial for rare cancers. Clin Cancer Res 2020;26(17):4454–9.
159. Patel SP, Mayerson E, Chae YK, et al. A phase II basket trial of Dual Anti-CTLA-4 and Anti-PD-1 Blockade in Rare Tumors (DART) SWOG S1609: high-grade neuroendocrine neoplasm cohort. Cancer 2021;127(17):3194–201.
160. Capdevila J, Teule A, López C, et al. 1157O A multi-cohort phase II study of durvalumab plus tremelimumab for the treatment of patients (pts) with advanced neuroendocrine neoplasms (NENs) of gastroenteropancreatic or lung origin: the DUNE trial (GETNE 1601). Ann Oncol 2020;31:S770–1.
161. Xu JX, Wu DH, Ying LW, et al. Immunotherapies for well-differentiated grade 3 gastroenteropancreatic neuroendocrine tumors: a new category in the World Health Organization classification. World J Gastroenterol 2021;27(47):8123–37.
162. Rudin CM, Pietanza MC, Bauer TM, et al. Rovalpituzumab tesirine, a DLL3-targeted antibody-drug conjugate, in recurrent small-cell lung cancer: a first-in-human, first-in-class, open-label, phase 1 study. Lancet Oncol 2017;18(1):42–51.
163. Johnson ML, Zvirbule Z, Laktionov K, et al. Rovalpituzumab tesirine as a maintenance therapy after first-line platinum-based chemotherapy in patients with extensive-stage SCLC: results from the phase 3 MERU study. J Thorac Oncol 2021;16(9):1570–81.

164. Blackhall F, Jao K, Greillier L, et al. Efficacy and safety of rovalpituzumab tesirine compared with topotecan as second-line therapy in DLL3-high SCLC: results from the phase 3 TAHOE study. J Thorac Oncol 2021;16(9):1547–58.
165. Uprety D, Remon J, Adjei AA. All that glitters is not gold: the story of rovalpituzumab tesirine in SCLC. J Thorac Oncol 2021;16(9):1429 33.
166. Jin N, Lubner SJ, Mulkerin DL, et al. A phase II trial of a histone deacetylase inhibitor panobinostat in patients with low-grade neuroendocrine tumors. Oncologist 2016;21(7):785–786g.
167. Balasubramaniam S, Redon CE, Peer CJ, et al. Phase I trial of belinostat with cisplatin and etoposide in advanced solid tumors, with a focus on neuroendocrine and small cell cancers of the lung. Anticancer Drugs 2018;29(5):457.
168. Schmitz RL, Weissbach J, Kleilein J, et al. Targeting hdacs in pancreatic neuroendocrine tumor models. Cells 2021;10(6):1408.
169. Wanek J, Gaisberger M, Beyreis M, et al. Pharmacological inhibition of class IIA HDACs by LMK-235 in pancreatic neuroendocrine tumor cells. Int J Mol Sci 2018;19(10):3128.
170. Koga S, Onishi H, Masuda S, et al. PTPN3 is a potential target for a new cancer immunotherapy that has a dual effect of T cell activation and direct cancer inhibition in lung neuroendocrine tumor. Transl Oncol 2021;14(9):101152.
171. Matlac DM, Hadrava Vanova K, Bechmann N, et al. Succinate mediates tumorigenic effects via succinate receptor 1: potential for new targeted treatment strategies in succinate dehydrogenase deficient paragangliomas. Front Endocrinol (Lausanne) 2021;12:129.
172. Ullrich M, Richter S, Seifert V, et al. Targeting cyclooxygenase-2 in pheochromocytoma and paraganglioma: focus on genetic background. Cancers (Basel) 2019;11(6).
173. Pang Y, Lu Y, Caisova V, et al. Targeting NAD+/PARP DNA repair pathway as a novel therapeutic approach to SDHB-mutated cluster I pheochromocytoma and paraganglioma. Clin Cancer Res 2018; 24(14):3423–32.
174. Kamihara J, Hamilton KV, Pollard JA, et al. Belzutifan, a potent HIF2α inhibitor, in the Pacak–Zhuang syndrome. N Engl J Med 2021;385(22):2059–65.
175. Chen W, Hill H, Christie A, et al. Targeting renal cell carcinoma with a HIF-2 antagonist. Nature 2016; 539(7627):112–7.
176. Caisova V, Li L, Gupta G, et al. The significant reduction or complete eradication of subcutaneous and metastatic lesions in a pheochromocytoma mouse model after immunotherapy using mannan-BAM, TLR ligands, and anti-CD40. Cancers (Basel) 2019;11(5):654.
177. Marotta V, Zatelli MC, Sciammarella C, et al. Chromogranin A as circulating marker for diagnosis and management of neuroendocrine neoplasms: more flaws than fame. Endocr Relat Cancer 2018;25(1): R11–29.
178. Sabari JK, Julian RA, Ni A, et al. Outcomes of advanced pulmonary large cell neuroendocrine carcinoma stratified by RB1 loss, SLFN11 expression, and tumor mutational burden. Am Soc Clin Oncol 2018;36(15_suppl):e20568.

Gastroenteropancreatic Neuroendocrine Tumor Diagnosis: DOTATATE PET/CT

Asha Kandathil, MBBS, DMRD, MD[a,*],
Rathan M. Subramaniam, MD, PhD, MPH, MBA, FRSN, FSNMMI, FRANZCR[b,c]

KEYWORDS

• Neuroendocrine tumor (NET) • Gastroenteropancreatic NET (GEP-NET) • ^{68}Ga DOTATATE PET/CT • SSTR

KEY POINTS

- ^{68}Ga-DOTATATE PET/computed tomography (CT) is indicated for localization and initial tumor staging in somatostatin receptor (SSTR) expressing gastroenteropancreatic neuroendocrine tumors (GEP-NETs).
- Increased sensitivity and specificity of SSTR imaging over anatomic imaging results in management change in up to 40% of patients.
- ^{68}Ga-DOTATATE PET/CT is a prerequisite for selecting patients for SSTR-targeted peptide receptor radionuclide therapy.
- National Comprehensive Cancer Network (NCCN) guidelines consider SSTR imaging with ^{68}Ga-DOTATATE PET/CT appropriate for staging and assessment of receptor status of GEP-NETs.

INTRODUCTION

Neuroendocrine neoplasms (NENs) arise in secretory cells of the diffuse neuroendocrine system, most commonly involving the gastrointestinal (GI) tract and pancreas. NENs include well-differentiated, indolent neuroendocrine tumors (NETs) and rapidly progressing neuroendocrine carcinomas (NECs). There has been a global increase in the incidence of NETs, with a disease prevalence of approximately 170,000 patients in the United States. Gastroenteropancreatic-NETs (GEP-NETs) comprise 55% to 70% of all NETs with tumors arising in the small intestine (30.8%), rectum (26.3%), colon (17.6%), pancreas (12.1%), and appendix (5.7%).[1–3] Carcinoid tumors of the GI tract originate from enterochromaffin cells, and pancreatic NETs (pNETs) arise in the islets of Langerhans or precursors in the ductal epithelium.[4] Although most GEP-NETs are sporadic, occasionally, these tumors can be part of inherited familial syndromes, including multiple endocrine neoplasia type 1 (MEN-1), tuberous sclerosis Von-Hippel Lindau syndrome, and neurofibromatosis type 1. There is a 3.6-fold increased risk of NET with a family history of NET in a first-degree relative.[2,4]

Tumors may be hormonally functioning or nonfunctioning. Serotonin and other vasoactive substances secreted by metastatic midgut carcinoids result in the typical carcinoid syndrome characterized by flushing, diarrhea, and right-sided valvular heart disease. pNETs may rarely present with clinical syndromes (insulinoma syndrome, gastrinoma syndrome, glucagonoma syndrome, and so forth) due to the production of a variety of peptide hormones. Insulinoma, the most common functioning pNET, presenting with the "Whipple triad" of symptomatic hypoglycemia, blood glucose level less than 50 mg/dL, and relief

[a] Department of Radiology, University of Texas Southwestern Medical Center, 5323 Harry Hines Boulevard, Dallas, TX 75390-9316, USA; [b] Duke University Medical Center, Department of Radiology, 2301 Erwin Road Box 3808, Durham, NC 27710, USA; [c] Department of Medicine, Otago Medical School, University of Otago, First Floor, Dunedin Hospital, 201 Great King Street, Dunedin 9016, New Zealand
* Corresponding author.
E-mail address: Asha.Kandathil@UTSouthwestern.edu

PET Clin 18 (2023) 189–200
https://doi.org/10.1016/j.cpet.2022.11.001
1556-8598/23/

of symptoms with ingestion of glucose is usually solitary lesions, smaller than 2 cm with very low malignant potential. Gastrinomas, which cause the Zollinger–Ellison syndrome, are potentially malignant. Atrophic gastritis is associated with multiple small Type 1 gastric NET. Type 2 solitary gastric NET, which causes the Zollinger–Ellison syndrome, is rare. Duodenal NETs are small lesions in the first or second part of the duodenum. NETs of the small intestine may be multifocal and have a high tendency to metastasize to the liver, mesenteric nodes, and peritoneum with the indolent progression of metastatic disease. Colonic NETs are rarely functional, large at diagnosis, and often metastatic. Rectal NETs are small tumors with a relatively low malignant potential but, once metastatic, can progress rapidly.[5]

The clinical behavior of GEP-NETs is determined by tumor grade measured by the proliferative activity according to the Ki-67 index and tumor differentiation. Low-grade (grade 1 [G1]) tumors have Ki-67 index $\leq$2%, intermediate-grade (G2) tumors have Ki-67 index 3% to 20%, and high-grade (G3) tumors have Ki-67 index greater than 20%. Poorly differentiated NECs usually have a Ki-67 greater than 55%.[6] Regardless of size or stage, well-differentiated G1 and G2 NENs are termed NETs, and poorly differentiated NENs are termed NECs. From a study on 154 patients with GEP-NET, Panzuto and colleagues report that the most important negative prognostic factors are a pancreatic site of the primary tumor, poor tumor differentiation, and the presence of distant metastases.[7]

European Society for Medical Oncology (ESMO) clinical practice guidelines recommend evaluating SSTR expression, proliferative activity, growth rate, and disease extent of NETs.[8] A comprehensive evaluation of a patient with suspected NET includes an assessment of symptoms to determine if the NET is secreting hormones and whether there is a hereditary predisposition. Imaging is performed to assess the organ of origin, assign stage, and determine somatostatin receptor (SSTR) expression. Biopsy determines tumor differentiation and grade. Cross-sectional abdominal imaging with computed tomography (CT) or MR imaging scans plays a key role in assessing the location and extent of GEP-NETs. According to NCCN guidelines, evaluation with SSTR imaging is appropriate for staging and assessing receptor status.[9] Prognosis is highly variable, but some patients with inoperable metastases survive for many years on treatment with good quality of life. Most localized tumors are amenable to resection. Patients with low-grade metastatic NETs are often treated with monthly long-acting somatostatin analog (SSA) injections; however, many patients receive several different therapies, including peptide receptor radionuclide therapy (PRRT) during the course of their illness.[10]

Somatostatin Receptors

High-density expression of SSTRs in NETs forms the basis of SSTR imaging with DOTATATE PET/CT. GEP-NETs express SSTR-2a abundantly, followed by SSTR-3 and -1. SSTR expression correlates inversely with tumor grade, with high expression in low-grade tumors and the lowest expression in high-grade or poorly differentiated tumors. A recent study, however, showed that 26% of the 163 included patients with high-grade GEP-NETs were strongly positive for SSTR-2a. Conversely, poorly differentiated, proliferative NECs have low SSTR-2a expression.

In general, DOTATATE PET/CT is preferred for imaging low-grade GEP-NETs which express SSTRs, and Fluorine 18- Fluorodeoxy glucose (^{18}F-FDG) PET imaging is preferred for imaging high-grade GEP-NETs which lose SSTR expression but have high metabolic activity[11,12] (**Fig. 1**).

Somatostatin Receptor Imaging

Functional imaging based on tumor SSTR expression was historically performed using indium-111 (^{111}In)-pentetreotide scintigraphy (OctreoScan). However, due to better sensitivity and specificity, decreased radiation dose, and shorter imaging protocol of SSTR PET, the American College of Radiology (ACR)[13] and the Society of Nuclear Medicine and Molecular Imaging (SNMMI)[14] recommend that SSTR PET should replace ^{111}In-pentetreotide in all indications in which ^{111}In-pentetreotide was previously being used. ^{68}Ga-DOTATATE, ^{64}Cu-DOTATATE, ^{68}Ga-DOTATOC, and ^{68}Ga-DOTANOC have been used for SSTR PET imaging.

^{68}Ga-DOTATATE combines SSA peptide Tyr3-octreotide with gallium-68 and the DOTA chelator (tetraazacyclododecane-tetraacetic acid). ^{68}Ga-DOTATOC combines Tyr3-octreotate, and ^{68}Ga-DOTANOC combines l-Nal3—octreotide with gallium-68 and the DOTA chelator.[15] ^{68}Ga-DOTATATE binds exclusively to SSTR2 with a 10-fold higher affinity than both ^{68}Ga-DOTATOC and ^{68}Ga-DOTANOC. In addition, ^{68}Ga DOTATOC has an affinity for SSTR-2 and some affinity for SSTR-5, and ^{68}Ga-DOTANOC has an affinity for SSTR-2, -5, and -3[16].

DOTATATE can also be labeled with ^{64}Cu produced in a cyclotron. ^{64}Cu-DOTATATE PET/CT is a diagnostic alternative for ^{68}Ga-DOTATATE PET/CT in centers that do not have a ^{68}Ga

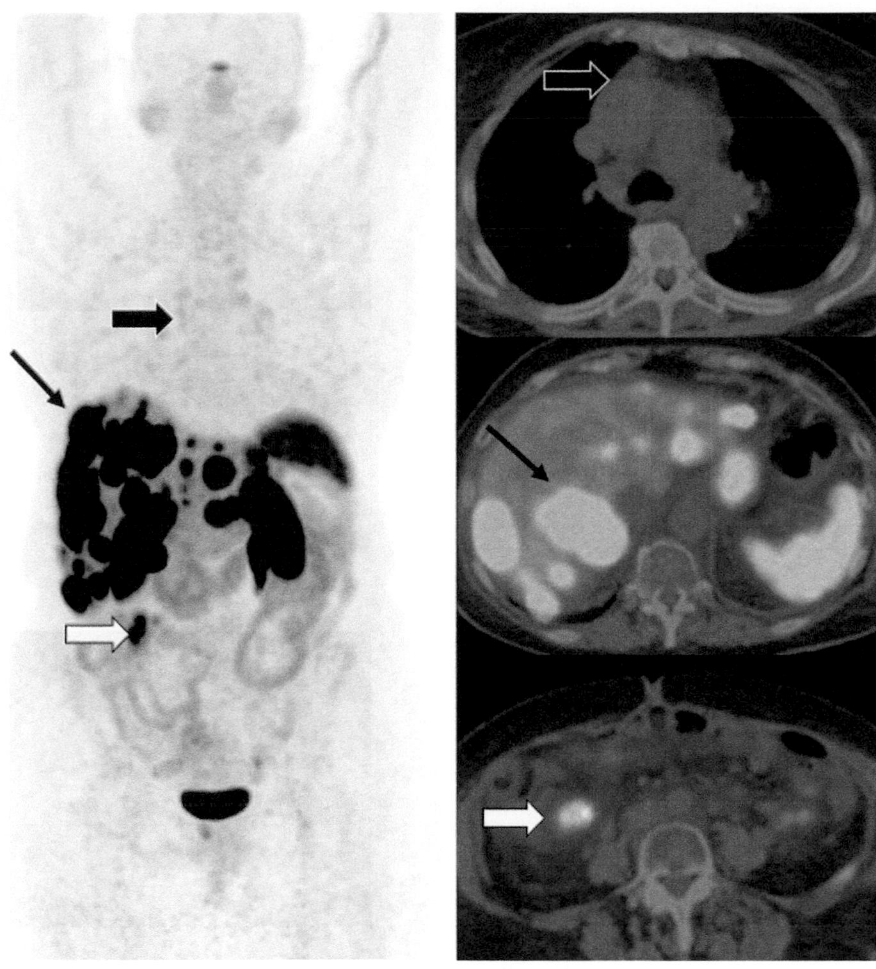

Fig. 1. An 84-year-old woman with metastatic ileal carcinoid. ^{68}Ga-DOTATATE PET/CT demonstrates a DOTATATE -avid mass in the terminal ileum (*broad white arrow*) and multiple liver metastases (*thin black arrows*). Note mildly Dotatate-avid reactive mediastinal nodes (*broad black arrow*).

generator.[17] ^{68}Ga-DOTATATE and ^{64}Cu-DOTATATE injections are FDA-approved for localization of SSTR positive NETs in adult patients (**Fig. 2**).

^{68}Ga-DOTATATE PET/CT

Preparation

Before SSTR-PET/CT, patients should be instructed to discontinue short-acting SSAs 12 hours before the study. SSTR-PET/CT should be scheduled 3 to 4 weeks after long-acting SSAs to avoid potential SSTR blockade.[13] A prospective study by Aalbersberg and colleagues, however, showed that lanreotide administration immediately before SSTR-PET did not significantly affect normal organ and tumor uptake.[18]

Physiologic biodistribution

The highest physiologic uptake is in the spleen. Kidneys, bladder, liver, adrenal glands, pituitary gland, thyroid gland, pancreas, stomach, small intestine, prostate gland, and uterus also have moderate to high uptake. Mild uptake is present in the parotid and submandibular glands, thymus, muscles, bones, and occasionally cervicothoracic sympathetic ganglia[19] (**Fig. 3**).

Interpretation

Focal tracer uptake, unexplained by physiologic biodistribution or higher than organ background uptake, is considered pathologic, particularly if there is a correlating abnormality on the CT portion of PET/CT. There may be intralesional heterogeneity of SSTR expression, with some areas of good uptake and others without uptake.[13] The degree of SSTR expression can be assessed visually and semi-quantitatively. Modified Krenning score is used to assess SSTR expression qualitatively; level 0, no uptake; 1, very low uptake; 2, uptake $\leq$ liver; 3, uptake greater than liver; and 4, uptake greater than spleen. SSTR expression

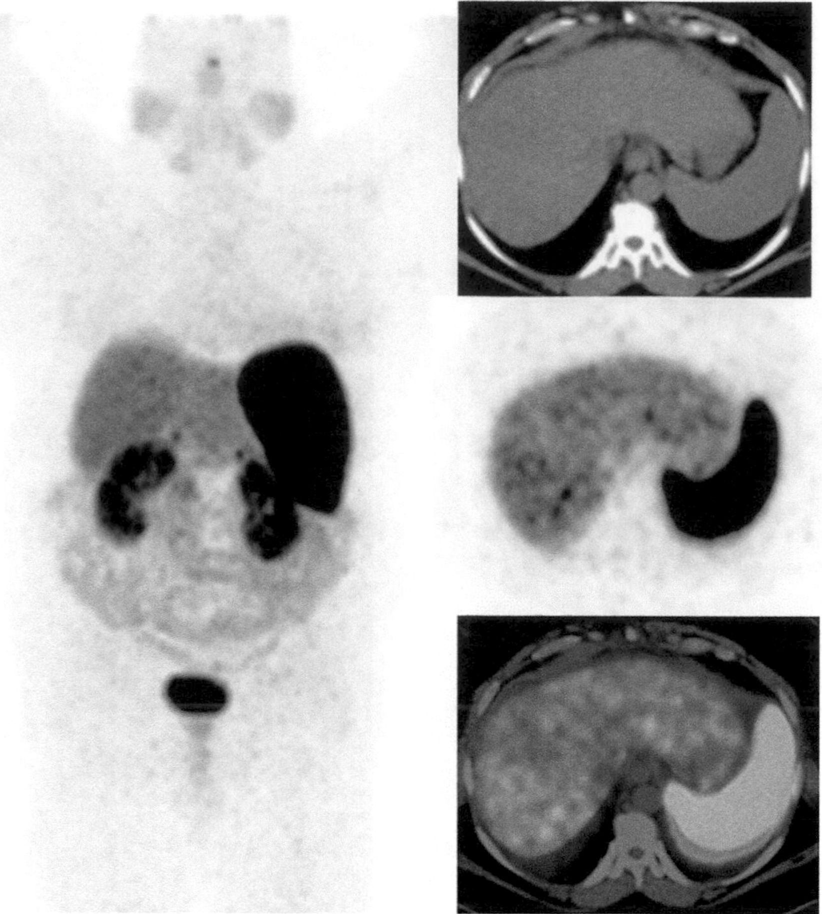

Fig. 2. ^{64}Cu- DOTATATE PET/CT.

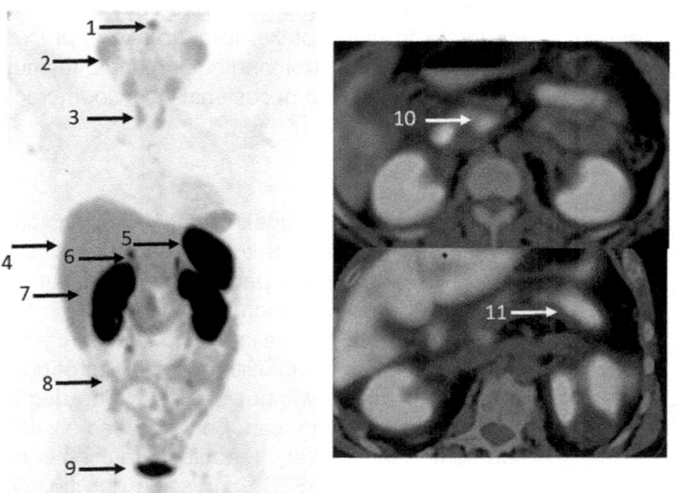

Fig. 3. ^{68}Ga-DOTATATE PET/CT: Normal biodistribution. (1) pituitary gland, (2) salivary glands, (3) thyroid gland, (4) liver, (5) spleen, (6) adrenal glands, (7) kidneys, (8) bowel, (9) bladder, (10) uncinate process of pancreas, and (11) tail of pancreas.

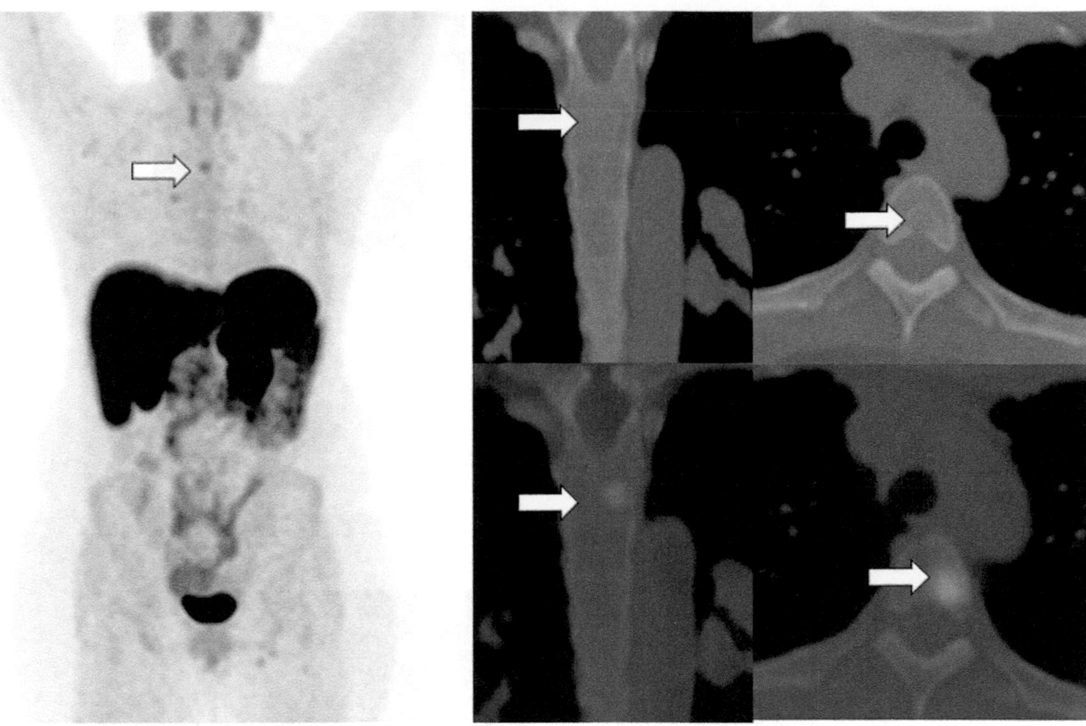

Fig. 4. A 34-year-old man with incidental DOTATATE uptake in a vertebral hemangioma (*broad white arrow*).

is assessed semi-quantitatively with standardized uptake value (SUV) measurements. An increase or decrease in SUV-based measurements should not be used to assess response. Instead, disease progression or response should be assessed by the development of new lesions or the disappearance of known lesions.[20] There may be false-positive and false-negative radiotracer uptake.

False-Positive Uptake

Physiologic uptake in the head/uncinate process or tail of the pancreas, splenules, splenosis, or heterotopic pancreas can mimic NET. Osteoblasts express SSTR-2. Osteoblastic activity related to the normal growth plate, degenerative bone and joint disease, fibrous dysplasia, fractures, and vertebral hemangiomas will have low-intensity uptake. However, it can be correctly diagnosed based on typical CT features (**Fig. 4**, false positive).

SSTR-2 expression by white blood count (WBCs) leads to low-intensity uptake in inflammatory lesions such as post-radiation or postsurgical changes, prostatitis, and reactive lymphadenopathy, including sarcoidosis and tuberculosis. Various non-NETs such as pheochromocytoma, paraganglioma, neuroblastoma, schwannoma, meningioma, and mesenchymal tumor-causing oncogenic osteomalacia have high intensity of uptake. ^{68}Ga-DOTATATE PET/CT is indicated in the evaluation of pheochromocytoma, paraganglioma, neuroblastoma, and atypical meningiomas (**Fig. 5**).

Variable SSTR expression is also seen in medullary thyroid cancer, Merkel cell carcinoma, small cell carcinoma, esthesioneuroblastoma, and differentiated thyroid cancer. Other tumors such as breast cancer, gastric cancer, colorectal cancer, melanoma, lymphoma, hepatocellular carcinoma, renal cell carcinoma, small cell and non-small cell lung cancer, sarcoma, and glioblastoma multiforme are also known to express SSTR. Knowledge of imaging appearance and pattern of spread of various neoplasms is essential for accurate interpretation[21] (**Fig. 6**).

False-Negative Uptake

Poorly differentiated tumors with low SSTR expression may result in false-negative SSTR PET. However, these tumors often show high metabolic activity on ^{18}F FDG-PET/CT (**Fig. 7**). Decreased SSTR expression may be seen following recent chemotherapy, radiation therapy, embolization, or PRRT. Small lesions below the resolution of PET/CT may not be detected. Tumor uptake may be obscured by uptake in inflammatory tissue or areas of high physiologic uptake, such as in the uncinate process or tail of the

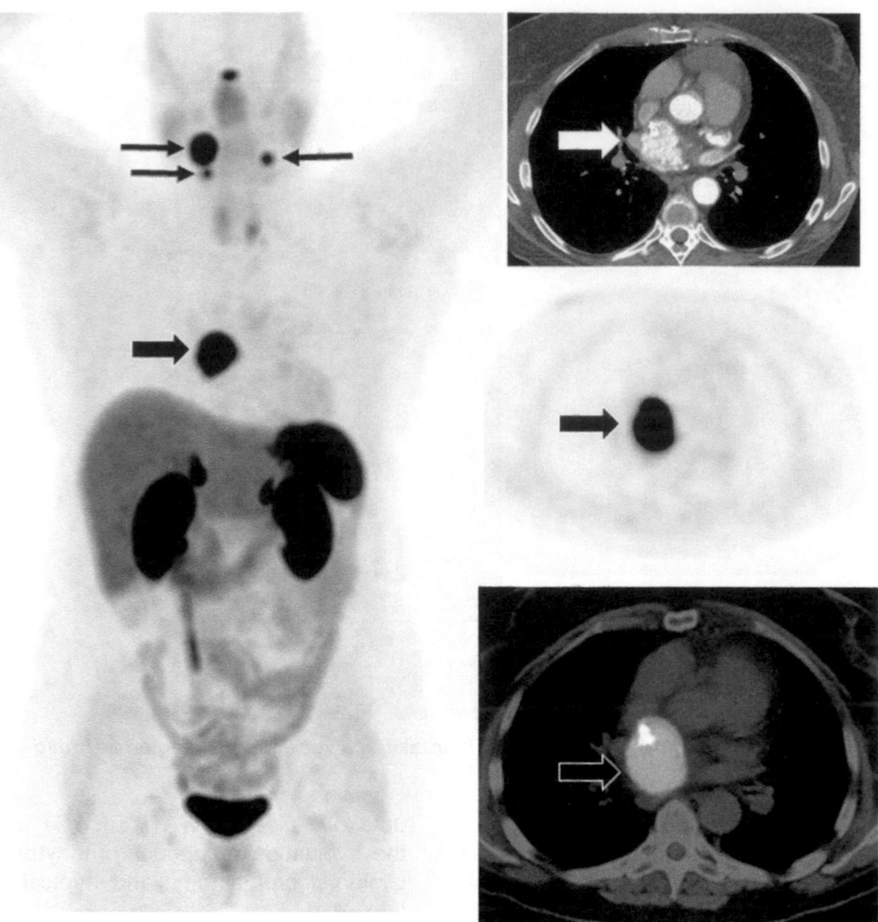

Fig. 5. A 54-year-old man with MEN-1 syndrome. ^{68}Ga-DOTATATE PET/CT demonstrates intense DOTATATE uptake (*broad black arrows*) in the enhancing (*broad white arrow*) mediastinal paraganglioma. Note multiple DOTATATE-avid paragangliomas in the neck (*thin black arrows*).

pancreas. In addition, there may be misregistration between CT and PET images due to motion, resulting in false-negative radiotracer uptake.[13]

Role of ^{68}Ga-DOTATATE PET/CT in Gastroenteropancreatic-Neuroendocrine Tumor

^{68}Ga-DOTATATE PET/CT is indicated for identification of primary tumor in patients with strong clinical suspicion and laboratory evidence of NET, in patients with known NET metastasis, and patients with MEN. It can also be used to evaluate lesions suggestive of NET on conventional imaging but is not amenable to biopsy. ^{68}Ga-DOTATATE PET/CT is also indicated for initial tumor staging in patients with biopsy-proven NET and the selection of patients for octreotide hormonal therapy or SSTR-targeted PRRT.[13,14]

Primary tumor

^{68}Ga-SSTR-PET/CT has reported a sensitivity of 88% to 93% and specificity of 88% to 95% for most well-differentiated NENs with a lower sensitivity of 68% and specificity of 52% for gastrinoma and NEN of unknown primary.[22] Insulinomas have low levels of SSTR-2 and may not be detected on ^{68}Ga-DOTATATE -PET/CT.[23] Nickel and colleagues, however, found that ^{68}Ga-DOTATATE -PET/CT detected 90% of insulinomas in their study cohort and suggested that ^{68}Ga-DOTATATE -PET/CT should be considered for localization of insulinomas when other imaging studies are negative.[24] In a retrospective review, Chauhan and colleagues identified the primary tumor on ^{68}Ga-DOTATATE-PET/CT in 17 of 38 (45%) patients with unknown primary. They found that higher grade (G3) tumors had a lower mean SUV than lower grade (G1 and G2) tumors. Treatment with long-acting SSTR agonists did not affect mean SUV in this patient population.[1] In a study of 38

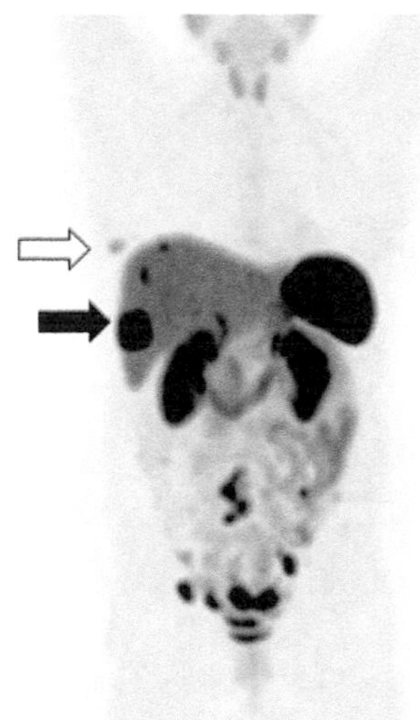
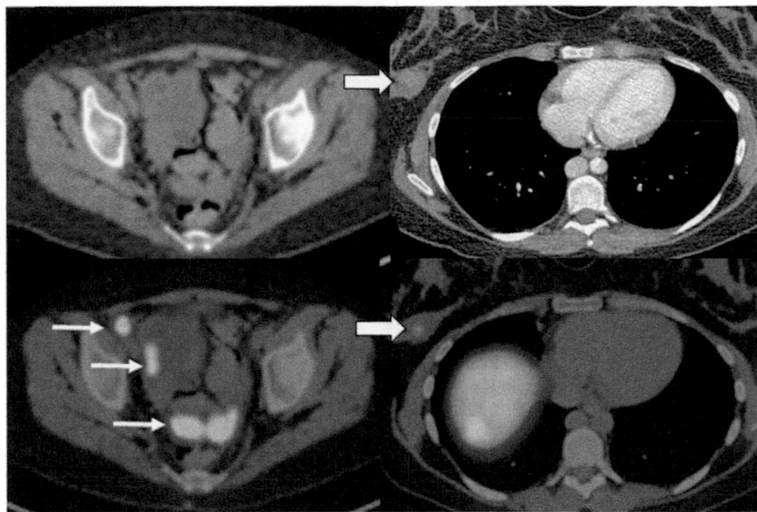

Fig. 6. A 40-year-old woman with postoperative recurrence of appendiceal neuroendocrine tumor. ^{68}Ga-DOTATATE PET/CT demonstrates multiple DOTATATE-avid peritoneal metastases (*thin white arrows*) and liver metastases (*broad black arrow*). Note mild DOTATATE uptake in a biopsy-proven fibroadenoma in the right breast (*broad white arrows*).

NET patients with cancer of unknown primary, ^{68}Ga-DOTATATE PET/CT had a higher sensitivity of 94% and accuracy of 87% compared with contrast-enhanced CT (ceCT), which had a sensitivity of 63% and accuracy of 68%. Most confirmed primary tumors were located in the ileum and pancreas.[25] A systematic review and meta-analysis on the use of SSTR PET/CT imaging for the detection of pNET found that ^{68}Ga-DOTATATE-PET/CT had pooled sensitivity of 79.6% and specificity of 95%, with pooled detection rate for the primary lesion of 81% on patient-based analysis and 92% for lesion-based analysis[26] (**Fig. 8**).

In a prospective study in patients with MEN-1 syndrome, ^{68}Ga-DOTATATE-PET/CT detected more lesions and metastases with change in management compared with (111)In-pentetreotide single photon emitting computerized tomography (SPECT)/CT and CT scan.[27]

Staging

An analysis of SEER data from 2010 to 2014 by Trikalinos and colleagues observed that 9% of patients with NENs had lung metastases, 77% had liver metastases, 7% had bone metastases, and 6% had brain metastases. Patients with bone or brain metastases had worse survival.[28] Tumor, node metastasis staging (TNM) staging system, which varies with the site of the primary NET tumor, is used to determine disease extent, therapeutic management, and prognosis.[29,30] In a

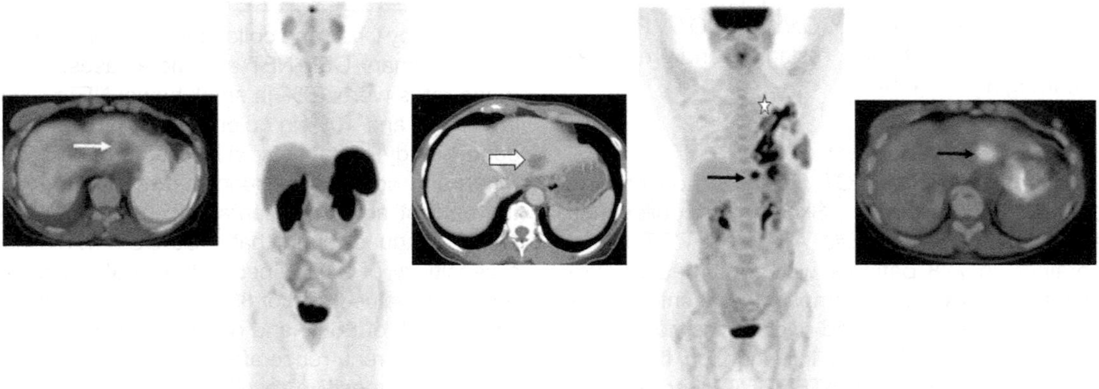

Fig. 7. A 60-year-old woman with metastatic high-grade neuroendocrine tumor. The liver metastasis (*broad white arrow*) is not avid (*thin white arrow*) on the ^{68}Ga-DOTATATE PET/CT but is avid (*thin black arrows*) on the ^{18}F FDG-PET/CT. Note incidental FDG uptake (*star*) in inflammatory changes around ruptured left breast implant.

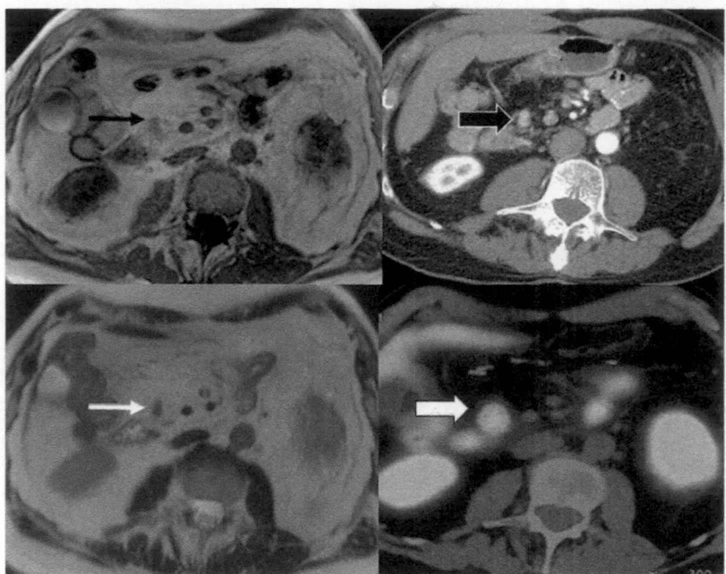
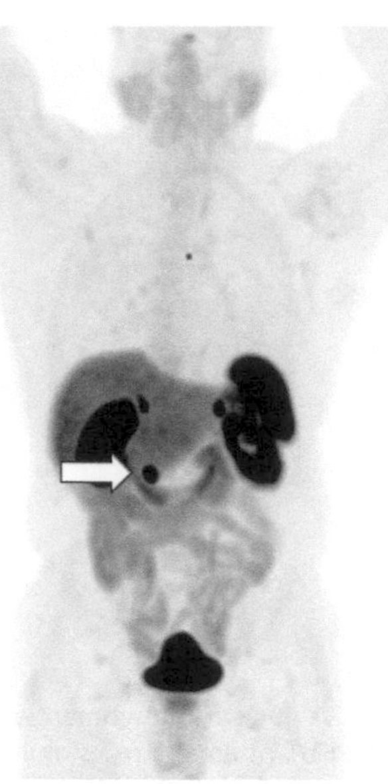

Fig. 8. A 70-year-old man with incidentally detected pancreatic nodule on CT (*broad black arrow*) which is isointense to muscle on T1W (*thin black arrow*) and T2W MR imaging sequences (*thin white arrow*). Endoscopic ultrasound guided biopsy was nondiagnostic. Intense uptake on ^{68}Ga-DOTATATE PET/CT (*broad white arrow*) is diagnostic of a pancreatic neuroendocrine tumor. No metastatic lesions were identified.

study on 154 patients with GEP-NET, Panzuto and colleagues found that 64.3% of patients had metastases at initial diagnosis, regardless of primary tumor site, with an overall 5-year survival rate of 77.5%. Patients with distant metastases, particularly non-hepatic metastases such as bone and lung lesions, had worse prognoses and shorter survival.[7] In a study evaluating the detection of extra-hepatic metastases in 54 NET patients, Albanus and colleagues found that ^{68}Ga-DOTATATE PET/ceCT had better sensitivity and specificity than stand-alone ceCT. Significantly more bone and lymph node metastases were identified on PET.[31] ^{68}Ga-SSR-PET/CT has a higher detection rate than conventional imaging.[26] ESMO guidelines recommend ^{68}Ga/^{64}Cu-DOTA-PET/CT imaging for NET staging, restaging, and preoperative imaging[8] (**Fig. 9**).

Impact on management

Additional SSTR PET/CT findings often change patient management.[32] Skoura and colleagues evaluated 1258 ^{68}Ga-DOTATATE PET/CT scans obtained in 728 patients with confirmed or suspected NENs and compared patient demographics, histology, and indications for ^{68}Ga-DOTATATE PET/CT and influence on the treatment plan. ^{68}Ga-DOTATATE PET/CT had a sensitivity of 97%, specificity of 95.1%, accuracy of 96.6%, a positive predictive value of 98.5%, and a negative predictive value of 90.4%. New SSTR PET/CT findings resulted in management change in 40.9% of patients.[33] In a retrospective analysis by Shell and colleagues of patients with carcinoid-like symptoms and negative anatomic imaging and endoscopy ^{68}Ga-DOTATATE- PET/CT detected NETs in both biochemically positive and biochemically negative patients resulting in management change and symptom improvement.[34] Another prospective study evaluating the detection of GEP-NETs and unknown primary site findings on ^{68}Ga-DOTATATE-PET/CT resulted in a change in management for 33% of patients compared with multiphasic CT and/or MR[27] (**Fig. 10**).

Tumor Recurrence

In a study by Chan and colleagues following resection of primary GEP-NET and metastases, recurrence rates were 18% in small bowel NETs, 26% in pNETs, and 10% in colon/rectum NETs.[35] In a cohort study of patients with resected GEP-NET, Singh and colleagues found that recurrence was the earliest among patients with pNETs.[36] Haug and colleagues found that ^{68}Ga-DOTATATE had a sensitivity of 94%, specificity of 89%, positive predictive value (PPV) of 85%, negative predictive value (NPV) of 96%, and accuracy of 91% in the detection of recurrence after curative resection of NETs. False-positive results were due to inflammatory changes, and false-negative results were due to high-grade tumors or small-size of metastases[37] NCCN guidelines recommend abdominal multiphasic CT or MR imaging for routine

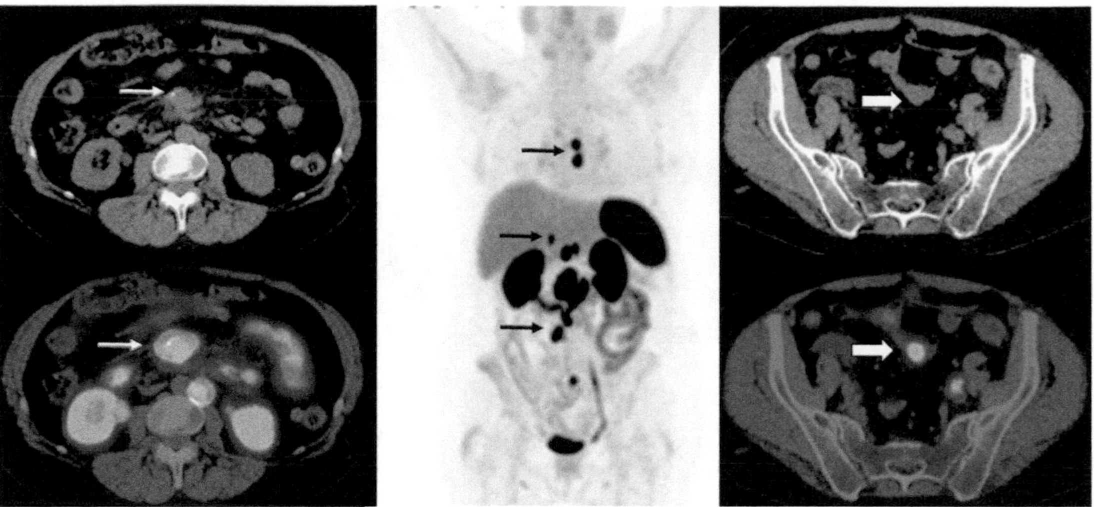

Fig. 9. An 80-year-old man with metastatic ileal carcinoid. ^{68}Ga-DOTATATE PET/CT demonstrates a DOTATATE-avid ileal tumor (*broad white arrow*), mesenteric nodal mass with calcification and adjacent fat stranding (*thin white arrow*) and multiple mediastinal and abdominal nodal metastases (*thin black arrow*).

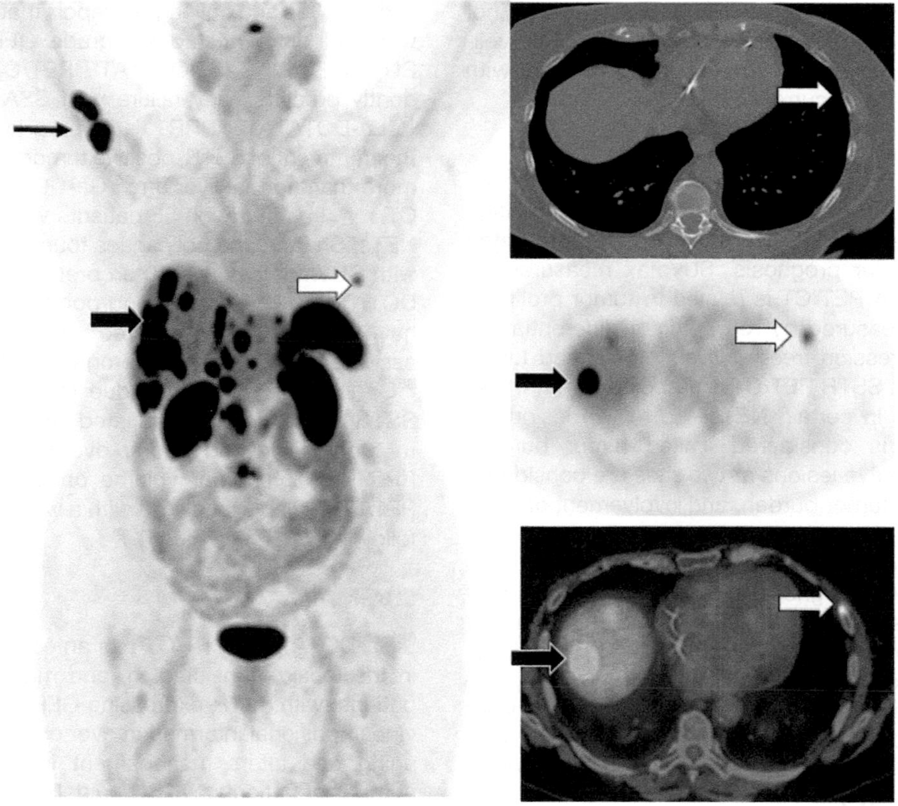

Fig. 10. A 52-year-old woman with metastatic neuroendocrine tumor. ^{68}Ga-DOTATATE PET/CT demonstrates multiple DOTATATE-avid liver metastases (*broad black arrow*). DOTATATE-avid bone metastases in the rib without corresponding changes on CT (*broad white arrow*) and right humerus (*thin black arrow*) were unexpected findings, associated with worse survival.

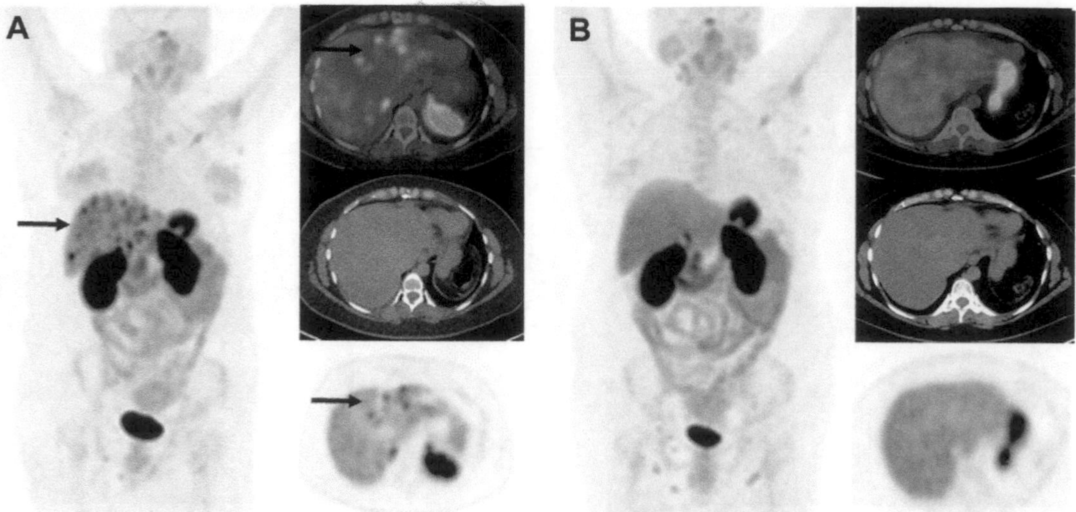

Fig. 11. A 42-year-old woman with metastatic neuroendocrine tumor, treated with ^{177}Lu-DOTATATE PRRT. (*A*) Pretreatment ^{68}Ga-DOTATATE PET/CT demonstrates multiple DOTATATE-avid liver metastases (*thin black arrow*) with uptake more than liver. (*B*) Post-treatment ^{68}Ga-DOTATATE PET/CT demonstrates marked decrease in DOTATATE-avid lesions. However, as the lesions are not adequately assessed on non-contrast-enhanced CT portion of PET/CT, contrast-enhanced CT or MR imaging is essential for therapeutic response assessment.

surveillance. Although SSTR-based imaging is not recommended for routine post-treatment surveillance, it is indicated for evaluating patients with known tumor recurrence.[9]

Prognostication

SSTR expression by GEP-NETs, as indicated by DOTATATE uptake, has a significant correlation with overall survival, with higher uptake associated with a better prognosis. SUVmax measured on ^{68}Ga DOTA-PET/CT is related to tumor proliferation as measured by Ki-67, tumor differentiation, and progression-free survival.[38] Increased tumor burden on SSTR PET/CT is associated with worse prognosis in certain NETs—up to five lesions at one site is considered limited tumor burden, more than five lesions at two sites are considered moderate tumor burden, and involvement of more than two sites is considered extensive tumor burden. A high overall tumor burden is associated with a worse prognosis.[20] In a prospective study of 184 patients total ^{68}Ga-DOTATATE-avid tumor volume of $\geq$7.0 mL was associated with higher odds of disease progression as defined by the development of a new lesion or growth of a known lesion and a ^{68}Ga-DOTATATE TV of $\geq$35.8 mL was associated with the increased risk of disease-specific death.[39]

Therapy selection

Findings on SSTR imaging can determine if patients are suitable for SSTR analog therapy or PRRT.[40] Lee and colleagues report that in patients with well-differentiated low-grade GEP-NET low SUVmax on ^{68}Ga- DOTATATE PET/CT independently predicts early failure with SSA therapy.[41] ^{177}Lu-DOTATATE PRRT is appropriate only for the treatment of SSTR-positive tumors with uptake more than normal liver on ^{68} Ga-DOTATATE PET/CT.[13,42] In a study on 55 patients with metastatic NETs, Sharma and colleagues found that patients with SUVmax below 13.0 on pretreatment ^{68} Ga-DOTATATE PET/CT respond poorly to PRRT and have worse progression-free survival.[43] Visually assessed intralesional heterogeneity on baseline ^{68}Ga-DOTATATE PET/CT due to heterogeneous SSTR expression is associated with shorter time to progression and poorer overall survival after PRRT.[44] High tumor volume on baseline SSTR PET/CT is also associated with a worse prognosis following PRRT[45] (**Fig. 11**).

SUMMARY

^{68}Ga-DOTATATE PET/CT has an established role in the localization, staging, and management of patients with SSTR-expressing GEP-NETs. It provides additional information over conventional imaging and alters management in a significant number of patients. NCCN guidelines, ACR practice parameters, and SNMMI appropriateness criteria consider ^{68}Ga-DOTATATE PET/CT appropriate for staging and receptor status assessment before SSA therapy and PRRT.

CLINICS CARE POINTS

- ^{68}Ga-DOTATATE PET/computed tomography (CT) is the standard of care for localization, staging, and management of patients with somatostatin receptor (SSTR)-expressing gastroenteropancreatic neuroendocrine tumors (GEP-NETs).
- ^{68}Ga-DOTATATE PET/CT has higher sensitivity and specificity than anatomic imaging. Additional findings detected on SSTR PET/CT alter management in a significant number of patients.
- SSTR expression as indicated by radiotracer uptake more than normal liver on ^{68}Ga-DOTATATE PET/CT is a prerequisite for PRRT.
- The degree and heterogeneity of SSTR expression and tumor volume on gallium-68 DOTATATE PET/CT have a significant correlation with overall survival.

DISCLOSURE

The authors have nothing to disclose.

REFERENCES

1. Chauhan A, Kohn E, Del Rivero J. Neuroendocrine tumors-less well known, often misunderstood, and rapidly growing in incidence. JAMA Oncol 2020; 6(1):21–2.
2. Cives M, Strosberg JR. Gastroenteropancreatic neuroendocrine tumors. CA Cancer J Clin 2018; 68(6):471–87.
3. Das S, Dasari A. Epidemiology, incidence, and prevalence of neuroendocrine neoplasms: are there global differences? Curr Oncol Rep 2021;23(4):43.
4. Frilling A, Akerström G, Falconi M, et al. Neuroendocrine tumor disease: an evolving landscape. Endocr Relat Cancer 2012;19(5):R163–85.
5. Deroose CM, Hindié E, Kebebew E, et al. Molecular imaging of gastroenteropancreatic neuroendocrine tumors: current status and future directions. J Nucl Med 2016;57(12):1949–56.
6. Sanli Y, Garg I, Kandathil A, et al. Neuroendocrine tumor diagnosis and management: (68)Ga-DOTATATE PET/CT. AJR Am J Roentgenol 2018;211(2): 267–77.
7. Panzuto F, Nasoni S, Falconi M, et al. Prognostic factors and survival in endocrine tumor patients: comparison between gastrointestinal and pancreatic localization. Endocr Relat Cancer 2005;12(4): 1083–92.
8. Pavel M, Öberg K, Falconi M, et al. Gastroenteropancreatic neuroendocrine neoplasms: ESMO Clinical Practice Guidelines for diagnosis, treatment and follow-up. Ann Oncol 2020;31(7):844–60.
9. Shah MH, Goldner WS, Benson AB, et al. Neuroendocrine and Adrenal Tumors, Version 2.2021, NCCN Clinical Practice Guidelines in Oncology. J Natl Compr Canc Netw 2021;19(7):839–68.
10. Khan MS, Pritchard DM. Neuroendocrine tumours: what gastroenterologists need to know. Frontline Gastroenterol 2022;13(1):50–6.
11. Remes SM, Leijon HL, Vesterinen TJ, et al. Immunohistochemical expression of somatostatin receptor subtypes in a panel of neuroendocrine neoplasias. J Histochem Cytochem 2019;67(10):735–43.
12. Yu J, Li N, Li J, et al. The correlation between [(68) Ga]DOTATATE PET/CT and cell proliferation in patients with GEP-NENs. Mol Imaging Biol 2019; 21(5):984–90.
13. Subramaniam RM, Bradshaw ML, Lewis K, et al. ACR practice parameter for the performance of gallium-68 DOTATATE PET/CT for neuroendocrine tumors. Clin Nucl Med 2018;43(12):899–908.
14. Hope TA, Bergsland EK, Bozkurt MF, et al. Appropriate use criteria for somatostatin receptor PET imaging in neuroendocrine tumors. J Nucl Med 2018; 59(1):66–74.
15. Antunes P, Gini M, Zhang H, et al. Are radiogallium-labelled DOTA-conjugated somatostatin analogues superior to those labelled with other radiometals? Eur J Nucl Med Mol Imaging 2007;34(7):982–93.
16. Reubi JC, Schär JC, Waser B, et al. Affinity profiles for human somatostatin receptor subtypes SST1-SST5 of somatostatin radiotracers selected for scintigraphic and radiotherapeutic use. Eur J Nucl Med 2000;27(3):273–82.
17. Johnbeck CB, Knigge U, Loft A, et al. Head-to-Head comparison of (64)Cu-DOTATATE and (68)Ga DOTATOC PET/CT: a prospective study of 59 patients with neuroendocrine tumors. J Nucl Med 2017; 58(3):451–7.
18. Aalbersberg EA, de Wit-van der Veen BJ, Versleijen MWJ, et al. Influence of lanreotide on uptake of (68)Ga-DOTATATE in patients with neuroendocrine tumours: a prospective intra-patient evaluation. Eur J Nucl Med Mol Imaging 2019; 46(3):696–703.
19. Ozguven S, Filizoğlu N, Kesim S, et al. Physiological biodistribution of (68)Ga-DOTA-TATE in normal subjects. Mol Imaging Radionucl Ther 2021;30(1): 39–46.
20. Park S, Parihar AS, Bodei L, et al. Somatostatin receptor imaging and theranostics: current practice and future prospects. J Nucl Med 2021;62(10): 1323–9.
21. Hofman MS, Lau WF, Hicks RJ. Somatostatin receptor imaging with 68Ga DOTATATE PET/CT: clinical

utility, normal patterns, pearls, and pitfalls in interpretation. Radiographics 2015;35(2):500–16.
22. Refardt J, Hofland J, Wild D, et al. New directions in imaging neuroendocrine neoplasms. Curr Oncol Rep 2021;23(12):143.
23. Papotti M, Bongiovanni M, Volante M, et al. Expression of somatostatin receptor types 1-5 in 81 cases of gastrointestinal and pancreatic endocrine tumors. A correlative immunohistochemical and reverse-transcriptase polymerase chain reaction analysis. Virchows Arch 2002;440(5):461–75.
24. Nockel P, Babic B, Millo C, et al. Localization of insulinoma using 68Ga-DOTATATE PET/CT scan. J Clin Endocrinol Metab 2017;102(1):195–9.
25. Kazmierczak PM, Rominger A, Wenter V, et al. The added value of (68)Ga-DOTA-TATE-PET to contrast-enhanced CT for primary site detection in CUP of neuroendocrine origin. Eur Radiol 2017; 27(4):1676–84.
26. Bauckneht M, Albano D, Annunziata S, et al. Somatostatin receptor PET/CT imaging for the detection and staging of pancreatic NET: a systematic review and meta-analysis. Diagnostics (Basel) 2020;10(8):598.
27. Sadowski SM, Millo C, Cottle-Delisle C, et al. Results of (68)Gallium-DOTATATE PET/CT scanning in patients with multiple endocrine neoplasia type 1. J Am Coll Surg 2015;221(2):509–17.
28. Trikalinos NA, Tan BT, Amin M, et al. Effect of metastatic site on survival in patients with neuroendocrine neoplasms (NENs). An analysis of SEER data from 2010 to 2014. BMC Endocr Disord 2020;20(1):44.
29. Rindi G, Klöppel G, Couvelard A, et al. TNM staging of midgut and hindgut (neuro) endocrine tumors: a consensus proposal including a grading system. Virchows Arch 2007;451(4):757–62.
30. Yang M, Zeng L, Zhang Y, et al. TNM staging of pancreatic neuroendocrine tumors: an observational analysis and comparison by both AJCC and ENETS systems from 1 single institution. Medicine (Baltimore) 2015;94(12):e660.
31. Albanus DR, Apitzsch J, Erdem Z, et al. Clinical value of (6)(8)Ga-DOTATATE-PET/CT compared to stand-alone contrast enhanced CT for the detection of extra-hepatic metastases in patients with neuroendocrine tumours (NET). Eur J Radiol 2015; 84(10):1866–72.
32. Ilhan H, Fendler WP, Cyran CC, et al. Impact of (68) Ga-DOTATATE PET/CT on the surgical management of primary neuroendocrine tumors of the pancreas or ileum. Ann Surg Oncol 2015;22(1):164–71.
33. Skoura E, Michopoulou S, Mohmaduvesh M, et al. The Impact of 68Ga-DOTATATE PET/CT imaging on management of patients with neuroendocrine tumors: experience from a national referral center in the United Kingdom. J Nucl Med 2016;57(1):34–40.
34. Shell J, Keutgen XM, Millo C, et al. 68-Gallium DOTATATE scanning in symptomatic patients with negative anatomic imaging but suspected neuroendocrine tumor. Int J Endocr Oncol 2018; 5(1):IJE04.
35. Chan H, Zhang L, Choti MA, et al. Recurrence patterns after surgical resection of gastroenteropancreatic neuroendocrine tumors: analysis from the national comprehensive cancer network oncology outcomes database. Pancreas 2021;50(4):506–12.
36. Singh S, Chan DL, Moody L, et al. Recurrence in resected gastroenteropancreatic neuroendocrine tumors. JAMA Oncol 2018;4(4):583–5.
37. Haug AR, Cindea-Drimus R, Auernhammer CJ, et al. Neuroendocrine tumor recurrence: diagnosis with 68Ga-DOTATATE PET/CT. Radiology 2014;270(2): 517–25.
38. Mehta S, de Reuver PR, Gill P, et al. Somatostatin receptor SSTR-2a expression is a stronger predictor for survival than Ki-67 in pancreatic neuroendocrine tumors. Medicine (Baltimore) 2015;94(40):e1281.
39. Tirosh A, Kebebew E. The utility of (68)Ga-DOTATATE positron-emission tomography/computed tomography in the diagnosis, management, follow-up and prognosis of neuroendocrine tumors. Future Oncol 2018;14(2):111–22.
40. Hu Y, Ye Z, Wang F, et al. Role of somatostatin receptor in pancreatic neuroendocrine tumor development, diagnosis, and therapy. Front Endocrinol 2021;12:679000.
41. Lee H, Eads JR, Pryma DA. 68) Ga-DOTATATE Positron emission tomography-computed tomography quantification predicts response to somatostatin analog therapy in gastroenteropancreatic neuroendocrine tumors. Oncologist 2021;26(1):21–9.
42. Hope TA, Bodei L, Chan JA, et al. NANETS/SNMMI consensus statement on patient selection and appropriate use of (177)Lu-DOTATATE peptide receptor radionuclide therapy. J Nucl Med 2020; 61(2):222–7.
43. Sharma R, Wang WM, Yusuf S, et al. 68)Ga-DOTATATE PET/CT parameters predict response to peptide receptor radionuclide therapy in neuroendocrine tumours. Radiother Oncol 2019; 141:108–15.
44. Graf J, Pape U-F, Jann H, et al. Prognostic significance of somatostatin receptor heterogeneity in progressive neuroendocrine tumor treated with Lu-177 DOTATOC or Lu-177 DOTATATE. Eur J Nucl Med Mol Imaging 2020;47(4):881–94.
45. Durmo R, Filice A, Fioroni F, et al. Predictive and prognostic role of pre-therapy and interim 68Ga-DOTATOC PET/CT parameters in metastatic advanced neuroendocrine tumor patients treated with PRRT. Cancers (Basel) 2022;14(3):592.

Gastro-Enteric-Pancreatic Neuroendocrine Tumor Treatment: ^{177}Lu-DOTATATE

Yasemin Sanli, MD[a,*], Dilara Denizmen, MD[a], Rathan M. Subramaniam, MD, PhD, MPH, MBA[b,c]

KEYWORDS

• ^{177}Lu-DOTATATE • PRRT • Neuroendocrine tumors • GEP-NETs

KEY POINTS

- Better understanding of the tumor biology and intratumoral heterogeneity using ^{68}Ga DOTATATE and ^{18}FDG PET/CT imaging, in addition to pathological classifications, guide the clinical decision for ^{177}Lu-DOTA-TATE therapy in neuroendocrine tumors (NETs).
- Benefit of peptide receptor radionuclide therapy (PRRT) is better in patients with well-differentiated low-grade NETs (Grade 1/2) than high-grade NETs and NEC. Moreover, combined therapy of ^{177}Lu-DOTA-TATE and chemotherapy is promising for the aggressive subgroups even though more data are needed.
- Liver-dominant metastatic disease results in poor prognosis. Liver-targeted therapies may be better beneficial, accompanied with or without PRRT.
- Owing to the kidney and bone marrow being dose-limiting organs, sufficient bone marrow reserves and kidney functions are required for ^{177}Lu-DOTA-TATE therapy. Dose modification, preferably with a dosimetric approach, should be considered in patients with low glomerular filtration rates and poor liver function rather than standard dose schemes.

INTRODUCTION

Diagnosis of neuroendocrine tumors (NETs) has increased significantly over the past decade. Successful detection of metastatic diseases has been achieved through overexpressed somatostatin receptors (SSTRs) using Ga-68-DOTATATE PET-CT imaging.[1–5]

In peptide receptor radionuclide therapy (PRRT), ^{177}Lu is a β-emitting radionuclide linked to TATE by the linker DOTA for this theragnostic approach. ^{177}Lu-DOTATATE has been an important SSTR-based molecular targeted systemic radionuclide therapy modality in the clinical management of patients with metastatic, inoperable, SSTR-positive NETs, especially in the most common type Gastroenteropancreatic-neuroendocrine tumors (GEP-NETs).[5] Theragnostic applications using ^{177}Lu-DOTATATE are now included in clinical guidelines and approved by Food and Drug Administration (FDA) and European Medicines Agency (EMA) owing to its proven benefit, minimal adverse effects, and well tolerability, by NETTER-1 study, in this particular group of patients.[6]

This review aims to provide up-to-date information about the clinical use of ^{177}Lu-DOTATATE through a literature review.

ELIGIBILITY CRITERIA FOR ^{177}LU-DOTATATE THERAPY

According to the European Neuroendocrine Tumor Society, The North American Neuroendocrine Tumor Society, and Endocrine and Neuroendocrine

[a] Department of Nuclear Medicine, Istanbul Faculty of Medicine, Istanbul University, Millet Caddesi, Istanbul 34390, Turkey; [b] Dean's Office, Otago Medical School, University of Otago, Dunedin 9016, New Zealand; [c] Department of Radiology, Duke University, Durham, NC, USA

* Corresponding author.
E-mail address: yasemin.sanli@yahoo.com

PET Clin 18 (2023) 201–214
https://doi.org/10.1016/j.cpet.2022.11.002
1556-8598/23/

Cancers (ENETs, NANETs, and ESMO) Guidelines, PRRT is a therapeutic option in metastatic/inoperable, progressive, SSTR-positive NETs with homogeneous SSTR expression. Primary tumors and most metastatic lesions should have SSTR expression higher than liver on DOTA PET imaging before PRRT.[7–9] Well-differentiated histology and low grade(1/2) according to the WHO criteria,[10] which represents Ki-67 less than 20%, results in higher SSTR radiopharmaceutical uptake.[11] A patient's pathology report should meet those criteria to be included for ^{177}Lu DOTATATE therapy; however, patients with well-differentiated grade 3 neuroendocrine neoplasms (NEN) who have failed a trial of chemotherapy may be considered for PRRT, even though there are not enough data on response rates and survival in this subgroup.

For the treatment of midgut NETs, ESMO Guideline refers to PRRT as second-line therapy after disease progression on somatostatin analogue (SSA). Meanwhile, ENETs Guideline recommends using PRRT after SSA or as a third-line after progression on everolimus. NANET Guideline divides patients with NET into two groups: hormone-secreting and nonfunctional tumors. According to the guideline for hormone-secreting midgut NETs, PRRT can be used as second-line therapy after the progression of SSA. In contrast, second-line therapy options for nonfunctional tumors should be individualized between everolimus and PRRT, taking SSTR positivity into account.

Regarding pancreatic NETs, ENETs, and ESMO recommend PRRT after progression on approved therapies such as SSA, chemotherapy, and novel targeted drugs (everolimus, sunitinib), but for selected G1/2 NETs, it might have an earlier use according to ENETs. NANETs do not define exact therapy timing because of the lack of trials and availability of many other therapeutic options other than PRRT.

A meta-analysis, published in 2019, compared PRRT and everolimus in advanced primitive neuro-ectodermal tumors (pNETs) revealed that PRRT has better disease control rate (DCR), objective response rate (ORR), and progression free survival (PFS) than everolimus (81% vs 73%, $P < 0.001$), (47% vs 12%, $P < 0.001$), (median PFS 25.7 vs 14.7 months, $P < 0.001$), whereas causing less grade 3 or 4 hematotoxicity (5% vs. 11%) and nephrotoxicity (1% vs. 2.5%). Even though we need more data, this study can be guided to make therapy choices in advanced pNETs.[12]

Because of the possible hematological and kidney toxicity as an adverse event of radionuclide therapy, patients should have sufficient bone marrow reserves and creatinine clearance. Patients should also have Karnofsky Performance Status greater than 50 and an expected survival of more than 3 months.[7–9]

When the proliferative index of the NETs (Ki-67 expression) rises, SSTR expression and uptake on ^{68}Ga-DOTATATE PET-CT of the tumors generally decrease, whereas ^{18}FDG-PET-CT uptake increases.[8,13] Therefore, (18)F-fluorodeoxyglucose (^{18}FDG) PET/CT is required to detect lesions of patients with higher grade NETs, and increased avidity of FDG is associated with poor prognosis. In contrast, high SSTR uptake is correlated with a relatively good prognosis which can be predicted by SSTR imaging before PRRT.[11,13–15] In addition, a recent study revealed that for risk stratification of all NEN patients, FDG PET is superior to histologic grading.[16] Combining these two imaging modalities before PRRT can provide extensive knowledge about the heterogeneity and character of the tumor; changing uptake values can be of use to help plan an ideal therapeutic option.[17,18] NETPET grading system, developed by Chan and colleagues,[19] calculated based on FDG and SSTR avidity of the tumor, is prognostic for survival and helps to decide between PRRT and chemotherapy.

Exclusion Criteria

^{177}Lu-DOTATATE is known to be a generally well-tolerated treatment option, but a group of patients is not favorable to undergoing this therapy. PRRT is contraindicated for pregnant patients and patients with ongoing lactation as all Radionuclide therapies. Grade 3–4 cardiac impairment, inability to comprehend PRRT due to a psychiatric or neurological disorder, and severe hepatic impairment (total bilirubin >3x upper limit or both an albumin <25 g/L and pro-thrombin time increased >1.5 ULN) as a result of the predictable toxicity of treatment count as absolute contraindications of PRRT according to the ENETs Guideline.[7] Moderate to severe right heart valvular disease, hematological impairment (Hb < 8 g/dL, platelets $<75 \times 10^9$/L, white blood cell [WBC] $< 10^9$/L), and contrast-enhancing lesions on CT or MR imaging that lack SSTR expression, which 18F-FDG PET/CT can confirm if available are also in the contraindications list. The guideline also adds that contraindications can be waived based on the patient's status.

Although ENETs Guideline acknowledges creatinine clearance lower than 50 mL/min as a contraindication for therapy, NANETs Guideline does not consider an absolute cut-off and offers to check for hydronephrosis pretreatment for all patients to prevent kidneys from extensive irradiation. Both guidelines agree that even patients on dialysis may be treated with PRRT with dose reduction and dosimetry.

NANETs and ESMO Guidelines also offer the use of positively charged amino acids, such as lysine and arginine, co-infusion with therapy to reduce renal irradiation and decrease the risk due to the competitive inhibition of reabsorption at the proximal tubule.

NANETs Guideline warns doctors treating patients with mesenteric or peritoneal diseases with PRRT due to the risk of escalating the desmoplastic process and causing bowel obstruction. To prevent this, prophylactic steroids in short courses can be used after each cycle. In addition, due to the tumor's potential heterogeneity, NANETs suggest using both FDG and SSTR PET/CT imaging before considering PRRT for G3 tumors to ensure all lesions are SSTR positive.

Clinical Trials

One of the first wide-ranging phase 2 studies were published in 2008, which reported the toxicity and efficacy of Lu-DOTA-TATE treatment (**Table 1**) in over 504 patients, including 458 GEP-NETs. Patients were treated with four cycles of each 7.4 GBq Lu-177 DOTA-TATE therapy up to 29.6 GBq cumulative dose in 6 to 10 weeks intervals. Grade 3–4 hematologic toxicity occurred at 3.6%, whereas three patients developed myelodysplastic syndrome (MDS), two patients had nonfatal liver toxicity, and six were hospitalized within 2 days after treatment due to a hormone-related crisis. Efficacy analysis made on 310 patients revealed complete response (CR), partial response (PR), ORR, median PFS, and median overall survival (OS) from the start of treatment as 2%, 28%, 46%, 40 months, and 46 months.[20]

The IEO prospective phase 1–2 trial published in 2011 also evaluated the toxicity and efficacy of 51 unresectable or metastatic SSTR2-positive NETs; 39 were GEP-NETs, whereas 94.6%were well-differentiated NETs, and 56.8% had a Ki-67 $\leq$ 20%. Twenty-one patients in group 1 received smaller doses per cycle to a median cumulative activity of 26.4 GBq, and 30 patients in group 2 received more per cycle to 25.2 GBq. As for hematological toxicity, only one patient had grade 3 thrombocytopenia and leucopenia. Grade 3–4 renal toxicity did not occur. The objective tumor response rate was 29.4% (15/51), whereas 13 were GEP-NETs. Seventeen patients with GEP-NET had SD, whereas 9 had PD. Higher administered cumulative activity and more progressive tumors at baseline had better responses to PRRT. Although median OS was not reached, the probability of 36 months of OS was 68%.[21]

Another study published in 2013 evaluated the efficacy and safety of Lu-DOTA-TATE, especially in 52 advanced G1-2 pancreatic NETs divided patients into two subgroups receiving mean dosages of 17.8 GBq (26 patients) and 25.5 GBq (26 patients) cumulative activities according to their underlying toxicity developing risk. Only one patient in the reduced dose group developed grade 3 renal toxicity, and no grade 3–4 hematological toxicity occurred. CR, PR, and SD were 12%, 27%, and 46%, respectively, in full-dose group, whereas 4%, 15%, and 58%, respectively, in reduced dose group. Median PFS was significantly longer in the full-dose group (20 months vs not reached), which can be considered recommended dosage, although median OS curves were not significantly different.[22] In 2016 long-term safety results of the same group were published. The Median PFS of the full-dose group was 53.5 months. The median OS of the reduced dose group was 63.8 months, yet it was not reached for the full-dose group. Also, this study revealed that patients whose FDG PET scans were positive before PRRT end up with significantly shorter metabolic progression-free survival (mPFS) (21.1 vs 68.7 months [$P < 0.0002$]) regardless of the total activity.[23]

The first US phase 2 study was published in 2014; 37 grade 1/2 progressive SSTR (+) patients were treated with 7.4 GBq activity per cycle every 6 to 9 weeks up to 29.6 GBq cumulative dose; 19 of them received all four cycles. An eighty percent of patients have nausea or vomiting during infusion, but no acute toxicity was observed. Seven patients developed grade 2/3 hematotoxicity, and 6 (85.7%) had a chemotherapy history, making prior chemotherapy a statistically significant risk factor ($P = 0.036$). Although grade 1/2/3 hepatotoxicity has occurred in five patients, there was no significant correlation between hepatic function and pretreatment hepatic metastasis even in patients with high baseline aspartate alanine aminotransferase, alanine aminotransferase, alkaline phosphatase (AST, ALT, and ALP). No grade 3/4 renal toxicity was reported. Thirty-two patients were evaluated radiologically, and 31% had a partial or minimal response, whereas 41% had stable disease and 28% progressed. Median PFS for patients who received all four cycles was 16.5 months, whereas all patients had 16.1 months.

Response to treatment was found significantly ($P = 0.04$) correlated with hepatic involvement of the disease. Even though statistical significance was not reached, patients with less than 50% hepatic involvement had longer median PFS values than those with extensive liver involvement.

Table 1
Studies reporting ^{177}Lu-DOTATATE therapy efficacy and adverse events in GEP-NETs

		Origin of Tumor								Adverse Events					Imaging Response					Survival	
Author, Year	*N*	GEP-NET	Others	Grade 1–2 (%)	Dosage per Cycle	Treatment Interval (Weeks)	Cumulative Dose (Median GBq)	Bone Marrow Absorbed Dose (Gy)	Renal Absorbed Dose (Gy)	Hematologic (G3–4)	MDS	AL	Renal Toxicity	Liver Toxicity	CR%	PR%	TRR%	SD%	DCR%	Median PFS (Months)	Median OS (Months)
Kwekkeboom et al,[20] 2008	310	310	0	nm	7.4 GBq x 4	6–10	27.8–29.6	-	-	3.6%	3	-	-	2	2	28	46	35	-	32	46
Bodei et al,[21] 2011, Group 1	21	39	12	28	3.7–5.18 × 6	6–9	26.4	0.8–1.3	15–37	4.7%	-	-	-	-	2	27	55	27	-	36	nr
Bodei et al,[21] 2011, Group 2	30			72	5.18–7.4 × 4	6–9	25.2	0.5–0.9	8–32	0%	-	-	-	-							
Sansovini et al,[22] 2013, Group 1	26	All PNET	0	84.6	5.1 × 5	6–8	25.5	-	-	-	-	-	-	-	12	27	-	46	85	nr	nr
Sansovini[22] 2013, Group 2	26	All PNET	0	80.7	3.5 × 5	6–8	17.8	-	-	-	-	-	1	-	4	14	-	58	77	20	nr
Delpassand et al,[24] 2014	32	32	0	100	7.4 × 4	6–9	29.6 (max)	-	-	12.5%	-	-	-	3	23	28	31	41	-	16.1	nr
Paganelli et al,[25] 2014–20, FD	25	25	0	72	5.5 × 5	6–8	25.7	-	-	-	-	-	-	-	nm	nm	4	80	84	59.8	97.6
Paganelli et al,[25] 2014–20, RD	18	18	0	72	3.7 × 5	6–8	18.4	-	-	-	-	-	-	-	nm	nm	11	72	83	59.8	71
Sabet et al,[27] 2015	61	All SINET	0	100	7.9 × 4	10–14	27.2	-	-	8.2%	-	-	-	-	-	13.1	44.2	47.5	91.8	33	61
Sansovini, 2016, Group 1	28	All PNET	0	nm	5.5 × 5	6–8	25.9	-	-	-	-	-	-	-	10.7	23.7	-	42.9	85.7	53.4	nr
Sansovini, 2016, Group 2	32	All PNET	0	nm	3.7 × 5	6–8	18.5	-	-	-	-	-	1	-	3.1	15.6	-	59.4	78.1	21.7	63.8
Strosberg et al,[33] 2017, NETTER-1	116	All Midgut NET	0	100	7.4 × 4	8	29.6	-	-	12%	1	-	-	-	0.9	16.8	18	-	-	nr	nr

Strosberg et al,[6] 2021, NETTER-1 Final Analysis	101	All Midgut NET	0	100	7.4 × 4	8	29.6	-	-	12%	1	-	6	-	-	-	-	-	-	nm	48
Zandee, 2018	34	Functioning PNET	0	nm	7.4 × 4	6–10	26.4	-	-	12%	1	-	-	5	2.9	55.9	-	23.6	78.3	18.1	nm
Satapathy et al,[30] 2020	40	25	15	92.5	6–7.4 × 4	8–12	27	-	-	8%	-	-	-	4%	nm	30	-	55	-	48	81
Kudo et al,[32] 2021	15	13	2	100	7.4 × 4	8	29.6	0.631	20.7	53.4%	-	-	-	-	6.7	46.7	-	33.3	-	nr	nr
Parghane et al,[31] 2021, Group 1	23	All GEPNET	0	100	7.4 × 4	8–10	22.2	-	-	-	-	-	-	-	4.3	34.8	-	52.3		nr	nr
Parghane et al,[31] 2021, Group 2	34	All GEPNET	0	97	7.4 × 4	8–10	27.45	-	-	-	-	-	-		0	26.5	-	70.5		nr	nr

Abbreviations: CR, complete response; DCR, disease control rate; N, number of patients included in the statistical analysis; nm, not mentioned; nr: not reached; OS, overall survival; PFS, progression free survival; PR, partial response; SD, stable disease; TRR, tumor response rate.

Pretreatment FDG positivity was correlated with patient death ($P = 0.03$), although significance was not reached, FDG-negative patients were found to have longer PFS ($P = 0.2$). In addition, patients were reported to have a better quality of life and improved performance status after ^{177}Lu-DOTATATE therapy.[24]

In another prospective phase 2 study published in 2014, 43 patients with advanced, well-differentiated, SSTR-positive gastrointestinal NETs received five cycles of PRRT. Although 25 of them received 5.5 GBq per cycle to a cumulative activity of 25.7 GBq (22.2–27.8); 18 patients with a high probability of developing hematotoxicity and nephrotoxicity received 3.7 GBq per cycle to a total of 18.4 GBq (14.4–20.4) cumulative activity at intervals of 6 to 8 weeks. CR or PR was reached in one patient in the high-dose group and two in the low-dose group. An eighty percent of the high-dose group and 72% of the low-dose group had stable disease, whereas the disease control rate was 84% and 83% for the two groups, respectively. No significant differences were found between the two groups regarding PFS; the median PFS was 36 months. FDG-negative patients had longer PFS than those with positive scans ($P = 0.025$), whereas DCR did not show a statistically significant difference. No treatment requiring major toxicity (Grade 3) or serious adverse events was seen, but patients who received reduced doses had lower ratios of (Grade 1/2) hematologic toxicities.[25] In 2020, late toxicity, PFS, and OS of the same cohort were published as an IRST phase 2 study of a 10-year follow-up. The median PFS of the two groups was identical at 59.8 months, whereas the median OS was 71 months in the low-dose group and 97.6 months in the high-dose group which was not significantly different. Patients who have lymph node limited progression had a longer median PFS of 110.2 months than the ones with hepatic lesions at 36.8 months, and grades 3, 2, and 1 tumor burden showed a median PFS of 46.2, 30.9, and 100.2 months, which makes hepatic lesions and tumor burden are prognostic markers. Median PFS for FDG PET/CT negative patients was 66.5 months, whereas 30.4 for positive patients. Thus FDG positivity is a prognostic marker for the first 5 years of follow-up. No unresolved or late toxicity has occurred in either group.[26]

Another retrospective phase 2 study published in 2015 evaluated the efficacy and safety of PRRT on patients with unresectable advanced G1–2 small intestinal NETs. Sixty-one patients received four cycles of mean 7.9 GBq activity. Five patients had Grade 3 hematotoxicity, whereas none had grade 3–4 nephrotoxicity. PR, MR, SD, and PD were 13.1%, 31.1%, 47.5%, and 8.2%; DCR was 91.8%. Median PFS and OS were calculated as 33 and 61 months. High baseline plasma chromogranin-A levels and functionality of the tumor were the independent predictors of shorter PFS, whereas longer survival was significantly associated with ORR ($P = 0.005$).[27]

In 2018, a retrospective study described the safety and efficacy of 34 metastatic functioning pNET patients who were treated with four cycles of 7.4 GBq PRRT. DCR and mPFS were found at 78% and 18.1 months, respectively. In addition, uncontrolled symptoms had a reduction in 71% of patients. Grade 3–4 hematological toxicity occurred in 12% of them. Three patients experienced a hormonal crisis, and the authors advised taking precautions specific to the type of tumor and secreted hormones.[28] In another phase 2 study published in December 2020, 47 SSTR positive, Ki-67 less than 20%, 46 NET patients, including 33 GEP-NETs, received 75 to 150 mCi per cycle four times every 8 to 12 weeks, called full induction therapy, 46 received all for cycles and 34 of them who reached stable disease or had a response to PRRT received additional maintenance therapy with 50 to 100 mCi every 6 months with a median of 3.5 cycles up to 4 years or until progression. In the midgut NET subgroup, median PFS was 47.7, and pancreatic NETs were 36.5. In other types, 23.9 months was not statistically significant, yet the estimated median OS was significantly longer in MNETs than in others ($P = 0.039$). Grade 1 NETs reached a median PFS of 47.7 months, whereas grade 2 (**Fig. 1**) was 29 months. Significantly longer PFS was achieved in patients who received PRRT right after progression on SSA compared with patients treated with other methods(48.9 vs 25.5 months [$P = 0.04$]). However, those were mostly MNETs. Based on RECIST criteria, DRR and SD were found at 5% and 80% in midgut NETs, 69.2% and 7.7% in pNETs, and 35.7% and 57.2% in other NETs. Also, longer PFS was reached than in the NETTER-1 trial, which only performed induction therapy (28.4 vs 47.7 months).[29]

A retrospective study was published in 2020, evaluating the role of PRRT as the first-line therapy in 45 metastatic NET patients; 40 were included in the statistical analyses, and 25 were GEP-NETs. Patients received 27 GBq median cumulative dose and capecitabine for each cycle. Grade 3–4 anemia and leucopenia were 2%, whereas neutropenia and hepatotoxicity were 4%. PR, SD, PD, and mPFS for all patients were 30%, 55%, 15%, and 48 months, whereas for GEP-NETs 48%, 44%, 8%, respectively. Current guidelines

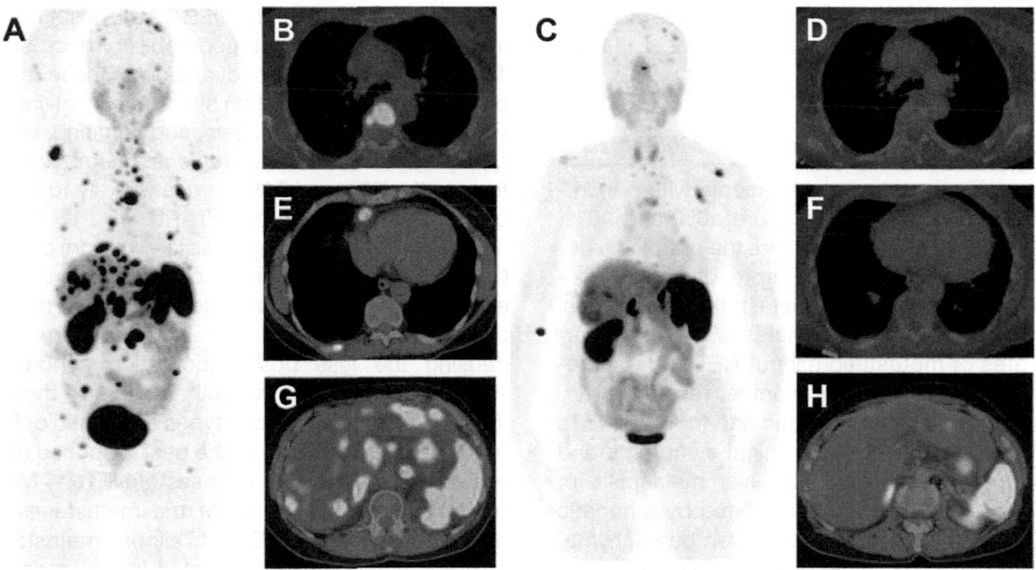

Fig. 1. A 64-year-old woman who has diagnosed metastatic grade 2 cecum NET (Ki-67:%10) underwent ^{68}Ga-DOTA-TATE PET/CT (*A, B, E, G*) for therapy response. The patient had a history of cecal primary mass resection, liver segment 5–6 metastasectomy and long-acting sandostatin therapy. PET/CT images showed increased somatostatin receptor expression in the both lobes of liver and extensive bone metastases. After diagnosing multiple liver and bone metastases, the patient received four cycles of ^{177}Lu-DOTA-TATE treatment (cumulative dose 31.6 GBq). Partial response was detected in skeletal and liver metastases on follow-up (*C, D, F, H*) images. The patient has been stable for 8 months after two additional cycles of PRRT with no additional symptom.

recommend SSA as a first-line treatment with 69% DCR and 14.3 months PFS, according to the PROMID trial. Conversely, this study showed 85% in all patients and 92% in GEP-NETs, which is promising for the future even though we need comprehensive data to be certain.[30]

In 2021, 57 unresectable GEP-NET patients were treated with 7.4 GBq Lu-DOTATATE4-5 cycles of neoadjuvant surgery; 26.3% became resectable after therapy which was found to be associated with primary tumors site-size and FDG uptake, lymph node-liver metastasis.40% of patients had PR or CR, whereas 2-year OS was 92.1%, and mPFS was not reached. No major toxicity was observed.[31] A single-arm, multicenter, phase 1/2 study published in 2021 evaluated the efficacy and safety of ^{177}Lu-DOTATATE in 15 Japanese patients; five midgut, eight pancreatic, and two lung with SSTR-positive, progressive, metastatic, or locally advanced unresectable NETs with a Ki-67 index $\leq$20%. Patients received four therapies of 7.4 GBq^{177}Lu-DOTATATE every 8 weeks and IM 30 mg sustained-release octreotide every 4 weeks for 60 weeks from the first therapy for symptom relief. For all patients, ORR was 53%, CR was 6.7%, PRs were 46.7%, stable disease was 33.3%, and progressive disease was 6.7%. ORR for patients with midgut NET was found to be 60%. At 52 weeks, PFS rate was 80%. As adverse effects, 73% of patients had nausea, 47% had higher than Grade 3 lymphopenia, and 7% had leucopenia.[32]

The first randomized controlled phase 3 trial was published in 2014; the NETTER-1 trial, which compared ^{177}Lu-DOTATATE (four cycles of 7.4 GBq every 8 weeks) combined low-dose octreotide (30 mg) group with high-dose octreotide group (60 mg every 4 weeks) in patients with well-differentiated, progressive M-NET. The response rate was 18% in the PRRT group and 3% in the octreotide LAR group, whereas the estimated PFS rate in 20 months was 65.2% and 10.8%. Less than 10% had significant myelosuppression in the PRRT group, whereas none of the patients in the control group experienced it. PRRT group had a 79% lower risk of death or progression than the control.[33] According to the promising results of the NETTER-1 trial, EMA and FDA approved the clinical use of ^{177}Lu-DOTATATE in 2017 and 2018. In 2021 final data of the same cohort was published, and the median OS was 48 months versus 36.3 months in PRRT and control groups. During 76.3 months of median follow-up in the ^{177}Lu-DOTATATE group, no new events occurred, but grade 3 or worse adverse events were observed in 3%, whereas 2 of 111 patients developed MDS.[6]

Locoregional Therapies for Liver Metastasis

The 5-year survival rates of patients with pancreatic NETs and midgut NETS are 40% and 90%, respectively. On the other hand, the prognosis deteriorates as the disease spreads.[34] Approximately 25% of NETs are metastatic at diagnosis, and 80% develop liver metastases.[35] Median survival rates of metastatic midgut NET and pancreatic NETs are 56 and 24 months, respectively.[36] The most common metastatic site for GEP-NETs is the liver, which causes clinical symptoms and leads to a poor prognosis. Liver metastasis of NETs is very hypervascular and fed by a hepatic artery in contrast to healthy liver parenchyma, which blood supply is provided by the portal venous system that makes liver-targeted therapies the treatment of choice when liver-dominant disease burden is present.[37] Locoregional therapies are generally indicated for patients with G1–2 NETs with predominant hepatic metastasis and who suffer from secretory syndromes resistant to medical therapy or can be used to control tumor growth.[38] Patients with low-volume lymph node, bone, or lung metastases can also be considered. The main target of these therapies is uplifting the quality of a patient's life while causing minimal damage to the healthy liver parenchyma.

Curative surgery is the recommended first-line treatment, yet patients who are not eligible for resection should have hepatic arterial embolization therapies (TAE [transarterial embolization], TACE [transarterial chemoembolization], and TARE [transarterial radioembolization]) by ENETs and NANETs Guidelines.[8,39] Portal vein thrombosis, neuroendocrine carcinoma, predominant extrahepatic liver metastasis, liver insufficiency (bilirubin >1.5 times normal value or prothrombin time >75%), bilioenteric anastomosis, and poor general status are the general contraindications, whereas renal insufficiency (creatinine levels >1.5x) and multiple previous RF ablation are in the relative contraindications list.[38,40]

Radiofrequency ablation is suitable for inoperable patients with small metastasis (one metastasis <5 cm, three metastasis <3 cm, or sum of all metastasis <8 cm), yet its contraindicated for masses close to vital structures as it works through coagulation necrosis.

TAE protocol is based on causing cell death through hypoxia using various embolizing products. Lipiodol-based *TACE* and drug-eluting bead DEB-TACE is other interventional radiological methods, but DEB TACE has a higher incidence of biloma and hepatobiliary necrosis.[41] The most significant disadvantage of these therapies is a post-embolization syndrome involving fever, malaise, abdominal pain, and vomiting, which can occur after extensive regional therapies more frequently. TAE and TACE are less likely to cause chronic hepatotoxicity than TARE.

Yttrium-90TARE using glass (1–8 million) or resin (15–20 million) radioembolic microspheres are extensively used to treat patients with liver metastasis who have preserved liver function while causing the less post-embolization syndrome. Although selective internal radiation therapy (SIRT) is used in numerous types of hepatic or liver metastatic tumors, one of the best response rates is derived from liver metastases of NETs.[42] Multiplicity and different sites of the metastases do not interfere with TARE. Yet, bilobar metastases are recommended to be treated in two sessions 4 to 8 weeks apart to decrease the risk of complications.[43] Disadvantages of TARE are the necessity of mapping angiography and the potential of inducing chronic hepatotoxicity radiation-induced liver disease (RILD) after recurrent cycles. Side effects are abdominal pain, leukocytosis, and fewer and elevated liver enzymes. More severe complications include hepatic infarct, liver abscess, radiation-induced live disease, bowel ischemia, and pleural effusion.

A multicenter, retrospective study published in 2016 compared TAE, TACE, and TARE results of 151 metastatic NET patients (71 pancreas, 68 gut, and 16 others) and proved that TARE has a higher hazard ratio compared with TAE and TACE in OS rates (unadjusted cox model HR 2.1 $P = 0.02$; 48 months vs 33 months), whereas hepatic PFS (HPFS) does not significantly change between modalities. The study also showed that higher tumor burden and grade cause poor prognosis (shorter HPFS and OS).[44]

In a meta-analysis published in 2019, 1108 NET patients (662 pancreas, 164 small bowel) with liver metastases and surgical resection resulted in the best OS compared with regional therapies and chemotherapy.[45]

Combination of Transarterial Radioembolization and Peptide Receptor Radionuclide Therapy

As PRRT has less benefit in patients with bulky liver metastases, combining PRRT and TARE can be a good option while considering the potential risk of cumulative radiation-induced hepatotoxicity.[46] According to the European Association of Nuclear Medicine (EANM) Guidelines, patients with diffuse or unresectable complex liver metastases should be treated with systemic therapy first; liver-targeted treatment can be evaluated after progression.[39]

A retrospective study published in 2019 analyzed 44 patients who received TARE (median Y90 activity 1.67 GBq) after a median of 335 days PRRT (7.4–61.6 GBq); DCR 3 months after TARE was 91%; 65% of symptomatic patients responded to therapy, whereas grade 3–4 hematological and biochemical toxicity occurred in 10% of patients. The most common toxicities were lymphocytopenia (42%) and gamma glutamyl transferase (GGT) elevation (10%). One patient experienced the fatal radioembolization-induced liver disease. There was no correlation between toxicity, the time between TARE–PRRT, and cumulative activity administered in PRRT. The presence of extrahepatic disease ($P = 0.001$) and hepatic tumor load being greater than 75% ($P = 0.007$) is confirmed to be significantly negative prognostic factors for OS.[47]

In a previous retrospective study published in 2012, 23 liver-dominant metastatic NET patients with a history of ^{177}Lu-DOTA-octreotate (mean cumulative activity 31.8 GBq) who received Y-90 resin microspheres with the cumulative activity of 3.4 GBq. No grade 4 adverse events were observed, whereas grade 3 hyperbilirubinemia was 8.7%. The symptomatic response was observed in 80%, whereas the radiologic response was 30.4%. Patients with low Ki-67 (< %5) had longer OS ($P = 0.007$).[48] Both these studies support the short-term safety of additional radioembolization in patients with the progressive hepatic disease after PRRT.

A comparator study investigated the responses and side effects of 15 patients treated with SIRT and 12 with a combination of SIRT and PRRT with liver-dominant metastatic NET published in 2020. Treatment response and stable disease was 86.6% in the SIRT group while 66.6% in the combination group. Median OS was not statistically significant, yet the SIRT group had longer ($P = 0.217$; 34.9 vs 67.5 months). The most common side effect was temporary lymphopenia, although short-term high levels of lactate dehydrogenase (LDH), bilirubin, ALP, and aminotransferase were detected in 6.6% of the SIRT group, they were much higher in the combination therapy group. This might be according to the higher hepatic tumor load in the combination group. No grade 4 hepatotoxicity or hematotoxicity or nephrotoxicity occurred in both groups. Longer PFS and OS were achieved in the combination group compared with PRRT and SSA group with LM in the NETTER-1 study (PFS: 20 vs 27.2 months). They also observed significantly longer survival in combination groups that had previously received other locoregional therapies.[49]

The first phase 2 prospective study published in 2020 called HEPAR PLUS aimed to assess the efficacy and safety through a 6-month follow-up of radioembolization with holmium-166 (^{166}Ho)-loaded particles (target liver absorbed dose was 60 Gy) within 20 weeks after four cycles of 7.4 GBq PRRT in 30 patients (22 of them were GEP-NETs) with grade 1 and 2 NET who have bulky liver metastases. According to RECIST 1.1 criteria, liver-specific PR and stable disease were 43% and 50% at 3 months, whereas 47% and 37% at 6 months. The most frequent CTCAE grade 3–4 toxicities were increased GGT (54%), lymphocytopenia (23%), and abdominal pain (10%) in 6 months follow-up, whereas the highest biochemical toxicities were observed in 6 weeks. One patient had radioembolization-induced liver disease 6 weeks after treatment and died 4 months after radioembolization; this patient was also under methotrexate therapy for rheumatoid arthritis, a known hepatotoxic agent.[50]

Compared with the NETTER-1 study, greater tumor reduction was observed, which suggests that combined radioembolization and PRRT treatment is an effective therapy with acceptable side effects.

Combination of Peptide Receptor Radionuclide Therapy and Chemotherapy

As mentioned, NETs with high Ki-67 index tend to express less SSTR and have more glucose uptake and poor prognosis.[15–18, 23] Several phase II studies have been published based on combining the 5-fluorouracil (5-FU) prodrug capecitabine as a radiosensitizer in FDG-positive G1–3 NETs.

In 2014, a retrospective study was published assessing PRCRT (peptide receptor chemoradionuclide therapy) outcomes of 52 FDG and SSTR-positive inoperable, metastatic GEP-NET patients. Three-to-five cycles of LuTate spaced 6 to 8 weeks to a total of 6 to 10 GBq were administered. Continuous 5-FU infusion was started 4 days before the second PRRT cycle for up to 3 weeks. Median PFS was 48 months; 68% of patients had SD, whereas 28% had PR, and 2% showed CR. The most common adverse effect was hematological toxicity; only four patients had grade 3–4 toxicity.[51]

A retrospective cohort study was published in 2017, including 167 NET patients, of which 125 were GEP-NETs. Patients were separated into two groups; 88 were treated with PRCRT, and 79 had PRRT alone. Combination group showed better response to therapy than PRRT group for PR, SD, and PD (34%, 50.2%, 6.8%) versus (6.3%, 60.9%, 26.5%), respectively. Also, median OS and PFS were not reached in the combination group, whereas 48 months were in the PRRT group. Toxicity analysis showed no significant difference between the two groups.[52]

In 2021, a prospective phase II study evaluated 37 advanced GEP-NET patients with Ki-67 less than 55%, SSTR positive, FDG avid, and dihydropyrimidine dehydrogenase proficient. Patients received five cycles of 5.5 GBq PRRT every 8 weeks, and oral capecitabine was administered orally in intercycle periods. DCR, PR, and SD were found at 85%, 30%, and 55%, respectively. Median PFS was 31.4 months. Grade 3–4 hematological toxicity occurred in 16.2% of patients. They also compared results with the previous PRRT alone study and showed a longer PFS in the combination group (31.4 vs 21.2 months).[53]

Based on the data we have to date, combination therapy with capecitabine is likely to be preferable in the treatment strategy of FDG-positive GEP-NET patients with negligible toxicity and satisfactory treatment response and survival rates, even though randomized controlled studies including more patients are needed for a definite conclusion.

Dosimetry

As a consequence of the radionuclide therapies not only are targeted malignant mass affected by radiation exposure but other tissues such as bone marrow, kidneys, liver, salivary, lacrimal, and pituitary glands are also being irradiated. Dose-limiting organs are usually bone marrow and kidneys according to a potential risk of side effects.

The most common adverse event after ^{177}Lu-DOTA-TATE therapy is hematologic toxicity. Based on I-131 treatments, 2 Gy absorbed dose is considered the limit for bone marrow.[54] IV administration of Lu and bone marrow circulation of the radiopharmaceutical are the major reasons for toxicity.[55] A review article published in 2016 evaluated 16 articles to identify myelotoxicity risk and its association with other factors. The study revealed that 10% of 2225 patients experienced myelotoxicity, mostly on platelet levels, and then WBC and Hb, which were managed easily with dose modification. Only 1.4% of patients developed MDS/AL after PRRT, and combination therapies with capecitabine/temozolomide and PRRT did not increase that risk. At the same time, prior radiotherapy and chemotherapy, especially with alkylating agents, significantly increase the risk. Baseline cytopenia, prior chemoradiotherapy, impaired renal function, and age greater than 70 years were associated with myelotoxicity risk.[56]

Even though a prospective study published in 2018 calculated bone marrow absorbed doses through blood sample-based dosimetry and found no correlation between absorbed dose and dosimetry[57]; a planar image-based dosimetry study for bone marrow after PRRT calculated the mean absorbed dose for 24 GBq as 0.64 Gy and found absorbed dose correlated with a decrease in Hb ($P < 0.01$), WBC ($P = 0.01$), and PLT ($P < 0.01$) counts in 2016.[58] Another bone marrow dosimetry study published in 2019 also found decreased platelet counts after PRRT significantly correlated with bone marrow absorbed doses; also, bone marrow absorbed doses were higher in patients with bone metastases as far as planar and hybrid methods demonstrated the same result, patients without bone metastases correlated with the planar method. In contrast, bone metastatic individuals were shown to have been best associated with the hybrid method.[59]

Even though blood-based dosimetry is the most common method, image-based dosimetry seems to be a more reliable option. EANM dosimetry guideline recommends collecting 2 or 3 images in the first 48 hours, and at least one more image is required for estimation. For SPECT-CT-based methods, EANM advises avoiding skeletal metastatic regions or adjusting for spill-in counts.[55]

Kidney

Lu-SSTR is mostly excreted from the kidneys, whereas uptake from proximal tubular cells increases the absorbed radiation doses, which may result in acute (renal failure) or chronic radiation nephropathy (parenchymal loss), which puts the kidneys in dose-limiting organ status.[60] Amino acid co-infusion is a widely used method aiming to reduce radiation exposure by competitively inhibiting the uptake of radiopharmaceuticals from tubular mega line receptors. Commonly known absorbed dose limit for kidneys is 23 to 28 Gy, which was obtained from external beam radiation studies and is unsuitable for 177-Lu therapies.[61,62] Recent studies indicate that kidneys can tolerate more than the standard 23 Gy absorbed dose and more than usually administered in four cycles of 7.4 GBq.[63–65] Even mean absorbed doses are calculated between 0.54 and 1.00 Gy/GBq in previous studies.[66,67] Patient's renal function, co-infused amino acid solutions, and tumor burden are the main reasons for different renal absorbed doses gained with the same amount of activity which makes it hard to determine a single dose and therapy cycle suitable for everyone. Previous studies have demonstrated that planar image-based dosimetry techniques overestimate the absorbed doses and SPECT-CT-based techniques are more reliable for calculation.

SUMMARY

^{177}Lu-DOTA-TATE therapy is a highly effective therapy in metastatic, well-differentiated, SSTR-positive GEP-NETs with mostly tolerable adverse effects. Guidelines generally refer to PRRT as a second-line therapy after SSA in gastroenteric and second- or third-line therapy in pancreatic NETs to improve survival rates and quality of life. Although we do not have sufficient data, ^{177}Lu-DOTA-TATE therapy may also have a role in high-grade NET therapy, mostly in combination with other treatments such as chemotherapy. The liver-dominant metastatic disease generally has poor outcomes and mostly requires liver-targeted therapies alone or in combination with PRRT depending on disease status.

CLINICS CARE POINTS

- Neuroendocrine tumors (NETs) are a rare, heterogeneous group of tumors and show overexpression of somatostatin receptors (SSTRs).
- High FDG uptake in metastatic lesions is associated with poor prognosis. In contrast, high SSTR uptake is correlated with a relatively good prognosis which can be predicted by SSTR imaging before peptite receptor radionuclide therapy (PRRT).
- ^{177}Lu-DOTATATE is highly effective and generally well-tolerated treatment option in metastatic/inoperable, progressive, SSTR-positive NETs with homogeneous SSTR expression.

DISCLOSURE

None.

REFERENCES

1. Dasari A, Shen C, Halperin D, et al. Trends in the incidence, prevalence, and survival outcomes in patients with neuroendocrine tumors in the United States. JAMA Oncol 2017;3(10):1335–42.
2. Oronsky B, Ma PC, Morgensztern D, et al. Nothing but NET: a review of neuroendocrine tumors and carcinomas. Neoplasia 2017;19(12):991–1002.
3. Krenning EP, Kwekkeboom DJ, Oei HY, et al. Somatostatin receptor imaging of endocrine gastrointestinal tumors. Schweiz Med Wochenschr 1992; 122(17):634–7.
4. Reubi JC, Schaer JC, Waser B, et al. Expression and localization of somatostatin receptor SSTR1, SSTR2, and SSTR3 messenger RNAs in primary human tumors using in situ hybridization. Cancer Res 1994; 54(13):3455–9.
5. Sanli Y, Garg I, Kandathil A, et al. Neuroendocrine tumor diagnosis and management: (68)Ga-DOTATATE PET/CT. AJR Am J Roentgenol 2018;211(2): 267–77.
6. Strosberg JR, Caplin ME, Kunz PL, et al. (177)Lu-Dotatate plus long-acting octreotide versus high-dose long-acting octreotide in patients with midgut neuroendocrine tumours (NETTER-1): final overall survival and long-term safety results from an open-label, randomised, controlled, phase 3 trial. Lancet Oncol 2021;22(12):1752–63.
7. Hicks RJ, Kwekkeboom DJ, Krenning E, et al. ENETS consensus guidelines for the standards of care in neuroendocrine neoplasia: peptide receptor radionuclide therapy with radiolabeled somatostatin analogues. Neuroendocrinology 2017;105(3): 295–309.
8. Hope TA, Bodei L, Chan JA, et al. NANETS/SNMMI consensus statement on patient selection and appropriate Use of (177)Lu-DOTATATE peptide receptor radionuclide therapy. J Nucl Med 2020; 61(2):222–7.
9. Pavel M, Öberg K, Falconi M, et al. Gastroenteropancreatic neuroendocrine neoplasms: ESMO Clinical Practice Guidelines for diagnosis, treatment and follow-up. Ann Oncol 2020;31(7):844–60.
10. Inzani F, Petrone G, Rindi G. The New World Health Organization classification for pancreatic neuroendocrine neoplasia. Endocrinol Metab Clin North Am 2018;47(3):463–70.
11. Brunner P, Jörg AC, Glatz K, et al. The prognostic and predictive value of sstr2-immunohistochemistry and sstr2-targeted imaging in neuroendocrine tumors. Eur J Nucl Med Mol Imaging 2017;44(3):468–75.
12. Satapathy S, Mittal BR. 177Lu-DOTATATE peptide receptor radionuclide therapy versus Everolimus in advanced pancreatic neuroendocrine tumors: a systematic review and meta-analysis. Nucl Med Commun 2019;40(12):1195–203.
13. Sundin A, Sundin R, Baudin E, et al. ENETS consensus guidelines for the standards of care in neuroendocrine tumors: radiological, nuclear medicine & hybrid imaging. Neuroendocrinology 2017; 105(3):212–44.
14. Bahri H, Laurence L, Edeline J, et al. High prognostic value of 18F-FDG PET for metastatic gastroenteropancreatic neuroendocrine tumors: a long-term evaluation. J Nucl Med 2014;55(11):1786–90.

15. Binderup T, Knigge U, Loft A, et al. 18F-fluorodeoxyglucose positron emission tomography predicts survival of patients with neuroendocrine tumors. Clin Cancer Res 2010;16(3):978–85.
16. Binderup T, Knigge U, Johnbeck CB, et al. (18)F-FDG PET is superior to who grading as a prognostic tool in neuroendocrine neoplasms and useful in guiding PRRT: a prospective 10-year follow-up study. J Nucl Med 2021;62(6):808–15.
17. Has Simsek D, Kuyumcu S, Turkmen C, et al. Can complementary 68Ga-DOTATATE and 18F-FDG PET/CT establish the missing link between histopathology and therapeutic approach in gastroenteropancreatic neuroendocrine tumors? J Nucl Med 2014;55(11):1811-7.
18. Binderup T, Knigge U, Loft A, et al. Functional imaging of neuroendocrine tumors: a head-to-head comparison of somatostatin receptor scintigraphy, 123I-MIBG scintigraphy, and 18F-FDG PET. J Nucl Med 2010;51(5):704–12.
19. Chan DL, Pavlakis N, Schembri GP, et al. Dual somatostatin receptor/FDG PET/CT imaging in metastatic neuroendocrine tumours: proposal for a novel grading scheme with prognostic significance. Theranostics 2017;7(5):1149–58.
20. Kwekkeboom DJ, Herder WW, Kam BL, et al. Treatment with the radiolabeled somatostatin analog [177 Lu-DOTA 0, Tyr3] octreotate: toxicity, efficacy, and survival. J Clin Oncol 2008;26(13).
21. Bodei L, Cremonesi M, Grana CM, et al. Peptide receptor radionuclide therapy with ^{177}Lu-DOTATATE: the IEO phase I-II study. Eur J Nucl Med Mol Imaging 2011;38(12):2125–35.
22. Sansovini M, Severi S, Ambrosetti A, et al. Treatment with the radiolabelled somatostatin analog Lu-DOTATATE for advanced pancreatic neuroendocrine tumors. Neuroendocrinology 2013;97(4):347–54.
23. Sansovini M, Severi S, Ianniello A, et al. Long-term follow-up and role of FDG PET in advanced pancreatic neuroendocrine patients treated with 177Lu-D OTATATE. Eur J Nucl Med Mol Imaging 2017;44(3): 490–9.
24. Delpassand ES, Samarghandi A, Zamanian S, et al. Peptide receptor radionuclide therapy with 177Lu-DOTATATE for patients with somatostatin receptor-expressing neuroendocrine tumors: the first US phase 2 experience. Pancreas 2014;43(4):518–25.
25. Paganelli G, Sansovini M, Ambrosetti A, et al. 177 Lu-Dota-octreotate radionuclide therapy of advanced gastrointestinal neuroendocrine tumors: results from a phase II study. Eur J Nucl Med Mol Imaging 2014;41(10):1845–51.
26. Paganelli G, Sansovini M, Nicolini S, et al. (177)Lu-PRRT in advanced gastrointestinal neuroendocrine tumors: 10-year follow-up of the IRST phase II prospective study. Eur J Nucl Med Mol Imaging 2021; 48(1):152–60.
27. Sabet A, Dautzenberg K, Haslerud T, et al. Specific efficacy of peptide receptor radionuclide therapy with (177)Lu-octreotate in advanced neuroendocrine tumours of the small intestine. Eur J Nucl Med Mol Imaging 2015;42(8):1238–46.
28. Zandee WT, Brabander T, Blažević A, et al. Symptomatic and radiological response to 177Lu-DOTATATE for the treatment of functioning pancreatic neuroendocrine tumors. J Clin Endocrinol Metab 2019;104(4):1336–44.
29. Sistani G, Sutherland DEK, Mujoomdar A, et al. Efficacy of (177)Lu-dotatate induction and maintenance therapy of various types of neuroendocrine tumors: a phase II registry study. Curr Oncol 2020;28(1): 115–27.
30. Satapathy S, Mittal BR, Sood A, et al. Peptide receptor radionuclide therapy as first-line systemic treatment in advanced inoperable/metastatic neuroendocrine tumors. Clin Nucl Med 2020;45(9): e393–9.
31. Parghane RV, Bhandare M, Chaudhari V, et al. Surgical feasibility, determinants, and overall efficacy of neoadjuvant (177)Lu-DOTATATE PRRT for locally advanced unresectable gastroenteropancreatic neuroendocrine tumors. J Nucl Med 2021;62(11): 1558–63.
32. Kudo A, Tateishi U, Yoshimura R, et al. Safety and response after peptide receptor radionuclide therapy with (177) Lu-DOTATATE for neuroendocrine tumors in phase 1/2 prospective Japanese trial. J Hepatobiliary Pancreat Sci 2022;29:487–99.
33. Strosberg J, El-Haddad G, Wolin E, et al. Phase 3 trial of 177Lu-Dotatate for midgut neuroendocrine tumors. New Engl J Med 2017;376(2):125–35.
34. Frilling A, Modlin IM, Kidd M, et al. Recommendations for management of patients with neuroendocrine liver metastases. Lancet Oncol 2014;15(1): e8–21.
35. Riihimaki M, Hemminki A, Sundquist K, et al. The epidemiology of metastases in neuroendocrine tumors. Int J Cancer 2016;139(12):2679–86.
36. Yao JC, Hassan M, Phan A, et al. One hundred years after "carcinoid": epidemiology of and prognostic factors for neuroendocrine tumors in 35,825 cases in the United States. J Clin Oncol 2008;26(18): 3063–72.
37. Lehrman ED, Fidelman N. Liver-directed therapy for neuroendocrine tumor liver metastases in the era of peptide receptor radionuclide therapy. Semin Intervent Radiol 2020;37(5):499–507.
38. Dermine S, Palmieri LJ, Lavolé J, et al. Non-pharmacological therapeutic options for liver metastases in advanced neuroendocrine tumors. J Clin Med 2019; 8(11).
39. Pavel M, O'Toole D, Costa F, et al. ENETS consensus guidelines update for the management of distant metastatic disease of intestinal, pancreatic,

bronchial neuroendocrine neoplasms (NEN) and NEN of unknown primary site. Neuroendocrinology 2016;103(2):172–85.
40. de Baere T, Deschamps F, Tselikas L, et al. GEP-NETS update: interventional radiology: role in the treatment of liver metastases from GEP-NETs. Eur J Endocrinol 2015;172(4):R151–66.
41. Bhagat N, Reyes DK, Lin M, et al. Phase II study of chemoembolization with drug-eluting beads in patients with hepatic neuroendocrine metastases: high incidence of biliary injury. Cardiovasc Intervent Radiol 2013;36(2):449–59.
42. Turkmen C, Ucar A, Poyanlı A, et al. Initial outcome after selective intraarterial radionuclide therapy with yttrium-90 microspheres as salvage therapy for unresectable metastatic liver disease. Cancer Biother Radiopharm 2013;28(7):534–40.
43. Roche A, Girish BV, Baere T, et al. Prognostic factors for chemoembolization in liver metastasis from endocrine tumors. Hepatogastroenterology 2004; 51(60):1751–6.
44. Chen JX, Rose S, White SB, et al. Embolotherapy for neuroendocrine tumor liver metastases: prognostic factors for hepatic progression-free survival and overall survival. Cardiovasc Interv Radiol 2017; 40(1):69–80.
45. Kacmaz E, Heidsma CM, Besselink MGH, et al. Treatment of liver metastases from midgut neuroendocrine tumours: a systematic review and meta-analysis. J Clin Med 2019;8(3).
46. Strosberg J, Hendifar A, Yao JC, et al. Impact of liver tumor burden on therapeutic effect of 177Lu-dotatate treatment in NETTER-1 study. Ann Oncol 2018; 29:viii471.
47. Braat A, Ahmadzadehfar H, Kappadath SC, et al. Radioembolization with (90)Y resin microspheres of neuroendocrine liver metastases after initial peptide receptor radionuclide therapy. Cardiovasc Intervent Radiol 2020;43(2):246–53.
48. Ezziddin S, Meyer C, Kahancova S, et al. 90Y Radioembolization after radiation exposure from peptide receptor radionuclide therapy. J Nucl Med 2012; 53(11):1663–9.
49. Yilmaz E, Engin MN, Ozkan ZG, et al. Y90 selective internal radiation therapy and peptide receptor radionuclide therapy for the treatment of metastatic neuroendocrine tumors: combination or not? Nucl Med Commun 2020;41(12):1242–9.
50. Braat A, Bruijnen RCG, Rooij RV, et al. Additional holmium-166 radioembolisation after lutetium-177-dotatate in patients with neuroendocrine tumour liver metastases (HEPAR PLuS): a single-centre, single-arm, open-label, phase 2 study. Lancet Oncol 2020;21(4):561–70.
51. Kashyap R, Hofman MS, Michael M, et al. Favourable outcomes of (177)Lu-octreotate peptide receptor chemoradionuclide therapy in patients with FDG-avid neuroendocrine tumours. Eur J Nucl Med Mol Imaging 2015;42(2):176–85.
52. Ballal S, Yadav MP, Damle NA, et al. Concomitant 177Lu-DOTATATE and capecitabine therapy in patients with advanced neuroendocrine tumors: a long-term-outcome, toxicity, survival, and quality-of-life study. Clin Nucl Med 2017;42(11):e457–66.
53. Nicolini S, Bodei L, Bongiovanni A, et al. Combined use of 177Lu-DOTATATE and metronomic capecitabine (Lu-X) in FDG-positive gastro-entero-pancreatic neuroendocrine tumors. Eur J Nucl Med Mol Imaging 2021;48(10):3260–7.
54. Lassmann M, Hänscheid H, Chiesa C, et al. EANM Dosimetry Committee series on standard operational procedures for pre-therapeutic dosimetry I: blood and bone marrow dosimetry in differentiated thyroid cancer therapy. Eur J Nucl Med Mol Imaging 2008;35(7):1405–12.
55. Sjögreen Gleisner K, Chouin N, Gabina PM, et al. EANM dosimetry committee recommendations for dosimetry of 177Lu-labelled somatostatin-receptor- and PSMA-targeting ligands. Eur J Nucl Med Mol Imaging 2022;49(6):1778–809.
56. Kesavan M, Turner JH. Myelotoxicity of peptide receptor radionuclide therapy of neuroendocrine tumors: a decade of experience. Cancer Biother Radiopharm 2016;31(6):189–98.
57. Garske-Román U, Sandström M, Baron KF, et al. Prospective observational study of 177Lu-DOTA-octreotate therapy in 200 patients with advanced metastasized neuroendocrine tumours (NETs): feasibility and impact of a dosimetry-guided study protocol on outcome and toxicity. Eur J Nucl Med Mol Imaging 2018;45(6):970–88.
58. Svensson J, Rydén T, Hagmarker L, et al. A novel planar image-based method for bone marrow dosimetry in (177)Lu-DOTATATE treatment correlates with haematological toxicity. EJNMMI Phys 2016;3(1):21.
59. Hagmarker L, Svensson J, Rydén T, et al. Bone marrow absorbed doses and correlations with hematologic response during 177Lu-DOTATATE treatments are influenced by image-based dosimetry method and presence of skeletal metastases. J Nucl Med 2019;60(10):1406–13.
60. Vegt E, Jong M, Wetzels JFM, et al. Renal toxicity of radiolabeled peptides and antibody fragments: mechanisms, impact on radionuclide therapy, and strategies for prevention. J Nucl Med 2010;51(7): 1049–58.
61. Dawson LA, Kavanagh BD, Paulino AC, et al. Radiation-associated kidney injury. Int J Radiat Oncol Biol Phys 2010;76(3 Suppl):S108–15.
62. Emami B, Lyman J, Brown A, et al. Tolerance of normal tissue to therapeutic irradiation. Int J Radiat Oncol Biol Phys 1991;21(1):109–22.
63. Sandstrom M, Garske-Román U, Granberg D, et al. Individualized dosimetry of kidney and bone marrow

in patients undergoing 177Lu-DOTA-octreotate treatment. J Nucl Med 2013;54(1):33–41.
64. Sundlöv A, Gustafsson J, Brolin G, et al. Feasibility of simplifying renal dosimetry in 177Lu peptide receptor radionuclide therapy. EJNMMI Phys 2018; 5(1):1–19.
65. Sundlöv A, Sjögreen-Gleisner K, Svensson J, et al. Individualised (177)Lu-DOTATATE treatment of neuroendocrine tumours based on kidney dosimetry. Eur J Nucl Med Mol Imaging 2017;44(9): 1480–9.
66. Cremonesi M, Ferrari ME, Bodei L, et al. Correlation of dose with toxicity and tumour response to (90)Y- and (177)Lu-PRRT provides the basis for optimization through individualized treatment planning. Eur J Nucl Med Mol Imaging 2018;45(13):2426–41.
67. Marin G, Vanderlinden B, Karfis I, et al. A dosimetry procedure for organs-at-risk in 177Lu peptide receptor radionuclide therapy of patients with neuroendocrine tumours. Physica Med 2018;56:41–9.

Gastro-Enteric-Pancreatic Neuroendocrine Tumor Treatment

Actinium-225-DOTATATE and Combined Therapies

Swayamjeet Satapathy, MD, Kunal Ramesh Chandekar, MD, Chandrasekhar Bal, MD, DSc*

KEYWORDS

• Peptide receptor radionuclide therapy • PRRT • Targeted alpha therapy • ^{225}Ac-DOTATATE
• Neuroendocrine tumors • GEP-NETs • Capecitabine • Temozolomide

KEY POINTS

- Lutetium-177-DOTATATE is currently the only Food and Drug Administrations (FDA)-approved agent for somatostatin receptor-(SSTR)-positive advanced gastro-entero-pancreatic neuroendocrine tumors; however, objective radiological response occurs less frequently.
- Actinium-225-DOTATATE, an alpha-particle emitter (physical $t_{1/2}$ = ~10 days; linear energy transfer = ~100 keV/μm), produces more blunt-ended double-stranded DNA breaks that are difficult to repair and hence, results in more efficient tumor killing; an objective response rate of >50% is reported.
- Further, the shorter path length of these alpha particles (~40 to 90 μm) spares the surrounding healthy tissue resulting in relatively fewer toxicities.
- Combination therapies with chemotherapeutic agents, such as capecitabine ± temozolomide, have shown improved outcomes, especially in the setting of higher grade and dual SSTR-positive, fluorodeoxyglucose-positive tumors.

INTRODUCTION

Gastro-enteric-pancreatic neuroendocrine tumors (GEP-NETs), although a rare group of tumors, have shown a rising burden over the decades, with the age-adjusted incidence rate increasing 6.4-fold from 1975 to 2015.[1] The 2019 World Health Organization (WHO) classification categorizes neuroendocrine neoplasms (NENs) of the digestive system into well-differentiated GEP-NETs and poorly differentiated neuroendocrine carcinomas (NECs). Genomic characteristics are being increasingly utilized for differentiating these two entities with mutations in MEN1, DAXX, and ATRX favoring a diagnosis of well-differentiated NETs and mutations in TP53 and RB1 favoring NECs. The GEP-NETs are further categorized into three grades depending on the mitotic rate and Ki-67 index: Grade 1—<2 mitoses/2 mm^2, Ki-67 index <3%; Grade 2—2 to 20 mitoses/2 mm^2, Ki-67 index 3% to 20%; and Grade 3—>20 mitoses/2 mm^2, Ki-67 index >20%.[2]

Although treatment of localized GEP-NETs is usually surgical resection, locally advanced inoperable or metastatic GEP-NETs require systemic therapies. Somatostatin analogs (SSAs) are widely used as first-line treatment of advanced GEP-NETs, whereas targeted and cytotoxic

Department of Nuclear Medicine, All India Institute of Medical Sciences, Ansari Nagar, New Delhi 110029, India
* Corresponding author.
E-mail address: csbal@hotmail.com

PET Clin 18 (2023) 215–221
https://doi.org/10.1016/j.cpet.2022.11.004
1556-8598/23/

chemotherapeutic agents are reserved for more progressive disease.[3] However, the clinical and financial toxicities associated with these treatment modalities often present a challenge for the patients. In this setting, Peptide Receptor Radionuclide Therapy (PRRT) has been established as a viable treatment option for such patients.[3] Most of the NETs progress slowly over the years; however, the aggressiveness varies according to the primary site. Although metastatic small intestinal NETs have an indolent course, metastatic gastric and rectal NETs often have rapid progression.[4] On the contrary, NECs have an overall worse prognosis and treatment options are mostly limited to platinum-based chemotherapy.[5]

Peptide Receptor Radionuclide Therapy

The rationale for the use of PRRT in GEP-NETs is based on the increased somatostatin receptor (SSTR) expression on the tumor cells.[6] The PRRT agents typically consist of a beta-emitting radionuclide linked to a peptide (SSTR agonist, eg, TOC-Tyr3 Octreotide or TATE-Tyr3Octreotate) by means of a chelator (DOTA). The binding of the agents to the SSTRs on the tumor cell membrane leads to internalization, thereby enabling the delivery of the beta-emitting radionuclides and causing cellular damage.[7] Lutetium-177 (^{177} Lu)-DOTATATE is currently the only FDA-approved PRRT for advanced/unresectable GEP-NETs. The approval was based on the NETTER-1 trial which enrolled 229 patients with progressive, well-differentiated, metastatic SSTR-positive mid-gut NET. The patients were randomly assigned (1:1) to 4 cycles of intravenous ^{177}Lu-DOTATATE 7·4 GBq (200 mCi) every 8 weeks plus intramuscular octreotide long-acting release (LAR) 30 mg (^{177}Lu-DOTATATE group) or high-dose octreotide LAR 60 mg every 4 weeks (control group). The trial met the primary endpoint with the progression-free survival (PFS) rate at 20 months being 65.2% (95% confidence interval [CI]: 50.0 to 76.8) in the ^{177}Lu-DOTATATE group vs 10.8% (95% CI: 3.5 to 23.0) in the control group (hazard ratio [HR]: 0.21; 95% CI: 0.13 to 0.33). Further, treatment with ^{177}Lu-DOTATATE also resulted in significantly higher objective radiological response (ORR) rate than high-dose octreotide LAR (18% vs 3%). ^{177}Lu-DOTATATE was also seen to be well-tolerated with grade 3/4 neutropenia, thrombocytopenia, and lymphopenia occurring in only 1%, 2%, and 9% of patients, respectively.[8] In a subsequent final analysis, the secondary endpoint, that is, median overall survival (OS) was 48·0 months (95% CI: 37·4 to 55·2) in the ^{177}Lu-DOTATATE group versus 36·3 months (95% CI: 25·9 to 51·7) in the control group (HR: 0·84, 95% CI: 0·60 to 1·17). Although the improvement of 11.7 months was clinically relevant, the non-significant results were attributed to a high proportion of patients (36%) in the control group crossing over and receiving subsequent PRRT.[9]

Existing Challenges to Peptide Receptor Radionuclide Therapy

Despite encouraging results observed in the NETTER-1 trial, few challenges persist. ^{177}Lu, being a beta-emitter with relatively lower linear energy transfer (LET) (~0.2 keV/μm), mostly causes single-stranded DNA breaks that are easier to repair.[10,11] This can account for a substantial proportion of patients not achieving ORR in the form of complete or partial response, as evident from the results of the NETTER-1 trial.[8] Another challenge to the use of PRRT in well-differentiated metastatic GEP-NETs is the presence of disease heterogeneity. Although tumor grade is routinely assessed from a single-site biopsy, the behavior of multiple metastatic sites could be different and affect treatment outcomes.[12] Such a scenario, therefore, sets out the rationale for using dual tracer PET/computed tomography (CT) with ^{68}Ga-based SSTR analogs and 2-deoxy-2-[^{18}F]-fluoro-D-glucose-PET/CT (^{18}F-FDG-PET/CT). Although routine ^{18}F-FDG-PET/CT is only recommended for grade 3 NENs, few studies have shown its prognostic significance in grade 1/2 tumors.[13,14] The proposed NETPET score, stratifying well-differentiated GEP-NETs by their relative SSTR/FDG expression, has been shown to be significantly associated with PRRT outcomes.[14] Thus, there is a scope for further improvement in PRRT outcomes. The strategies for the same include targeted alpha therapy (TAT), initiating PRRT earlier in the course of disease, and combination therapies.

Targeted Alpha Therapy

Actinium-225 (^{225}Ac) is an alpha-particle emitter with a half-life of ~10 days and a substantially higher LET of ~100 keV/μm. This enables it to produce blunt-ended double-stranded DNA breaks, which are difficult to repair. This coupled with its effectiveness in hypoxic tumor microenvironment results in more efficient tumor killing. Further, the shorter path length of the alpha particles (~40 to 90 μm) not only spares the surrounding healthy tissue resulting in relatively fewer toxicities, but is also particularly suited for bone-predominant micrometastatic disease.[10,11]

Chan and colleagues[15] compared the in-vitro radiobiological characteristics of PRRT using bismuth-213 (^{213}Bi, a daughter radionuclide in ^{225}Ac decay) and ^{177}Lu using the CA20948 cell line. Cell survival after exposure to ^{213}Bi-DOTATATE showed a linear-exponential relation with the absorbed dose, whereas that after exposure to ^{177}Lu-DOTATATE showed the characteristic curvature of the linear-quadratic model. 10% cell survival of CA20948 was reached at 3 Gy with ^{213}Bi-DOTATATE compared with 18 Gy for ^{177}Lu-DOTATATE, translating to a 6-factor advantage in cell killing. This advantage was shown to be even higher for ^{225}Ac-PRRT in another in-vitro study by Graf and colleagues[16] using SSTR-expressing AR42 J cells. The ED50 value for ^{225}Ac-DOTATOC was calculated to be 14 kBq/mL after 48 h of incubation, whereas it was 10 MBq/mL for ^{177}Lu-DOTATOC (~700-folds higher).

Apart from these in-vitro findings, the initial results with in-vivo ^{225}Ac-based PRRT have been promising. Miederer and colleagues[17] studied the bio-distribution, toxicity, and therapeutic efficacy of ^{225}Ac-DOTATOC in nude mice bearing AR42 J rat pancreas NET xenografts. They observed that ^{225}Ac-DOTATOC effectively accumulated in the xenograft NETs (radioactivity concentration at 30 min: ~10%/injected dose/g) and reduced tumor growth. Further, improved efficacy was observed with ^{225}Ac-DOTATOC compared with ^{177}Lu-DOTATOC. The highest non-toxic dose of ^{225}Ac-DOTATOC (20 kBq/mouse) when compared with ^{177}Lu-DOTATOC (1 MBq/mouse) resulted in significantly lower post-therapy mean tumor weight ($0.12 \text{ g} \pm 0.11$ g vs $0.52 \text{ g} \pm 0.38$ g, respectively, $p < 0.01$).

Ballal and colleagues[18] reported the first clinical experience with ^{225}Ac-DOTATATE TAT in GEP-NET patients who had exhausted or were refractory to ^{177}Lu-DOTATATE. In a prospective study, the authors recruited 32 patients with metastatic GEP-NETs who were having stable (14/32) or progressive disease (18/32) on ^{177}Lu-DOTATATE therapy. Systemic TAT was performed in the patients with intravenous ^{225}Ac-DOTATATE (100 kBq/kg body weight per cycle) over 1-5 cycles at intervals of 8 weeks. The morphological response assessed in 24/32 patients showed objective response in 62.5% patients with no event of disease progression or death during the median follow-up of 8 months (range 2 to 13 months). No grade 3/4 hematotoxicity, nephrotoxicity or hepatotoxicity was observed. Further, the patients had remarkable improvement in their quality-of-life with the endocrine symptoms, gastrointestinal symptoms, and disease-related worries declining significantly after ^{225}Ac-DOTATATE therapy ($p \leq 0.001$).

The same group of authors followed this up with a long-term outcome study comprising 91 patients of metastatic GEP-NETs treated with ^{225}Ac-DOTATATE (100 to 120 kBq/kg per cycle, median four cycles, range 1 to 10 cycles). Over a median follow-up of 24 months (range: 5 to 41 months), the median PFS and OS were not reached with 24-month PFS probability of 67.5% and 24-month OS probability of 70.8%. Notably, the ORR rate was 50.6%, whereas the disease control rate was 79.8%. Interestingly, the OS was not affected by the status of prior PRRT, thereby suggesting improved survival outcomes with ^{225}Ac-DOTATATE, even in ^{177}Lu-DOTATATE-refractory patients.[19]

Despite encouraging efficacy results with ^{225}Ac-based TAT, the data pertaining to its long-term safety profile are rather limited. The Heidelberg group reported 5-year follow-up data of hematological and renal toxicity after ^{225}Ac-DOTATOC therapy in 39 patients. Grade ≥3 acute hematological toxicities were observed at single treatment activities >40 MBq or repeated cycles of >20 MBq ^{225}Ac-DOTATOC at intervals of 4 months. No case of secondary myeloproliferative disease was noted. The average eGFR-loss per year was 8.4 mL/min (9.9%) and treatment-related kidney failure occurred in 2/39 (5%) patients after an interval of >4 years. The authors concluded that treatment activities of up to ~20 MBq per cycle administered at 4-months intervals and cumulative activities of up to 60 to 80 MBq could be considered safe and avoided grade 3/4 hematotoxicities.[20] Another report also highlighted a case of thyroid dysfunction developing one month after completion of four cycles of ^{225}Ac-DOTATATE therapy in a patient with NET. This was attributed to thyroiditis developing due to higher LET from alpha radiation, which got accumulated in the thyroid gland due to physiological SSTR expression.[21]

Initial studies with systemic TAT in GEP-NETs have mostly focused on patients who are refractory to beta-emitter PRRT. However, given the observed efficacy and safety profiles in this setting, it is reasonable to expect even better outcomes with the institution of TAT earlier in the disease course. This was shown in a recent report wherein a 46-year-old patient with grade 2 rectal NET and extensive nodal, hepatic, and skeletal metastases was treated upfront with 6 cycles of ^{225}Ac-DOTATATE (100 kBq/kg per cycle) at 8 weeks' intervals. The patient showed excellent symptomatic, biochemical, and radiological response with no grade 3/4 adverse events. In view of the radiobiological characteristics associated with alpha particles, the authors concluded that the first-line use of ^{225}Ac-DOTATATE presented a novel strategy for metastatic GEP-NETs, particularly those with high skeletal disease burden.[22] Subsequently, in a phase 1 trial, Delpassand and colleagues[23] also evaluated the role of TAT in PRRT-naïve patients using another alpha emitter, lead-212 (^{212} Pb). At the recommended phase 2 dose (RP2D) regimen consisting of 4 cycles of 2.50 MBq/kg of ^{212}Pb-DOTAMTATE administrated intravenously at 8-week intervals, the ORR was 80%.

Combination Therapies

Despite being one of the more effective therapeutic options for metastatic/inoperable NETs, PRRT often results in symptomatic relief and disease control rather than cure. Also, literature on the efficacy of PRRT in high grade (WHO Grade 3) tumors is relatively scarce. Grade 2 and 3 NETs are more complex, have rapid proliferative rates and heterogeneous SSTR expression, resulting in limited response to PRRT. However, recent retrospective studies have shown that even in high grade tumors, PRRT can provide modest objective response rates (31% to 42%) and disease control rates (69% to 78%) provided they are SSTR-analogue avid.[24–26] To potentiate the effect of PRRT, especially in Grade 2 or 3 tumors, combination therapy with radiosensitizing and other chemotherapeutic agents has gained popularity.

5-fluorouracil (5-FU) and its oral pro-drug, capecitabine have been successfully used as radiosensitizers for EBRT owing to their inhibitory action on thymidylate synthase, which is an important enzyme for DNA synthesis.[27] Early studies established that the addition of 5-FU infusion or oral capecitabine as radiosensitizers to ^{177}Lu-DOTATATE therapy in patients with inoperable/metastatic, progressive, well-differentiated NETs did not increase the toxicity of radiopeptide therapy while achieving high tumor control and disease stabilization rates.[28–30] In a pioneering phase 2 study, Claringbold and colleagues[30] enrolled 33 patients with inoperable and progressive, SSTR-positive well-differentiated NETs and administered 7.8 GBq ^{177}Lu-octreotate 8-weekly, with concomitant oral capecitabine (1,650 mg/m^2 per day) for 14 days during each cycle. The combination was seen to be safe with minimal transient myelosuppression and no nephrotoxicity. Notably, the median absorbed dose to the kidneys and liver were 2.4 Gy per cycle and 4.8 Gy per cycle, respectively, with the cumulative absorbed doses being less than the toxic thresholds. The ORR was 24% with the 20-month PFS probability being close to 90%. To put in context, the 20-month PFS probability in the NETTER-1 trial was 65.2%.[8]

Concomitant capecitabine plus temozolomide (an alkylating agent) has also been evaluated as radiosensitizer. In a prospective phase 2 trial by Claringbold and colleagues,[31] grade 1 or 2, metastatic/inoperable, progressive pancreatic NETs (pNETs) were treated with combination of ^{177}Lu-Octreotate-Capecitabine-Temozolomide radiopeptide chemotherapy. ^{177}Lu-Octreotate was administered at a fixed dose of 7.9 GBq per cycle for 4 cycles, 8 weeks apart. Five days before radiopeptide administration, oral capecitabine (1500 mg/m^2) was started and continued for 14 days. Temozolomide (200 mg/m^2) was given in the last 5 days of each 14-day capecitabine period. Combination radiopeptide chemotherapy was highly effective with an ORR of 80% and median PFS of 48 months. However, this combination was found to have slightly higher toxicity with grade 3 thrombocytopenia and anemia being reported in 10% of the patients each, and one patient also developing myelodysplastic syndrome 4 years after treatment.

The role of concomitant radiosensitizing chemotherapy was further established by Ballal and colleagues[19] in a large retrospective comparative analysis of 167 patients. Here, the authors evaluated the efficacy and safety of low-dose capecitabine administered concomitantly with ^{177}Lu-DOTATATE (group 1, n = 88) and compared it to ^{177}Lu-DOTATATE therapy alone (group 2, n = 76). Capecitabine was administered orally at a dose of 1250 mg/m^2 on days 0-14 of each PRRT cycle. The study reported the combination therapy to be safe with significantly higher rates of objective response (34% vs 6.3%) compared with ^{177}Lu-DOTATATE therapy alone. Further, patients receiving combination therapy achieved longer OS and PFS (median not reached vs 48 months each) compared with those receiving ^{177}Lu-DOTATATE mono-therapy. It is noteworthy that capecitabine was used here as a radiosensitizer and administered regardless of the tumor grade.[32] Based on these findings, the authors also used concomitant capecitabine (2 g/day) with ^{225}Ac-DOTATATE on days 0-14 of each cycle to sensitize to the downstream beta-emissions in the decay scheme of ^{225}Ac.

Combination Therapy in First-Line Setting

So far, the use of PRRT has been limited to progressive disease settings, wherein patients have failed treatment with first-line SSAs. Given the overwhelmingly positive results, it is reasonable to expect even better outcomes with the institution of PRRT earlier in the disease course.[33] This can be further improved with the addition of radiosensitizing low-dose chemotherapy. A single-center retrospective study from India, comprising 76 patients, evaluated the efficacy and safety of first-line systemic ^{177}Lu-DOTATATE plus radiosensitizing low-dose capecitabine (1250 mg/m^2 per day orally on days 0 to 14 of each PRRT cycle) and compared the results with first-line octreotide LAR. ^{177}Lu-DOTATATE plus low-dose capecitabine achieved significantly higher ORR (38% vs 15%), higher disease control rate (88% vs 67%), and longer median PFS (54 months vs 16 months) compared with octreotide LAR in treatment-naive patients with advanced, grade 1/2 GEP-NETs. This benefit was observed at the cost of no additional grade 3/4 toxicity.[34]

Areas for Further Research

Further clinical studies are needed to assess the long-term safety and survival outcomes of ^{225}Ac-DOTATATE as well as combination strategies in larger patient cohorts. Long-term safety signals such as delayed nephrotoxicity and treatment-related myeloid neoplasms need to be particularly addressed. Randomized trials comparing ^{225}Ac-DOTATATE versus ^{177}Lu-DOTATATE in PRRT-naïve patients and allowing for a crossover design are also necessary to determine the optimum treatment sequence in these patients. Further, the role of concomitant radiosensitizing chemotherapy with ^{225}Ac-based PRRT remains to be definitively established in adequately powered future trials. Apart from radiosensitization, strategies for alternate combination therapy (drugs that improve delivery of radiopharmaceutical and/or tumor perfusion or increase the density of SSTR expression on tumor cells) also need to be developed.

CLINICS CARE POINTS

- Actinium-225 (^{225}Ac)-DOTATATE, an alpha-particle emitter, has higher linear energy transfer and shorter tissue path length compared with the beta-emitting lutetium-177-DOTATATE.
- These superior radiobiological characteristics result in more double-stranded DNA breaks and hence, more efficient tumor cell killing with minimal toxicity to surrounding healthy tissues.
- Concomitant administration of chemotherapeutic agents like capecitabine and temozolomide with Peptide Receptor Radionuclide Therapy can have radiosensitizing as well as independent tumoricidal effects, and can result in improved outcomes.
- Further studies are needed to assess the long-term safety (particularly delayed nephrotoxicity and treatment-related myeloid neoplasms) and survival outcomes of ^{225}Ac-DOTATATE as well as combination strategies in larger patient cohorts.

DISCLOSURE

The authors have no commercial or financial conflict of interest. No funding was provided for the preparation of this article.

REFERENCES

1. Xu Z, Wang L, Dai S, et al. Epidemiologic trends of and factors associated with overall survival for patients with gastroenteropancreatic neuroendocrine tumors in the United States. JAMA Netw Open 2021;4:e2124750.
2. Nagtegaal ID, Odze RD, Klimstra D, et al. The 2019 WHO classification of tumours of the digestive system. Histopathology 2020;76:182–8.
3. Uri I, Grozinsky-Glasberg S. Current treatment strategies for patients with advanced gastroentero-pancreatic neuroendocrine tumors (GEP-NETs). Clin Diabetes Endocrinol 2018;4:16.
4. Cives M, Strosberg JR. Gastroenteropancreatic neuroendocrine tumors. CA Cancer J Clin 2018;68:471–87.
5. Rinke A, Gress TM. Neuroendocrine cancer, therapeutic strategies in G3 cancers. Digestion 2017;95:109–14.
6. Hofman MS, Lau WE, Hicks RJ. Somatostatin receptor imaging with ^{68}Ga DOTATATE PET/CT: clinical utility, normal patterns, pearls, and pitfalls in interpretation. Radiographics 2015;35:500–16.
7. Van Der Zwan WA, Bodei L, Mueller-Brand J, et al. GEP–NETs Update: radionuclide therapy in neuroendocrine tumours. Eur J Endocrinol 2015;172:R1–8.
8. Strosberg J, El-Haddad G, Wolin E, et al. Phase 3 trial of ^{177}Lu-DOTATATE for midgut neuroendocrine tumours. N Engl J Med 2017;376:125–35.
9. Strosberg JR, Caplin ME, Kunz PL, et al. ^{177}Lu-Dotatate plus long-acting octreotide versus high-dose long-acting octreotide in patients with midgut neuroendocrine tumours (NETTER-1): final overall survival and long-term safety results from an open-label, randomised, controlled, phase 3 trial. Lancet Oncol 2021;22:1752–63.

10. Kratochwil C, Giesel FL, Heussel CP, et al. Patients resistant against PSMA-targeting α-radiation therapy often harbor mutations in DNA damage-repair-associated genes. J Nucl Med 2020;61:683–8.
11. Tafreshi NK, Doligalski ML, Tichacek CJ, et al. Development of targeted alpha particle therapy for solid tumors. Molecules 2019;24:4314.
12. Basu S, Parghane RV, Kamaldeep, et al. Peptide receptor radionuclide therapy of neuroendocrine tumors. Semin Nucl Med 2020;50:447–64.
13. Zhang J, Liu Q, Singh A, et al. Prognostic value of ^{18}F-FDG PET/CT in a large cohort of patients with advanced metastatic neuroendocrine neoplasms treated with peptide receptor radionuclide therapy. J Nucl Med 2020;61:1560–9.
14. Chan DL, Pavlakis N, Schembri GP, et al. Dual somatostatin receptor/FDG PET/CT imaging in metastatic neuroendocrine tumours: proposal for a novel grading scheme with prognostic significance. Theranostics 2017;7:1149–58.
15. Chan HS, de Blois E, Morgenstern A, et al. In Vitro comparison of 213Bi- and 177Lu-radiation for peptide receptor radionuclide therapy. PLoS One 2017;12:e0181473.
16. Graf F, Fahrer J, Maus S, et al. DNA double strand breaks as predictor of efficacy of the alpha-particle emitter Ac-225 and the electron emitter Lu-177 for somatostatin receptor targeted radiotherapy. PLoS One 2014;9:e88239.
17. Miederer M, Henriksen G, Alke A, et al. Preclinical evaluation of the alpha-particle generator nuclide 225Ac for somatostatin receptor radiotherapy of neuroendocrine tumors. Clin Cancer Res 2008;14:3555–61.
18. Ballal S, Yadav MP, Bal C, et al. Broadening horizons with ^{225}Ac-DOTATATE targeted alpha therapy for gastroenteropancreatic neuroendocrine tumour patients stable or refractory to ^{177}Lu-DOTATATE PRRT: first clinical experience on the efficacy and safety. Eur J Nucl Med Mol Imaging 2020;47:934–46.
19. Ballal S, Yadav MP, Tripathi M, et al. Survival outcomes in metastatic gastroenteropancreatic neuroendocrine tumor patients receiving concomitant ^{225}Ac-DOTATATE targeted alpha therapy and capecitabine: a real-world scenario management based long-term outcome study. J Nucl Med 2022. https://doi.org/10.2967/jnumed.122.264043.
20. Kratochwil C, Apostolidis L, Rathke H, et al. Dosing ^{225}Ac-D122.264043. OTATOC in patients with somatostatin-receptor-positive solid tumors: 5-year follow-up of hematological and renal toxicity. Eur J Nucl Med Mol Imaging 2021;49:54–63.
21. Kavanal AJ, Satapathy S, Sood A, et al. Subclinical hypothyroidism after 225Ac-DOTATATE therapy in a case of metastatic neuroendocrine tumor: unknown adverse effect of PRRT. Clin Nucl Med 2022;47:e184–6.
22. Satapathy S, Sood A, Das CK, et al. Alpha before beta: exceptional response to first-line 225Ac-DOTATATE in a patient of metastatic neuroendocrine tumor with extensive skeletal involvement. Clin Nucl Med 2022;47:e156–7.
23. Delpassand ES, Tworowska I, Esfandiari R, et al. Targeted alpha-emitter therapy with ^{212}Pb-DOTAMTATE for the treatment of metastatic SSTR-expressing neuroendocrine tumors: first-in-human, dose-escalation clinical trial. J Nucl Med 2022;121:263230. jnumed.
24. Thang SP, Lung MS, Kong G, et al. Peptide receptor radionuclide therapy (PRRT) in European Neuroendocrine Tumour Society (ENETS) grade 3 (G3) neuroendocrine neoplasia (NEN) – a single-institution retrospective analysis. Eur J Nucl Med Mol Imaging 2017;45:262–77.
25. Zhang J, Kulkarni HR, Singh A, et al. Peptide receptor radionuclide therapy in Grade 3 neuroendocrine neoplasms: safety and survival analysis in 69 patients. J Nucl Med 2019;60:377–85.
26. Carlsen EA, Fazio N, Granberg D, et al. Peptide receptor radionuclide therapy in gastroenteropancreatic NEN G3: a multicenter cohort study. Endocr Relat Cancer 2019;26:227–39.
27. Rich TA, Shepard RC, Mosley ST. Four decades of continuing innovation with fluorouracil: current and future approaches to fluorouracil chemoradiation therapy. J Clin Oncol 2004;22:2214–32.
28. Van Essen M, Krenning EP, Kam BL, et al. Report on short-term side effects of treatments with 177Lu-octreotate in combination with capecitabine in seven patients with gastroenteropancreatic neuroendocrine tumours. Eur J Nucl Med Mol Imaging 2008;35:743–8.
29. Hubble D, Kong G, Michael M, et al. 177Lu-octreotate, alone or with radiosensitising chemotherapy, is safe in neuroendocrine tumour patients previously treated with high-activity 111In-octreotide. Eur J Nucl Med Mol Imaging 2010;37:1869–75.
30. Claringbold PG, Brayshaw PA, Price RA, et al. Phase II study of radiopeptide 177Lu-octreotate and capecitabine therapy of progressive disseminated neuroendocrine tumours. Eur J Nucl Med Mol Imaging 2011;38:302–11.
31. Claringbold PG, Turner JH. Pancreatic neuroendocrine tumor control: durable objective response to combination 177Lu-octreotate-capecitabine- temozolomide radiopeptide chemotherapy. Neuroendocrinology 2016;103:432–9.
32. Ballal S, Yadav MP, Damle NA, et al. Concomitant 177Lu-DOTATATE and capecitabine therapy in patients with advanced neuroendocrine tumours: a long-term outcome, toxicity, survival, and

quality-of-life study. Clin Nucl Med 2017;42: e457–66.

33. Satapathy S, Mittal BR, Sood A, et al. Peptide receptor radionuclide therapy as first-line systemic treatment in advanced inoperable/metastatic neuroendocrine tumors. Clin Nucl Med 2020;45: e393–9.

34. Satapathy S, Mittal BR, Sood A, et al. ^{177}Lu-DOTATATE plus radiosensitizing capecitabine versus octreotide long-acting release as first-line systemic therapy in advanced grade 1 or 2 gastroenteropancreatic neuroendocrine tumors: a single-institution experience. JCO Glob Oncol 2021;7: 1167–75.

Diagnosis and Treatment of Lung Neuroendocrine Neoplasms

Somatostatin Receptor PET Imaging and Peptide Receptor Radionuclide Therapy

Hyesun Park, MD[a,*], Rathan M. Subramaniam, MD[b,c]

KEYWORDS

• Lung carcinoid • Somatostatin receptor PET imaging • Peptide receptor radionuclide therapy

KEY POINTS

- ^{68}Ga-DOTA-0-Tyr3-Octreotate (DOTATATE) PET/CT is the modality of choice for lung carcinoid diagnosis, on which typical lung carcinoid usually shows intense uptake, whereas atypical lung carcinoid can demonstrate a variable degree of uptake, usually less uptake compared with typical lung carcinoid.
- 18F-fluorodeoxyglucose (^{18}F-FDG) PET/CT can identify higher-grade lung carcinoid with lack of SSTR expression, and dual tracer PET/CT using ^{18}F-FDG and ^{68}Ga-DOTATATE may help selecting the patients with lung carcinoid who would benefit from the peptide receptor radionuclide therapy (PRRT).
- PRRT using ^{177}Lu-labeled or ^{90}Y-labeled somatostatin analog (SSA) may be effective and safely used for advanced lung carcinoids with high SSTR expression, which progressed after SSA therapy.

INTRODUCTION

Neuroendocrine tumor (NET) is a heterogeneous group of malignancies originating from the neuroendocrine cells, most commonly originating from pancreatic-gastrointestinal tract and lung, with a wide range of pathologic condition from indolent to highly aggressive tumor biology. Neuroendocrine neoplasm of the lung comprises approximately 25% of all invasive lung neoplasms, with an increasing incidence of typical and atypical carcinoids mainly due to improvement of detection methods and increased awareness of the disease.[1,2]

According to 2021 World Health Organization (WHO) classification, neuroendocrine neoplasm of the lung can be categorized into 3 major categories: (1) precursor lesion–diffuse idiopathic neuroendocrine cell hyperplasia, (2) NET/carcinoid tumor not otherwise specified, including typical carcinoid/grade 1 NET and atypical carcinoid/grade 2 NET, and (3) neuroendocrine carcinomas (NECs) including small cell carcinoma and large cell NEC.[3] Typical and atypical carcinoids are categorized as a single group of tumors in the 2021 WHO classification, and subtype classification is based on morphology with mitoses and the presence of necrosis.[3] The Ki-67 proliferation index can help differentiate carcinoids from NEC, with an index value less than 5% for typical carcinoids and ranging from 9% to 18% for atypical

[a] Department of Radiology, Lahey Hospital and Medical Center, 41 Burlington Mall Road, Burlington, MA 01850, USA; [b] Department of Medicine, Otago Medical School, Dunedin, 01 Great King Street, Central Dunedin, Dunedin 9016, New Zealand; [c] Department of Radiology, Duke University, Davison Building, Durham, NC 27710, USA
* Corresponding author.
E-mail address: hyesun.park@lahey.org

PET Clin 18 (2023) 223–231
https://doi.org/10.1016/j.cpet.2022.11.005

carcinoids.[4] However, there is a lack of reproducible cutoffs of Ki-67 for typical versus atypical carcinoids, and the prognostic implication of the proliferation index is unclear.[4] Given the heterogeneity of tumor biology and the variety of treatment strategy for lung carcinoids, a multidisciplinary team approach including surgeons, medical and radiation oncologists, pathologists, and diagnostic/interventional radiologists are critical for the optimal management plan. This review provides updates on the diagnostic modality of lung carcinoids, including somatostatin receptor (SSTR) imaging. In addition, we will discuss treatment options, including the theragnostic approach to lung carcinoids in precision medicine.

Diagnosis of Lung Carcinoid

Chest CT—Chest CT is a mainstay of detecting and evaluating lung nodules. Typical and atypical lung carcinoids have similar imaging findings, presenting as a peripheral solitary nodule involving the segmental bronchus (57%), or a central solitary nodule involving the segmental or larger bronchus (43%).[5] Lung nodules can be associated with air trapping, bronchiectasis, or atelectasis. Other CT features suggesting lung carcinoid and atypical carcinoid include lobulated margin, high attenuation on contrast-enhanced CT (mean, 55.2 Hounsfield Unit [HU]; range, 34–73 HU), and presence of calcification that is often characterized as punctate, eccentric, or diffuse[5] (**Fig. 1**).

No specific staging system exists for pulmonary carcinoids because of the rare entity. Tumor, node, metastasis (TNM) staging has been applied to lung carcinoid staging, although it was originally designed for the staging of nonsmall cell lung cancer.[6] Previous studies showed that the TNM staging system of lung carcinoids could predict the clinical outcome in lung carcinoids,[7,8] which was mainly related to nodule size and lymph node involvement in disease. However, TNM staging is limited because the histologic grade of lung carcinoid is not considered in staging. Given the significant impact of histologic grade on the clinical outcome, an integrated classification system that incorporates histologic grade and anatomic/pathologic grade is needed for lung carcinoid staging.

SSTR imaging—SSTRs are cell membrane-bound, G-protein-coupled receptors that mediate intracellular signaling pathways involved in cell proliferation, differentiation, and angiogenesis.[9] SSTRs are highly expressed in NETs, up to 70% in lung typical carcinoids, and progressively decreased amounts in atypical carcinoids. Synthetic somatostatin analogs (SSAs) showing high binding affinity to SSTR 2, 3, and 5 are widely used for diagnostic and therapeutic procedures of NETs. Typical lung carcinoid usually shows intense uptake on SSTR imaging due to high expression of SSTR. However, atypical lung carcinoid can demonstrate a variable degree of uptake depending on the amount of SSTR expression in the cell membrane and usually shows less uptake compared with typical lung carcinoid. ^{111}In-labeled pentetreotide scan with SPECT/CT used to be a main SSTR imaging modality for the identification of SSTR-positive NETs. Compared with CT, ^{111}In or ^{99m}Tc-labeled pentetreotide scan with SPECT/CT showed higher sensitivity and diagnostic accuracy for the diagnosis of lung carcinoid.[9,10] However, octreotide scan has several limitations, including relatively slow pharmacokinetics, high-energy γ-emissions, and limited injectable activity to about 37–74 MBq (1–2 mCi), all resulting in low resolution of images.

Recently introduced new SSTR PET, including ^{68}Ga-labeled DOTATATE, provides better resolution and favorable dosimetry. ^{68}Ga-labeled DOTATATE PET/CT provides an estimation of SSTR density and functionality, detection of tumor heterogeneity, and information to select the patient

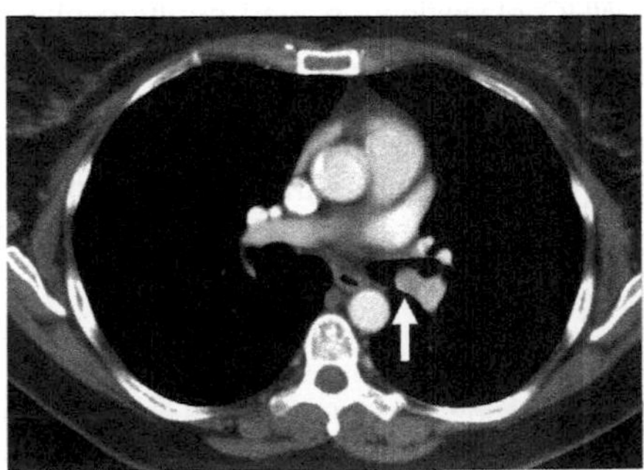

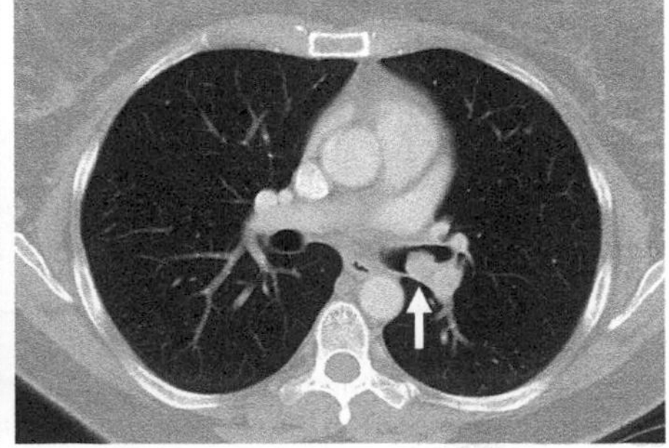

Fig. 1. A 46-year-old woman presented with hemoptysis. On chest CT, there was a 1.4-cm endobronchial mass within the left main bronchus with luminal narrowing (*arrows*). She underwent left bronchial sleeve resection and left lower lobe superior segmentectomy, and it was confirmed as atypical carcinoid with Ki-67 proliferation index is 5% to 10%.

cohort who would benefit from SSA or peptide receptor radionuclide therapy (PRRT). ^{68}Ga-labeled DOTATATE PET/CT was more sensitive for detecting typical or atypical carcinoids compared with CT only for staging, with upstage disease and change in management after PET/CT in 22.7% of patients, mainly due to hepatic metastasis, which was isodense to background liver parenchyma and marrow involvement or subtle osseous lesions, all of which are difficult to see on CT.[11] Many studies proved that ^{68}Ga-labeled DOTATATE PET/CT showed better diagnostic performance (ie, improved sensitivity and specificity) than octreotide scan for identifying NET.[12–14] According to the recently published study, ^{68} Ga labeled-SSTR PET/CT demonstrates excellent diagnostic performance in detecting distant metastases and intrathoracic lymph node metastases for TNM staging, especially in typical carcinoids[15] (**Figs. 2** and **3**).

One challenge of SSTR imaging for lung carcinoids is tumor heterogeneity of a wide range of SSTR expression and histologic grade across the tumor. Approximately 9% of typical and 27% of atypical carcinoids can demonstrate heterogeneous receptor positivity among metastatic lesions.[11] Lung carcinoids with a high proliferative index (ki-67 > 10%) would show mild or no uptake on ^{68}Ga-DOTATATE PET/CT, which would be difficult to identify the lesion.

^{18}F-FDG PET/CT—^{18}F-FDG PET/CT can help identify the relatively higher grade lung carcinoid with an increased metabolism of tumors. The FDG uptake in lung carcinoids may depend on histologic grade and tumor biology. Several studies showed that SUV_{max} of atypical lung carcinoids is significantly higher than typical carcinoids on ^{18}F-FDG PET/CT.[16,17] The difference in FDG uptake can be explained by the difference in Glucose transporter 1 (GLUT1) expression, which is closely related to malignancy between typical and atypical carcinoids (7% in typical carcinoids vs 21% in atypical carcinoids).[18,19]

Dual tracer PET/CT using ^{18}F-FDG and ^{68}Ga-DOTATATE has been proposed to evaluate NET. This approach can better reflect tumor heterogeneity in metastatic sites and predict the clinical outcome.[20] FDG-positive and SSTR-positive NET showed a worse prognosis than FDG-negative SSTR-positive NETs and worse clinical outcomes after PRRT.[21,22] Therefore, FDG can be used as an imaging biomarker to identify the NET patient group who would benefit from PRRT. In lung carcinoids, there is limited data regarding dual tracer use. A recent retrospective study by Zidan and colleagues[23] investigated the role of a combination of ^{18}F-FDG and ^{68}Ga-DOTATATE PET/CT in lung carcinoids (**Table 1**). In this study, 34% of all lung carcinoid patients (32% in typical carcinoids and 35% in atypical carcinoids) demonstrated sites of increased FDG uptake in both typical and atypical carcinoids, and 42% of these patients had one or more discordant FDG and DOTATATE uptake of lesions (ie, DOTATATE-negative and FDG positive). In addition, significant interpatient

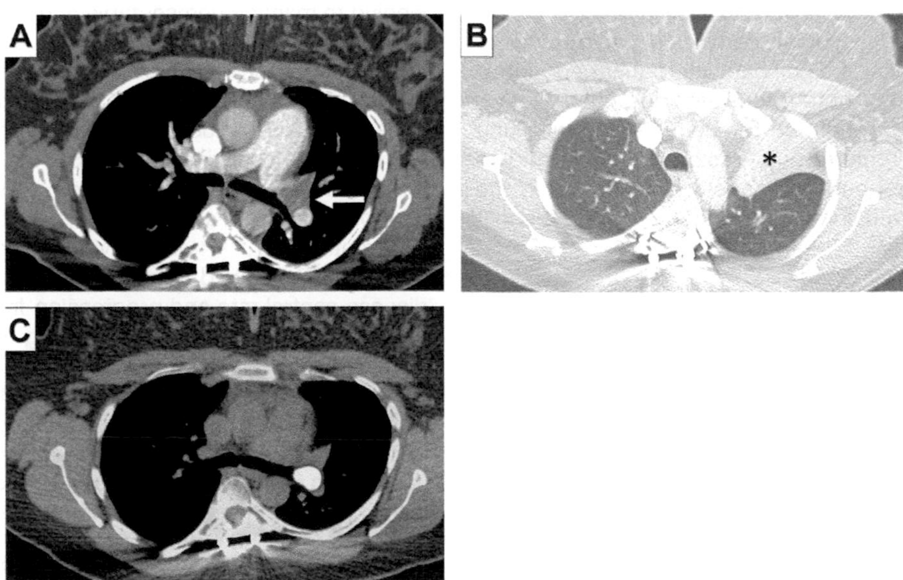

Fig. 2. A 40-year-old woman presented with dyspnea. (*A, B*) Chest CT showed a 1.5-cm endobronchial lesion in the left upper lobar bronchus (*arrow*), resulting in complete atelectasis (*asterisk*). (*C*) This lesion was intensely avid on 68Ga-DOTATATE PET/CT. The mass was biopsied and confirmed as typical carcinoid (Ki-67<1%).

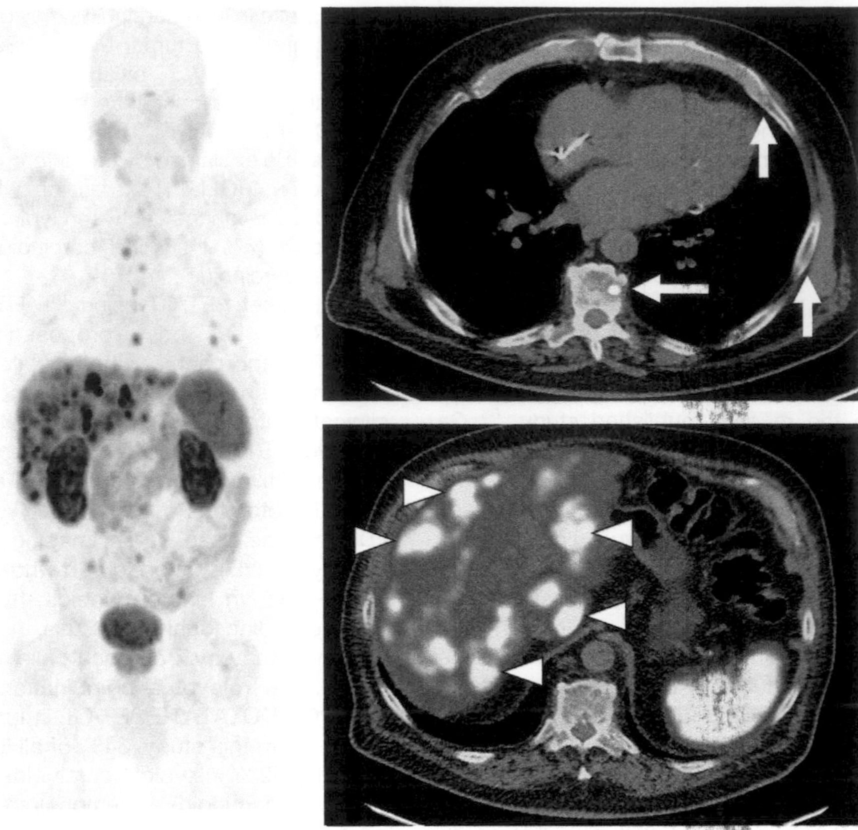

Fig. 3. A 79-year-old man with previous history of right middle lobe carcinoid, which was resected. On ^{68}Ga-DOTATATE PET/CT, there are multiple intense foci of uptake in the liver (*arrows*) and bone (*arrowheads*), consistent with positive SSTR expressing metastases.

tumor heterogeneity was found, with variable degrees of DOTATATE and FDG uptake in both typical and atypical carcinoids. According to these results of significant interpatient and intrapatient tumor heterogeneities, dual tracer imaging may be helpful to characterize the lung carcinoid regardless of histologic grade and to guide therapeutic management in selecting the patients with lung carcinoids who may benefit from PRRT[23] (**Figs. 4** and **5**).

Management of Lung Carcinoid

Localized disease—Surgery can be a curative option for localized lung carcinoids. An excellent clinical outcome can be achieved after resection of localized typical carcinoid, with 5-year and 10-year overall survival rates greater than 90%.[24] However, the prognosis of localized atypical carcinoid after surgery is less favorable, with 5-year overall survival of 70% and 10-year overall survival of 50%.[24] Adjuvant chemotherapy using platinum-based agents and etoposide can be considered after surgery of atypical carcinoids.[25,26]

Advanced/unresectable disease—It is challenging to manage unresectable and/or advanced lung carcinoids. There is a lack of evidence or consensus regarding the optimal treatment approaches for lung carcinoids, and most data are based on trials, including gastroenteropancreatic NETs. A previous trial showed SSA is beneficial for preventing disease progression in asymptomatic patients with advanced gastrointestinal or pancreatic NET.[27,28] In previous retrospective studies, SSA showed antitumor activity regarding disease control rate and progression-free survival (PFS) as first-line therapy for lung carcinoids without significant adverse events.[29,30] Therefore, the National Comprehensive Cancer Network recommends SSA for hormone-releasing lung carcinoids.[26] Targeted therapy using everolimus (rapamycin inhibitor) can improve PFS compared with placebo in advanced nonfunctional lung NETs (median PFS of 9.2 versus 3.6 months, hazard ratio, 0.50; 95% CI, 0.28–0.88). Tumor shrinkage was more commonly noted in patients who received everolimus compared with placebo (58% vs 13%) according to the lung subgroup

Table 1
Clinical outcome and safety profile of retrospective studies of lung carcinoid after peptide receptor radionuclide therapy

Reference	Total (n)	Lung Carcinoid (n)	PRRT	PFS (month)	OS (month)	Grade 3–4 Toxicity (n)
Sabet et al,[38] 2017	22	22	^{177}Lu-DOTATATE	27 (9–45)	42 (25–59)	3 (13.6%) hematotoxicity
Parghane et al,[39] 2017	19	19	^{177}Lu-DOTATATE	N/A	40 (13.1 –64.8)	None
Brabander et al,[40] 2017	610 for safety evaluation; 443 for efficacy evaluation	23	^{177}Lu-DOTATATE	20	52 (49–55)	61 (10%) hematotoxicity 10 (3%) hepatotoxicity 6 (1%) renal toxicity
Mirvis et al,[41] 2020	25	25	7 ^{90}Y-DOTATATE 18 ^{177}Lu-DOTATATE	17 (13–20)	42	1 (4%) hematotoxicity 1 (4%) pericarditis

study of phase III RADIANT-4 trial.[31,32] For locally advanced diseases, radiation therapy with or without platinum-based chemotherapy can be considered.[26] There are many ongoing trials investigating treatment options in advanced lung carcinoids, including the phase II LUNA trial evaluating the efficacy of the combination of everolimus plus pasireotide long-acting release in patients with well-differentiated lung or thymic carcinoids (NCT01563354) and phase III SPINET trial assessing the efficacy and safety of lanreotide (autogel/Depot) in patients with advanced well-differentiated, metastatic/unresectable SSTR-positive carcinoid (NCT02683941).

Peptide Receptor Radionuclide Therapy for Advanced Lung Carcinoid

Peptide receptor radionuclide therapy agents

Radiolabeled SSA is made up of 3 components: (1) a radionuclide isotope, either ^{90}Y or ^{177}Lu, (2) a

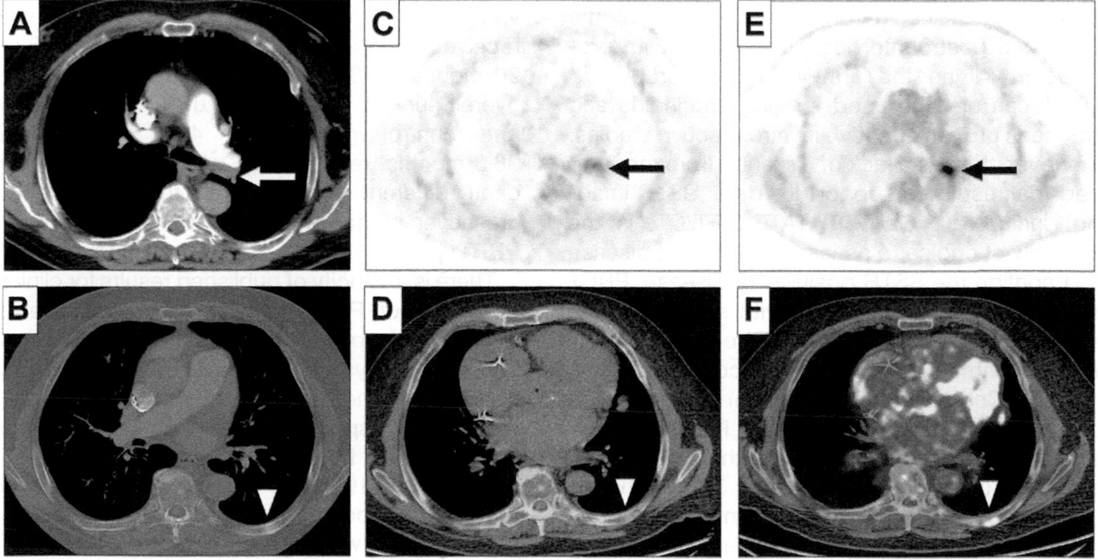

Fig. 4. A 69-year-old man with atypical carcinoid. On CT, there is a 1.7-cm left hilar nodule (*A*, *arrow*) and multiple sclerotic osseous lesions (*B*, *arrowheads*), which was mildly avid on ^{68}Ga-DOTATATE PET/CT (*C*, *D*) and intensely avid on ^{18}F-FDG PET/CT (*E*, *F*). (*arrow* in C and E, left hilar nodule; arrowhead in D and F, osseous lesion).

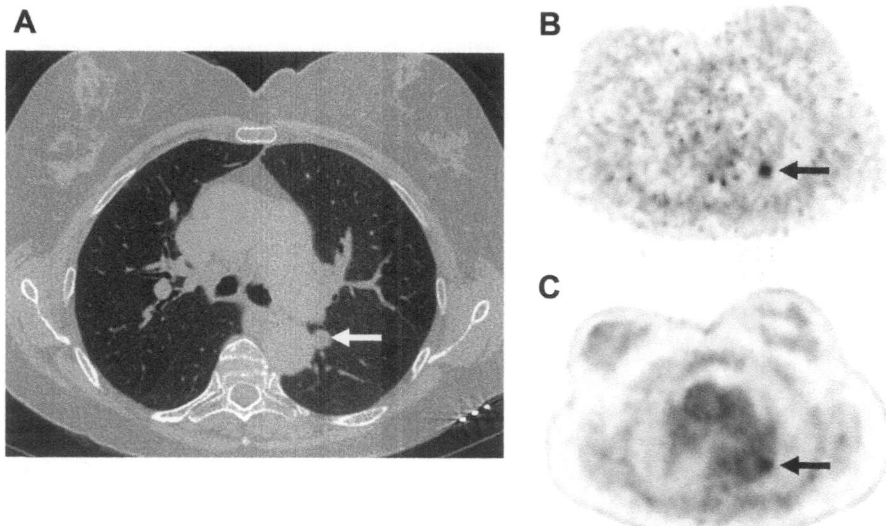

Fig. 5. (*A*) A 68-year-old woman with incidentally detected nodule in the left lower lobe superior segment (*arrow*). The nodule showed intense uptake on ^{68}Ga-DOTATATE PET/CT (*B*) and moderate uptake on ^{18}F-FDG PET/CT (*C*). The biopsy result showed low-grade neuroendocrine neoplasm (typical carcinoid).

ligand or carrier molecule (TOC or TATE), and (3) a DOTA chelator or linker that binds them together and stabilizes the complex.[33] Once radiolabeled SSA is injected into the patient's body, it binds to the SSTR at the membrane of the cells. Radiolabeled SSA is internalized into the cells once bound to the cell membrane receptor, releasing the radiolabeled peptides, which can deliver the radiation to the tumor cell.

Guideline of peptide receptor radionuclide therapy for lung carcinoid

Current guideline recommends PRRT for the advanced gastroenteropancreatic NET with progression during the first-line SSA therapy.[34,35] PRRT can also be used for lung carcinoids and has been proven effective in retrospective studies. However, there is a lack of evidence from randomized trial results to support the data. SSTR imaging, including ^{68}Ga-DOTATATE PET/CT, is the modality of choice to assess the extent of disease and confirm the SSTR positivity of disease. PRRT is not indicated for patients with significant disease sites with a lack of SSTR expression on imaging. Patients should have an acceptable renal function (Cr clearance >50 mL/min) and preserved bone marrow reserve to receive PRRT. Karnofsky's performance status greater than 50% or expected survival greater than 3 months is recommended for the PRRT candidate. Grade 1-2 hematotoxicity is usually acceptable; severe bone marrow dysfunction is a contraindication for PRRT. Other contraindications include severe hepatic or cardiac dysfunction and pregnancy.

Clinical outcome of peptide receptor radionuclide therapy in lung carcinoid

PRRT has been proven to be an effective treatment of lung NET with progression after the initial SSA therapy. Previous trial results evaluating the efficacy and safety of PRRT includes a majority of gastroenteropancreatic NETs, and few studies include lung carcinoid. In the NETTER-1 phase 3 trial of 229 patients with well-differentiated advanced gastroenteropancreatic NET, the group of patients who received 177-Lu DOTATATE showed markedly improved progression-free survival (PFS) compared with the other group who received long-acting octreotide alone (PFS at 20 months of 65.2% vs 10.8%).[36] However, the overall survival rate of the Lu-DOTATATE group and control group was 48.0 months and 36.3 months, respectively, which was not significantly different, potentially due to the high rate of crossover of patients in the control arm to the PRRT group.[37]

There is a paucity of published results for clinical outcomes of PRRT in lung carcinoid patients. Several retrospective studies or lung carcinoid subgroup analysis of NET trials showed favorable clinical outcomes with acceptable safety profiles with overall response rates of lung carcinoid after PRRT ranging from 13% to 30%, whereas PFS ranged from 19 to 28 months and OS ranged from 32 to 59 months.[38–41] In a retrospective study of 25 patients with advanced lung carcinoids (11 typical carcinoids, 11 atypical carcinoids, 3 unknown) treated with PRRT, the median PFS was 17 months, and the median OS was 42 months.[41]

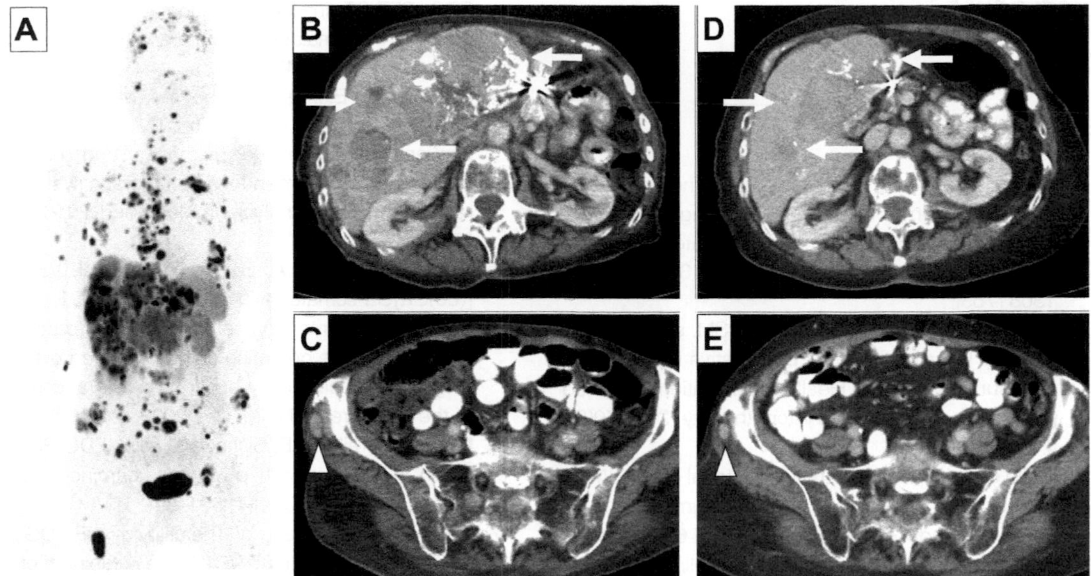

Fig. 6. A 73-year-old woman with history of atypical carcinoid in the lung, which was resected. (*A–C*) On ^{68}Ga-DOTATATE PET/CT, there are numerous metastases in the liver (*arrows*) and bone with soft tissue component (*arrowhead*), which are all intensely avid. Despite systemic therapy including long-acting octreotide and everolimus in addition to chemoembolization therapy to liver, there was progression of disease. The patient eventually underwent 4 cycles of PRRT using ^{177}Lu-DOTATATE. (*D, E*) After therapy, the liver lesions (*arrows*) and soft tissue components of the osseous lesions (*arrowhead*) have mildly decreased.

A high proliferation rate (ki-67 > 20) and the low uptake on SSTR imaging were associated with shorter PFS. This study proved that it could be effective in lung carcinoids even after previous heavy treatment. Another retrospective study of 22 patients with advanced lung carcinoids showed comparable clinical outcomes, with a median OS was 40 months.[40] No major toxicity, such as hematotoxicity or renal toxicity, has been reported in lung carcinoid patients after PRRT. According to these data, PRRT might be an effective treatment option for lung carcinoids with high-SSTR expression (**Fig. 6**). There is no consensus on the optimal timing to use PRRT in lung carcinoids due to a lack of data. If PRRT were reserved for a more advanced stage of disease, it would be less effective due to the progressive reduction of SSTR expression and the development of tumor mutation. Moreover, previous chemotherapy can negatively affect the treatment efficacy of SSTR. Future randomized trials are needed to better define the optimal treatment strategy for lung carcinoids, with combination or sequential treatment of PRRT with long-acting SSA or chemotherapy.

SUMMARY

Recent advances in SSTR PET/CT imaging and the development of PRRT changed the NET diagnosis and management paradigm. Lung carcinoid can be accurately diagnosed with ^{68}Ga-DOTATATE PET/CT, although there is significant tumor heterogeneity with variable degrees of SSTR expression in the primary site and metastases. ^{18}F-FDG and ^{68}Ga-DOTATATE dual tracer imaging can better characterize the tumor heterogeneity and help select the candidate for PRRT who would benefit from therapy. PRRT using ^{177}Lu-labeled or ^{90}Y-labeled SSA may be effective and safely used for advanced lung carcinoids.

CLINICS CARE POINTS

- There is increase in incidence of neuroendocrine tumor of the lung.
- Somatostatin receptor imaging, including 68Ga-DOTATATE PET/CT can be used for diagnosis of well-differentiated neuroendocrine tumor.
- Dual tracer imaging using 18F-FDG and 68Ga-DOTATATE can identify the tumor heterogeneity within the patients, which will help optimize the management.
- Peptide receptor radionuclide therapy shows promising outcome in advanced somatostatin receptor positive lung neuroendocrine tumors.

DISCLOSURE

None.

REFERENCES

1. Shah S, Gosain R, Groman A, et al. Incidence and survival outcomes in patients with lung neuroendocrine neoplasms in the United States. Cancers (Basel) 2021;13(8). https://doi.org/10.3390/cancers13081753.
2. Swarts DR, Rudelius M, Claessen SM, et al. Limited additive value of the Ki-67 proliferative index on patient survival in World Health Organization-classified pulmonary carcinoids. Histopathology 2017;70(3): 412–22.
3. WHO classification of Tumours Editorial Board, WHO classification of Tumours - Thoracic tumors, 5.
4. Pelosi G, Rindi G, Travis WD, et al. Ki-67 antigen in lung neuroendocrine tumors: unraveling a role in clinical practice. J Thorac Oncol 2014;9(3):273–84.
5. Meisinger QC, Klein JS, Butnor KJ, et al. CT features of peripheral pulmonary carcinoid tumors. AJR Am J Roentgenol 2011;197(5):1073–80.
6. Caplin ME, Baudin E, Ferolla P, et al. Pulmonary neuroendocrine (carcinoid) tumors: European Neuroendocrine Tumor Society expert consensus and recommendations for best practice for typical and atypical pulmonary carcinoids. Ann Oncol 2015;26(8):1604–20.
7. Dermawan JK, Farver CF. The prognostic significance of the 8th edition TNM staging of pulmonary carcinoid tumors: a single institution study with long-term follow-up. Am J Surg Pathol 2019;43(9): 1291–6.
8. Yoon JY, Sigel K, Martin J, et al. Evaluation of the prognostic significance of TNM staging guidelines in lung carcinoid tumors. J Thorac Oncol 2019; 14(2):184–92.
9. Righi L, Volante M, Tavaglione V, et al. Somatostatin receptor tissue distribution in lung neuroendocrine tumours: a clinicopathologic and immunohistochemical study of 218 'clinically aggressive' cases. Ann Oncol 2010;21(3):548–55.
10. Chiaravalloti A, Spanu A, Danieli R, et al. 111In-Pentetreotide SPECT/CT in pulmonary carcinoid. Anticancer Res 2015;35(7):4265–70.
11. Prasad V, Steffen IG, Pavel M, et al. Somatostatin receptor PET/CT in restaging of typical and atypical lung carcinoids. EJNMMI Res 2015;5(1):53.
12. Fallahi B, Manafi-Farid R, Eftekhari M, et al. Diagnostic fficiency of (68)Ga-DOTATATE PET/CT as ompared to (99m)Tc-Octreotide SPECT/CT andonventional orphologic odalities in euroendocrine umors. Asia Ocean J Nucl Med Biol 2019;7(2):129–40.
13. Jiang Y, Hou G, Cheng W. Performance of 68Ga-DOTA-SST PET/CT, octreoscan SPECT/CT and 18F-FDG PET/CT in the detection of culprit tumors causing osteomalacia: a meta-analysis. Nucl Med Commun 2020;41(4):370–6.
14. Deppen SA, Blume J, Bobbey AJ, et al. 68Ga-DOTATATE compared with 111In-DTPA-octreotide and conventional imaging for pulmonary and gastroenteropancreatic neuroendocrine tumors: a systematic review and meta-analysis. J Nucl Med 2016;57(6): 872–8.
15. Deleu AL, Laenen A, Decaluwé H, et al. Value of [(68)Ga]Ga-somatostatin receptor PET/CT in the grading of pulmonary neuroendocrine (carcinoid) tumours and the detection of disseminated disease: single-centre pathology-based analysis and review of the literature. EJNMMI Res 2022;12(1):28.
16. Moore W, Freiberg E, Bishawi M, et al. FDG-PET imaging in patients with pulmonary carcinoid tumor. Clin Nucl Med 2013;38(7):501–5.
17. Jiang Y, Hou G, Cheng W. The utility of 18F-FDG and 68Ga-DOTA-Peptide PET/CT in the evaluation of primary pulmonary carcinoid: a systematic review and meta-analysis. Medicine (Baltimore) 2019;98(10): e14769.
18. Mamede M, Higashi T, Kitaichi M, et al. [18F]FDG uptake and PCNA, Glut-1, and Hexokinase-II expressions in cancers and inflammatory lesions of the lung. Neoplasia 2005;7(4):369–79.
19. Ozbudak IH, Shilo K, Tavora F, et al. Glucose transporter-1 in pulmonary neuroendocrine carcinomas: expression and survival analysis. Mod Pathol 2009;22(5):633–8.
20. Chan DL, Pavlakis N, Schembri GP, et al. Dual somatostatin receptor/FDG PET/CT imaging in metastatic neuroendocrine tumours: proposal for a novel grading scheme with prognostic significance. Theranostics 2017;7(5):1149–58.
21. Alevroudis E, Spei ME, Chatziioannou SN, et al. Clinical utility of (18)F-FDG PET in neuroendocrine tumors prior to peptide receptor radionuclide therapy: a systematic review and meta-analysis. Cancers (Basel) 2021;13(8). https://doi.org/10.3390/cancers13081813.
22. Binderup T, Knigge U, Johnbeck CB, et al. (18)F-FDG PET is superior to WHO grading as a prognostic tool in neuroendocrine neoplasms and useful in guiding PRRT: a prospective 10-year follow-up study. J Nucl Med 2021;62(6):808–15.
23. Zidan L, Iravani A, Kong G, et al. Theranostic implications of molecular imaging phenotype of well-differentiated pulmonary carcinoid based on (68) Ga-DOTATATE PET/CT and (18)F-FDG PET/CT. Eur J Nucl Med Mol Imaging 2021;48(1):204–16.
24. Detterbeck FC. Management of carcinoid tumors. Ann Thorac Surg 2010;89(3):998–1005.
25. Ramirez RA, Thomas K, Jacob A, et al. Adjuvant therapy for lung neuroendocrine neoplasms. World J Clin Oncol 2021;12(8):664–74.

26. Shah MH, Goldner WS, Halfdanarson TR, et al. NCCN guidelines insights: neuroendocrine and adrenal tumors, version 2.2018. J Natl Compr Canc Netw 2018;16(6):693–702.
27. Caplin ME, Pavel M, Ćwikła JB, et al. Lanreotide in metastatic enteropancreatic neuroendocrine tumors. N Engl J Med 2014;371(3):224–33.
28. Rinke A, Müller HH, Schade-Brittinger C, et al. Placebo-controlled, double-blind, prospective, randomized study on the effect of octreotide LAR in the control of tumor growth in patients with metastatic neuroendocrine midgut tumors: a report from the PROMID Study Group. J Clin Oncol 2009;27(28):4656–63.
29. Bongiovanni A, Recine F, Riva N, et al. Outcome analysis of first-line somatostatin analog treatment in metastatic pulmonary neuroendocrine tumors and prognostic significance of (18)FDG-PET/CT. Clin Lung Cancer 2017;18(4):415–20.
30. Sullivan I, Le Teuff G, Guigay J, et al. Antitumour activity of somatostatin analogues in sporadic, progressive, metastatic pulmonary carcinoids. Eur J Cancer 2017;75:259–67.
31. Yao JC, Fazio N, Singh S, et al. Everolimus for the treatment of advanced, non-functional neuroendocrine tumours of the lung or gastrointestinal tract (RADIANT-4): a randomised, placebo-controlled, phase 3 study. Lancet 2016;387(10022):968–77.
32. Fazio N, Buzzoni R, Delle Fave G, et al. Everolimus in advanced, progressive, well-differentiated, non-functional neuroendocrine tumors: RADIANT-4 lung subgroup analysis. Cancer Sci 2018;109(1):174–81.
33. Hirmas N, Jadaan R, Al-Ibraheem A. Peptide receptor radionuclide therapy and the treatment of gastroentero-pancreatic neuroendocrine tumors: current findings and future perspectives. Nucl Med Mol Imaging 2018;52(3):190–9.
34. Hope TA, Bodei L, Chan JA, et al. NANETS/SNMMI consensus statement on patient selection and appropriate use of (177)Lu-DOTATATE peptide receptor radionuclide therapy. J Nucl Med 2020;61(2):222–7.
35. Bodei L, Mueller-Brand J, Baum RP, et al. The joint IAEA, EANM, and SNMMI practical guidance on peptide receptor radionuclide therapy (PRRNT) in neuroendocrine tumours. Eur J Nucl Med Mol Imaging 2013;40(5):800–16.
36. Strosberg J, El-Haddad G, Wolin E, et al. Phase 3 trial of (177)Lu-dotatate for midgut neuroendocrine tumors. N Engl J Med 2017;376(2):125–35.
37. Strosberg JR, Caplin ME, Kunz PL, et al. (177)Lu-Dotatate plus long-acting octreotide versus high-dose long-acting octreotide in patients with midgut neuroendocrine tumours (NETTER-1): final overall survival and long-term safety results from an open-label, randomised, controlled, phase 3 trial. Lancet Oncol 2021;22(12):1752–63.
38. Sabet A, Haug AR, Eiden C, et al. Efficacy of peptide receptor radionuclide therapy with (177)Lu-octreotate in metastatic pulmonary neuroendocrine tumors: a dual-centre analysis. Am J Nucl Med Mol Imaging 2017;7(2):74–83.
39. Parghane RV, Talole S, Prabhash K, et al. Clinical response profile of metastatic/advanced pulmonary neuroendocrine tumors to peptide receptor radionuclide therapy with 177Lu-DOTATATE. Clin Nucl Med 2017;42(6):428–35.
40. Brabander T, van der Zwan WA, Teunissen JJM, et al. Long-Term efficacy, survival, and safety of [(177)Lu-DOTA(0),Tyr(3)]octreotate in patients with gastroenteropancreatic and bronchial neuroendocrine tumors. Clin Cancer Res 2017;23(16):4617–24.
41. Mirvis E, Toumpanakis C, Mandair D, et al. Efficacy and tolerability of peptide receptor radionuclide therapy (PRRT) in advanced metastatic bronchial neuroendocrine tumours (NETs). Lung Cancer 2020;150:70–5.

Paragangliomas and Pheochromocytomas

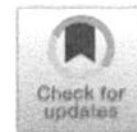

Positron Emission Tomography/Computed Tomography Diagnosis and Therapy

Charles Marcus, MD[a,*],
Rathan M. Subramaniam, MD, PhD, MPH, MBA, FRSN, FSNMMI, FRANZCR[b,c]

KEYWORDS

• Pheochromocytoma • Paraganglioma • ^{18}F-FDG • ^{68}Ga-DOTATATE • ^{18}F-FDOPA • ^{18}F-FDA

KEY POINTS

- PET/CT imaging of pheochromocytomas and paragangliomas outperforms Meta-Iodo-Benzyl-Guanidine (MIBG)-scintigraphy in most cases.
- Gallium-68-DOTATATE (^{68}Ga-DOTATATE) PET/CT outperforms other PET radiotracers in most patients and should be considered a modality for imaging evaluation when available.
- ^{18}F-fluorodeoxyglucose PET/CT may be useful in specific patient groups such as succinate dehydrogenase complex subunit B–associated disease.
- Treatment strategy often requires a multidisciplinary approach and ranges from local therapy to targeted radionuclide therapy.

INTRODUCTION

Pheochromocytomas and paragangliomas (PPGLs) are neuroendocrine tumors originating from the chromaffin cells of the adrenal medulla or extra-adrenal paraganglia. Histologically these tumors have similar characteristics, and the anatomic location is used to differentiate between the two, with pheochromocytomas localized to the adrenal gland and paragangliomas to the extra-adrenal paraganglia.[1] Most of these tumors are detected in the abdomen and pelvis and about 10% in the thorax. Data on the incidence of these tumors are limited.[2,3] The annual incidence is estimated to be 500 to 1600 cases per year[4] with 0.05% to 0.1% incidentally detected at autopsy.[5,6] Patient presentation can vary from asymptomatic to various presenting symptoms, including headaches, profuse sweating, palpitations, and hypertension.[7] These tumors are often detected incidentally during cross-sectional imaging in up to 57.6% of patients.[8,9]

PPGLs have the highest inheritability of any endocrine tumor type, and a small portion of these patients is also identified incidentally during genetic testing. Most PPGLs are characterized by their somatic or germline mutations. Hence, the current standard of care includes routine genetic testing for these patients, thereby improving our understanding of these tumors and enabling precise diagnosis, classification, and treatment. Germline mutations are seen in 35% to 40% of these

[a] Division of Nuclear Medicine and Molecular Imaging, Department of Radiology and Radiological Sciences, Emory University School of Medicine, 1364 Clifton Road Northeast, 1st Floor #E163, Atlanta, GA 30322, USA; [b] Department of Medicine, Otago Medical School, University of Otago, 1st Floor, Dunedin Hospital, 201 Great King Street, Dunedin 9016, New Zealand; [c] Duke University Medical Center, Department of Radiology, 2301 Erwin Road, Box 3808, Durham, NC 27710, USA
* Corresponding author.
E-mail address: cvmarcu@emory.edu

PET Clin 18 (2023) 233–242
https://doi.org/10.1016/j.cpet.2022.11.006

patients, and the remaining sporadic PPGLs exhibit somatic mutations in approximately one-third of the patients. Identification of these mutations is vital because these determine the treatment plan, follow-up frequency, and functional imaging selection. The categorization of these mutations defines the catecholamines secreted by these tumors, which in turn determines the symptom profile. These also have an impact on the selection of specific medications.[10] The severity of the disease can be ascertained by certain factors, such as tumor size (>5 cm), extra-adrenal location, dopaminergic phenotype, high Ki-67 index, succinate dehydrogenase subunit B (*SDHB*) mutation, and so forth.[11] A detailed review of the genetics and epigenetics of neuroendocrine neoplasms is provided in a separate section of this edition.

Imaging evaluation of PPGLs is usually performed after biochemical confirmation. Anatomic imaging, such as computed tomography (CT) and MRI are useful in the anatomic delineation of these tumors, which is crucial for surgical planning. Functional imaging methods target catecholamine metabolism, glucose metabolism, or tumor somatostatin receptor status. The overall performance of these modalities depends on the extent of disease, location, and genetic factors. This review will focus on the positron emission tomography/computed tomography (PET/CT) imaging and treatment of PPGLs.

Positron Emission Tomography/Computed Tomography Imaging of Pheochromocytoma and Paraganglioma

PET/CT imaging using an array of different radiotracers has been studied to evaluate PPGLs. These include ^{18}F-L-3,4-dihydroxyphenylalanine (^{18}F-DOPA), ^{18}F-dopamine (^{18}F-FDA), ^{18}F-fluorodeoxyglucose (^{18}F-FDG), and ^{68}Ga-DOTATATE. PET imaging using these radiotracers is superior to MIBG scintigraphy in evaluating these patients. MIBG still has a role in identifying patients suitable for ^{131}I-MIBG treatment.[12] PET/MRI using these tracers has been used to evaluate PPGLs and seems feasible, providing good quality images that may be especially useful in pediatric patients.[13] These radiotracers will be discussed in detail in the following sections (**Table 1**).

^{18}F-Fluorodeoxyglucose Positron Emission Tomography/Computed Tomography

The widely used oncologic PET radiotracer, ^{18}F-FDG, has a limited role in the routine evaluation of PPGLs in comparison with other radiotracers described subsequently. Its use is limited to specific groups of PPGLs, as described subsequently. The PPGL susceptibility gene clusters exhibit typical genotype–phenotype characteristics that influence molecular imaging characteristics. For example, cluster 1a PPGLs have a pseudohypoxic phenotype with increased aerobic glycolysis. Hence, these tumors are expected to demonstrate increased ^{18}F-FDG avidity and are better for staging and restaging these tumors. The ^{18}F-FDG uptake is significantly higher in cluster 1 tumors[14] than cluster 2 tumors (P = .002) or in tumors without mutations (P = .04).[15] ^{18}F-FDG uptake is more elevated in succinate dehydrogenase (SDH) complex[16] (**Fig. 1**), von Hippel-Lindau syndrome–related tumors than in multiple endocrine neoplasia type 2 tumors.[17] In SDHB-associated PPGLs, which have a higher propensity for metastatic disease, the patient level detection rate of ^{18}F-FDG is superior to ^{123}I-MIBG and ^{18}F-FDA PET/CT (100% vs 80% vs 88%, respectively).[18] ^{18}F-FDG uptake is higher in metastatic PPGLs and extra-adrenal disease. Normetanephrine secreting pheochromocytomas, paragangliomas, and nonsecreting paragangliomas demonstrate higher radiotracer uptake than metanephrine secreting pheochromocytomas and nonsecretory pheochromocytomas.[19] Hence, understanding these tumors' genetic characteristics and behavior before imaging can guide clinicians toward the most accurate molecular imaging method. A meta-analysis including 17 studies of metastatic PPGLs with germline mutations showed a pooled sensitivity and specificity of 85%, 55%, and 95%, 87% for ^{18}F-FDG PET/CT and ^{68}Ga-DOTATATE PET/CT, respectively.[20] A study comparing the detection rate of ^{68}Ga-DOTATATE PET/CT to ^{18}F-FDG PET/CT showed superior detection rates with ^{68}Ga-DOTATATE (96.4% vs 85.7%) with significantly higher tracer uptake in primary (P = .009) and metastatic disease (P = .033).[21] A study comparing the detection rates of 6 different imaging modalities in patients with sporadic pheochromocytoma showed superior detection rates with ^{18}F-DOPA PET/CT compared with ^{18}F-FDG PET/CT (100% vs 78.6%) with higher tracer uptake within the disease sites.[22] There have been reports of a correlation between brown adipose tissue (BAT) activation and poor outcome. Active BAT demonstrated on ^{18}F-FDG PET/CT is associated with decreased overall survival (HR 5.8; P = .02) irrespective of SDHB mutation. It has been hypothesized that increased stress in the patient due to circulating high norepinephrine levels results in BAT activation.[23,24] In patients undergoing ^{131}I-MIBG therapy, the ratio of pretreatment to posttreatment ^{18}F-FDG uptake is significantly different between responders and nonresponders, providing prognostic information.[25]

Table 1
Detection rates of different positron emission tomography/computed tomography radiotracers in evaluating pheochromocytoma and paragangliomas

Study	Diagnosis	^{68}Ga-DOTATATE	^{18}F-FDG	^{18}F-FDOPA	^{18}F-FDA	^{131}I/^{123}I-MIBG	CT/MRI
Janssen et al,[46] 2016	Sporadic metastatic PPGLs	98%	49%	75%	78%		82%
Archier et al,[27] 2016	Head and neck paragangliomas	100%		87%			80%
Janssen et al,[47] 2016	Head and neck paragangliomas	100%	63%	97%	29%		61%
Tan et al,[64] 2015	Metastatic PPGLs	92%	51%			16%	
Maurice et al,[65] 2012	Initial diagnosis of PPGL	100%				66%	77%
Timmers et al,[37] 2009	Nonmetastatic PGL		88%	81%	77%	77%	
Timmers et al,[37] 2009	Metastatic PGL		74%	45%	76%	57%	
Timmers et al,[37] 2009	SDHB-associated PGL		83%	20%	82%	57%	
Janssen et al,[44] 2015	SDHB-associated metastatic PPGLs	99%	86%	61%	52%		85%
Timmers et al,[37] 2009	Non-SDHB PGL		62%	93%	76%	59%	

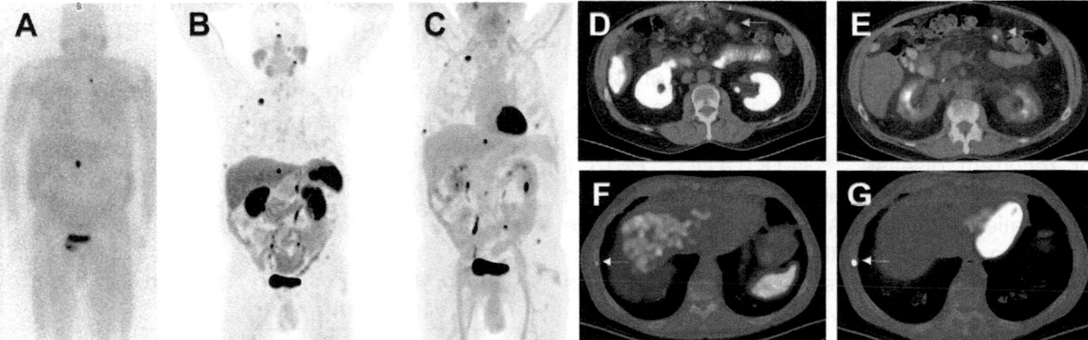

Fig. 1. A 69-year-old man with metastatic pheochromocytoma, likely SDHB-associated disease. ^{123}I-MIBG scan (*A*) showed a radiotracer avid skeletal lesion in the left clavicle and a preaortic lymph node. The patient received radiation therapy for the osseous lesion followed by 400 mCi ^{131}I-MIBG therapy. A follow-up ^{64}Cu-DOTATATE PET/CT (*B*, *D*, *F*) shows numerous radiotracer avid osseous lesions and a mesenteric nodule. ^{18}F-FDG PET/CT (*C*, *E*, *G*) shows similar radiotracer avid osseous lesions (*white arrows*) and mesenteric nodule (*yellow arrows*). Some of the lesions demonstrate more FDG avidity than somatostatin receptor avidity.

^{68}Ga-DOTATATE Positron Emission Tomography/Computed Tomography

^{68}Ga-DOTATATE PET/CT was first evaluated in patients with PPGL in the late 2000s and has demonstrated better performance attributed to the more specific nature of this radiotracer targeting the somatostatin receptors in these tumors rather than relying on tumor glucose metabolism, or catecholamine receptor and storage. The former mechanism lacks specificity, whereas the latter can be downregulated in dedifferentiated tumors. Compared with ^{18}F-FDG PET/CT, as described above, ^{68}Ga-DOTATATE PET/CT demonstrates radiotracer uptake in most of the lesions detected with a significantly higher lesion-to-background ratio. ^{18}F-FDG PET/CT has the disadvantage of decreased specificity. As expected, ^{18}F-FDG uptake is more elevated in aggressive or poorly differentiated diseases. In comparison, the previously preferred functional imaging modality using MIBG has significantly lower performance detecting PPGLs. In studies comparing these agents, ^{123}I/^{124}I-MIBG imaging detected one-third fewer lesions.[26] The detection rates of ^{68}Ga-DOTATATE PET/CT is superior to other PET radiotracers across different groups of PPGLs (see **Table 1**). In head and neck paragangliomas, ^{68}Ga-DOTATATE PET/CT has shown to be most valuable in the detection, especially in SDHD-associated tumors. The better sensitivity is attributed to the small size of many of these tumors that fail to concentrate other PET radiotracers.[27] As the evidence presented comparing different functional and anatomic imaging modalities, ^{68}Ga-DOTATATE PET/CT outperforms these techniques in detecting and localizing PPGLs. It should be considered for evaluating these patients when feasible. This observation has also been proven in the pediatric patient population, with ^{68}Ga-DOTATATE PET/CT showing higher sensitivity than ^{18}F-FDG PET/CT and ^{131}I-MIBG, suggesting that it may be the surveillance imaging of choice in patients with Von Hippel Lindau (VHL) and other familial syndromes.[28] In patients being evaluated for recurrent disease, ^{68}Ga-DOTATATE PET/CT findings affect the change in management in most patients (91%).[29] A notable exception is the evaluation of patients with polycythemia/paraganglioma syndrome, where the detection rate has been reported to be only 35%.[30]

^{18}F-L-3,4-Dihydroxyphenylalanine Positron Emission Tomography/Computed Tomography

^{18}F-DOPA localization to PPGLs is based on the capacity of these tissues to take up amino acids through amino acid transporters, especially LAT1,[31] decarboxylate and store them intracellularly. Normal radiotracer biodistribution includes uptake in the basal ganglia, pancreas, especially the uncinate process, and biliary and genitourinary tracts. Mild uptake has been reported in the bowel, liver, myocardium, and peripheral muscles.[32] ^{18}F-DOPA PET/CT is useful in evaluating nonmetastatic PGLs, especially in patients with non-SDHB–related PPGLs. In SDHx-related PGLs, it is hypothesized that the amino acid composition of the cell undergoes changes that reduce the radiotracer uptake. Patients with a false-negative result should be tested for these mutations.[33] A meta-analysis demonstrated a pooled sensitivity and specificity of 91% and 95% at the patient level and 79% and 95% at the lesion level. Improvement in sensitivity was noted SDHB gene mutations were excluded.[34] However, smaller studies have shown that this modality may be useful in evaluating SDH-mutation–related PPGLs, including SDH-D, SDH-B, and SDH-C.[35,36] A study demonstrated 93% detection rate in non-SDHB disease compared with 76%, 59% and 62% for ^{18}F-FDA PET/CT, ^{123}I-MIBG scintigraphy, and ^{18}F-FDG PET/CT, respectively. As discussed earlier, ^{18}F-FDG PET/CT has the highest detection rates in SDHB tumors (83%).[37] In head and neck PGLs, as discussed above, per lesion sensitivity of ^{18}F-DOPA PET/CT was only 67% compared with 100% with ^{68}Ga-DOTATOC PET/CT, although the per-patient detection rates were similar.[38] In patients with SDHD-related disease, the most common location of head and neck PGLs is along the vagus nerve, with most of these patients demonstrating multifocal disease, and ^{18}F-DOPA PET/CT can help management decisions.[39] MYC-associated factor X gene-related pheochromocytomas are extremely rare, and evaluation with ^{18}F-DOPA PET/CT has shown superior detection rates compared with conventional imaging, ^{68}Ga-DOTATATE PET/CT, and ^{18}F-FDG PET/CT.[40] Apart from localizing the disease, radiotracer uptake demonstrated on ^{18}F-DOPA PET/CT correlates with the biochemical secretory profile of pheochromocytomas.[41] In VHL patients with metastatic or sporadic PPGLs, ^{18}F-DOPA PET/CT is the functional imaging modality of choice, if available.[42]

^{18}F-Dopamine Positron Emission Tomography/Computed Tomography

^{18}F-FDA is a dopamine analog and a better surrogate for the norepinephrine transport system on cell membranes.[43] To evaluate the primary nonmetastatic PPGLs, ^{18}F-FDA PET/CT is comparable to the other PET radiotracers described above but less with CT and MRI. In patients with metastatic disease, the sensitivity (76%) is reported to be comparable to ^{18}F-FDG (74%) and superior to ^{18}F-DOPA (45%) and ^{123}I-MIBG (57%). In patients with SDHB-related disease, ^{18}F-FDG (83%) and ^{18}F-FDA (82%) have similar high sensitivities and are significantly better than ^{18}F-DOPA (20%) and ^{123}I-MIBG (57%).[37] However, another study showed that ^{68}Ga-DOTATATE (99%) demonstrated higher lesion detection rates than ^{18}F-FDA (52%) and ^{18}F-FDG (86%), respectively, in these patients.[44] A study detected more bone metastases with ^{18}F-FDA (90%), followed by bone scintigraphy (82%), CT/MRI (78%), and ^{18}F-FDG (76%) in these patients.[45] In sporadic metastatic PPGLs, ^{68}Ga-DOTATATE PET/CT seems to outperform ^{18}F-FDA PET/CT, with higher detection rates (98% vs 78%), and is considered the imaging modality of choice for evaluation.[46] Similarly, in head and neck paragangliomas, ^{68}Ga-DOTATATE PET/CT detects significantly more lesions than ^{18}F-FDA PET/CT ($P < .01$).[47]

Treatment of Pheochromocytoma and Paraganglioma

The treatment strategy for these patients often includes consensus from multiple medical teams. The treatment plan depends on various factors, including the patient's age, general condition, coexisting medical conditions, tumor characteristics such as local versus metastatic disease, sites involved, genetic and secretory profile, and imaging characteristics, including functional imaging findings. Surgical management is the treatment of choice for patients with a localized disease with appropriate perioperative medical management of functional PPGLs.[48]

Medical Management

Any invasive manipulation of functional tumors, including surgery, percutaneous ablation, and tissue sampling, can induce excessive catecholamine secretions, resulting in life-threatening hyperadrenergic symptoms. Therefore, these patients may need adequate prophylactic medical management before any intervention. Most guidelines recommend alpha-adrenergic blockers as the first medication of choice for one to 2 weeks before intervention to adequately control hyperadrenergic effects. A high fluid and sodium intake are also recommended to compensate for the decrease in blood volume, causing hypotension that may result after tumor removal. Close monitoring of these patients is crucial in the postoperative period because the blood pressure and heart rate can be labile. Biochemical testing is also essential to detect residual and recurrent/metastatic disease in the follow-up period.[49]

Surgical Management

In patients with localized disease, surgical resection is the treatment of choice. The principle of surgical resection is to completely resect the tumor with or without en bloc resection of adjacent structures and to avoid tumor rupture or spill to prevent recurrent disease. Minimally invasive surgical techniques are preferred in patients with small adrenal pheochromocytomas (<6 cm). In larger tumors, open resection is recommended to prevent tumor spill, recurrent disease, and complete tumor resection. In certain patients with a low risk of malignancy who have already undergone contralateral adrenalectomies, such as hereditary diseases and small tumors, partial adrenalectomy can be considered to prevent adrenal insufficiency. Open resection is generally preferred in paragangliomas unless the disease is small, well-circumscribed, and in an appropriate location for minimally invasive surgical techniques.[49] In some patients, such as those with head and neck paragangliomas (HNPGLs), preoperative embolization of vascular supply to these tumors may be necessary. The surgical window to approach these tumors must be carefully planned depending on the location of the tumor to prevent damage to adjacent vital structures such as the major vessels of the neck and cranial nerves. Surgical management is rarely considered in metastatic disease to reduce tumor volume and decrease secretory effects.[48]

Systemic Chemotherapy

Systemic chemotherapy is considered in patients with metastatic PPGLs and can help reduce and control the biochemical effects of these tumors. Cyclophosphamide/vincristine/dacarbazine (CVD) or temozolomide is the most common chemotherapy regimen. A systemic review and meta-analysis of 4 studies with 50 patients showed that patients treated with CVD showed complete response, partial response, and stable disease in 4%, 37%, and 14%, respectively. The biochemical response was seen in 14%, 40%, and 20%, respectively.[50] Temozolomide first-line treatment in metastatic PPGL has been reported in small studies. Temozolomide-based chemotherapy is effective in SDHB-associated metastatic PPGL attributed to the downregulation of O (6)-Methylguanine-DNA-methyltransferase (MGMT) expression.[51,52] However, another recent study showed no significant impact of SDHx mutations on tumor response to temozolomide.[53] Other agents studied in treating metastatic PPGL include tyrosine-kinase inhibitors and hypoxia-inducible factor 2 alpha inhibitors. Tyrosine-kinase inhibitors with an antiangiogenic effect, such as sunitinib,[54] and pazopanib[55] may help in decreasing tumor volume, preventing disease progression, and improving excess catecholamine-associated symptoms. However, these agents can have significant toxicity profiles, and patients may require additional medical management to counteract side effects related to hormonal excess.[56] Immunotherapy with pembrolizumab has been studied in these patients, with a phase 2 study showing response in 9% of patients with a progression-free survival of 6 months.[57] More clinical trials are required to understand the therapeutic effect of these agents as single-agent therapies or in combination with other chemotherapeutic agents.

Radiopharmaceutical Therapy

The 2 main targeted radionuclide therapies include ^{131}I-MIBG and somatostatin receptor-targeted radionuclide therapy. Patients with metastatic PPGLs that are MIBG positive can benefit from high-specific activity ^{131}I-MIBG. For patients who received at least one dose of the treatment, one-fourth showed a reduction in antihypertensive medication by half. In addition, 92% of the patients showed stable or partial response for 12 months. The median overall survival rate was 37 months.[58] Guidelines for the handling and administering of this therapeutic agent have been described by the European Association of Nuclear Medicine guidelines. Patients are prepared with adequate thyroid blockade to prevent hypothyroidism. Although medications such as calcium channel blockers and beta-blockers can interfere with the treatment, in some patients with significant catecholamine excess, it may be challenging to withdraw these medications. Therefore, it should be carefully reviewed and risk versus benefits weighed. The agent is administered as a slow intravenous infusion with optimal patient monitoring and supportive care. The administered activity can range between 100 and 300 mCi. Myelotoxicity is a dose-limiting side effect that should be carefully monitored. Radiation safety precautions should be carefully followed during and after treatment to prevent unnecessary radiation exposure to treating health-care workers and other individuals who may come in contact with the patient.[59]

With the wide success of peptide receptor radionuclide therapy (PRRT) in patients with metastatic neuroendocrine tumors refractory to somatostatin analog therapy, given the avid somatostatin receptor targeted radiotracer uptake on PET/CT imaging, as described above, PRRT has also found significant interest in treating patients with metastatic PPGLs. Pretreatment

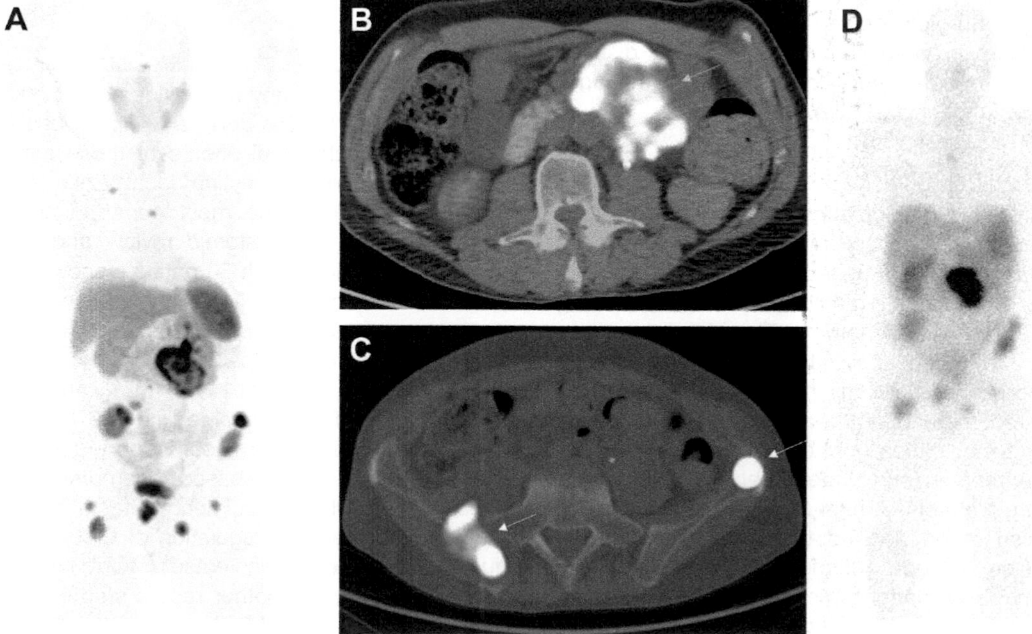

Fig. 2. A 57-year-old man with metastatic paraganglioma. ^{68}Ga-DOTATATE PET/CT (*A–C*) shows a large retroperitoneal mass (*yellow arrow*) with multiple radiotracer avid osseous lesions (*white arrows*). The patient was then treated with ^{177}Lu-PRRT. Posttreatment whole body scan (*D*) shows radiotracer uptake in the lesions seen on the pretherapy PET/CT.

medical management should be considered in patients with biochemically active tumors, as described above.[60] No large clinical trials are available comparing MIBG versus PRRT treatments. A small study suggests a trend toward better outcomes in patients treated with ^{177}Lu-PRRT.[61] A meta-analysis of 12 studies comprising 201 patients with advanced PPGLs, showed a response rate of 25% with an 84% disease control rate. Approximately two-thirds of the patients demonstrated clinical and biochemical responses. No significant difference was demonstrated between ^{90}Y-based and ^{177}Lu-based PRRT[62] (**Fig. 2**). ^{90}Y-PRRT is not widely available and is mostly confined to academic centers with local resources to acquire radiopharmaceuticals. Commercially available ^{177}Lu-PRRT is used off-label for these patients, and the regimen is like the PRRT of metastatic neuroendocrine tumors. Early studies suggest that alpha-emitter therapy with ^{225}Ac-DOTATATE may be effective in treating metastatic PGLs, even in patients who did not respond to ^{177}Lu-DOTATATE therapy. Larger prospective clinical trials are pertinent.[63]

SUMMARY

Molecular imaging evaluation of PPGLs depends on multiple factors, including localized versus metastatic disease and tumors' genetic and biochemical profiles. PET/CT imaging of these tumors outperforms MIBG scintigraphy in most cases. A few PET radiotracers have been studied in evaluating these patients with somatostatin receptor PET imaging has shown superior performance compared with other agents in most of these patients. ^{18}F-FDG PET/CT imaging is useful in select patients, such as those with SDHB-associated disease. Treatment strategy depends on multiple factors and necessitates a multidisciplinary approach. Most recently, targeted radionuclide therapy has demonstrated clinical and biochemical responses with significant disease control rates.

CLINICS CARE POINTS

- Patients with paragangliomas and pheochromocytomas need a multidisciplinary staging including imaging, clinical, genetic and biochemical evaluations.
- Recent advances in PET/CT imaging especially, somatostatin receptor PET/CT imaging out performs conventional imaging techniques and should be used when available.
- Knowledge of the molecular imaging patterns of these patients is important to choose the appropriate imaging technique that will benefit the patient.
- Targeted radionuclide therapy can be beneficial in patients with metastatic disease and should be considered in select patients.

DISCLOSURE

The authors have nothing to disclose.

REFERENCES

1. Neumann HPH, Young WF Jr, Eng C. Pheochromocytoma and paraganglioma. N Engl J Med 2019; 381(6):552–65.
2. Beard CM, Sheps SG, Kurland LT, et al. Occurrence of pheochromocytoma in Rochester, Minnesota, 1950 through 1979. Mayo Clin Proc 1983;58(12): 802–4.
3. Berends AMA, Buitenwerf E, de Krijger RR, et al. Incidence of pheochromocytoma and sympathetic paraganglioma in The Netherlands: a nationwide study and systematic review. Eur J Intern Med 2018;51:68–73.
4. Chen H, Sippel RS, O'Dorisio MS, et al. The North American Neuroendocrine Tumor Society consensus guideline for the diagnosis and management of neuroendocrine tumors: pheochromocytoma, paraganglioma, and medullary thyroid cancer. Pancreas 2010;39(6):775–83.
5. Lo CY, Lam KY, Wat MS, et al. Adrenal pheochromocytoma remains a frequently overlooked diagnosis. Am J Surg 2000;179(3):212–5.
6. McNeil AR, Blok BH, Koelmeyer TD, et al. Phaeochromocytomas discovered during coronial autopsies in Sydney, Melbourne and auckland. Aust N Z J Med 2000;30(6):648–52.
7. Lenders JW, Eisenhofer G, Mannelli M, et al. Phaeochromocytoma *Lancet* 2005;366(9486):665–75.
8. Gruber LM, Hartman RP, Thompson GB, et al. Pheochromocytoma characteristics and behavior differ depending on method of discovery. J Clin Endocrinol Metab 2019;104(5):1386–93.
9. Patel D, Phay JE, Yen TWF, et al. Update on pheochromocytoma and paraganglioma from the sso endocrine/head and neck disease-site work group. part 1 of 2: advances in pathogenesis and diagnosis of pheochromocytoma and paraganglioma. Ann Surg Oncol 2020;27(5):1329–37.
10. Talvacchio S, Nazari MA, Pacak K. Supportive management of patients with pheochromocytoma/paraganglioma undergoing noninvasive treatment. Curr

Opin Endocrinol Diabetes Obes 2022;29(3): 294–301.
11. Nolting S, Bechmann N, Taieb D, et al. Personalized management of pheochromocytoma and paraganglioma. Endocr Rev 2022;43(2):199–239.
12. Rufini V, Treglia G, Castaldi P, et al. Comparison of metaiodobenzylguanidine scintigraphy with positron emission tomography in the diagnostic work-up of pheochromocytoma and paraganglioma: a systematic review. Q J Nucl Med Mol Imaging 2013;57(2): 122–33.
13. Blanchet EM, Millo C, Martucci V, et al. Integrated whole-body PET/MRI with 18F-FDG, 18F-FDOPA, and 18F-FDA in paragangliomas in comparison with PET/CT: NIH first clinical experience with a single-injection, dual-modality imaging protocol. Clin Nucl Med 2014;39(3):243–50.
14. van Berkel A, Vriens D, Visser EP, et al. Metabolic subtyping of pheochromocytoma and paraganglioma by (18)f-fdg pharmacokinetics using dynamic PET/CT scanning. J Nucl Med 2019;60(6): 745–51.
15. Ansquer C, Drui D, Mirallie E, et al. Usefulness of FDG-PET/CT-Based Radiomics for the characterization and genetic orientation of pheochromocytomas before surgery. Cancers (Basel) 2020;12(9):2424.
16. van Berkel A, Rao JU, Kusters B, et al. Correlation between in vivo 18F-FDG PET and immunohistochemical markers of glucose uptake and metabolism in pheochromocytoma and paraganglioma. J Nucl Med 2014;55(8):1253–9.
17. Timmers HJ, Chen CC, Carrasquillo JA, et al. Staging and functional characterization of pheochromocytoma and paraganglioma by 18F-fluorodeoxyglucose (18F-FDG) positron emission tomography. J Natl Cancer Inst 2012;104(9):700–8.
18. Timmers HJ, Kozupa A, Chen CC, et al. Superiority of fluorodeoxyglucose positron emission tomography to other functional imaging techniques in the evaluation of metastatic SDHB-associated pheochromocytoma and paraganglioma. J Clin Oncol 2007;25(16):2262–9.
19. Tiwari A, Shah N, Sarathi V, et al. Genetic status determines (18) F-FDG uptake in pheochromocytoma/paraganglioma. J Med Imaging Radiat Oncol 2017; 61(6):745–52.
20. Kan Y, Zhang S, Wang W, et al. 68)Ga-somatostatin receptor analogs and (18)F-FDG PET/CT in the localization of metastatic pheochromocytomas and paragangliomas with germline mutations: a meta-analysis. Acta Radiol 2018;59(12):1466–74.
21. Xu S, Pan Y, Zhou J, et al. Integrated PET/MRI with 68Ga-DOTATATE and 18F-FDG in pheochromocytomas and paragangliomas: an initial study. Clin Nucl Med 2022;47(4):299–304.
22. Jha A, Patel M, Carrasquillo JA, et al. Sporadic primary pheochromocytoma: a prospective intraindividual comparison of six imaging tests (CT, MRI, and PET/CT Using (68)Ga-DOTATATE, FDG, (18)F-FDOPA, and (18)F-FDA). AJR Am J Roentgenol 2022;218(2):342–50.
23. Abdul Sater Z, Jha A, Hamimi A, et al. Pheochromocytoma and paraganglioma patients with poor survival often show brown adipose tissue activation. J Clin Endocrinol Metab 2020;105(4):1176–85.
24. Santhanam P, Treglia G, Ahima RS. Detection of brown adipose tissue by (18) F-FDG PET/CT in pheochromocytoma/paraganglioma: a systematic review. J Clin Hypertens (Greenwich) 2018;20(3): 615.
25. Nakazawa A, Higuchi T, Oriuchi N, et al. Clinical significance of 2-[18F]fluoro-2-deoxy-D-glucose positron emission tomography for the assessment of 131I-metaiodobenzylguanidine therapy in malignant phaeochromocytoma. Eur J Nucl Med Mol Imaging 2011;38(10):1869–75.
26. Chang CA, Pattison DA, Tothill RW, et al. 68)Ga-DOTATATE and (18)F-FDG PET/CT in Paraganglioma and Pheochromocytoma: utility, patterns and heterogeneity. Cancer Imaging 2016;16(1):22.
27. Archier A, Varoquaux A, Garrigue P, et al. Prospective comparison of (68)Ga-DOTATATE and (18)F-FDOPA PET/CT in patients with various pheochromocytomas and paragangliomas with emphasis on sporadic cases. Eur J Nucl Med Mol Imaging 2016;43(7):1248–57.
28. Jaiswal SK, Sarathi V, Malhotra G, et al. The utility of (68)Ga-DOTATATE PET/CT in localizing primary/metastatic pheochromocytoma and paraganglioma in children and adolescents - a single-center experience. J Pediatr Endocrinol Metab 2021;34(1): 109–19.
29. Skoura E, Priftakis D, Novruzov F, et al. The impact of Ga-68 DOTATATE PET/CT imaging on management of patients with paragangliomas. Nucl Med Commun 2020;41(2):169–74.
30. Han S, Suh CH, Woo S, et al. Performance of (68) Ga-DOTA-Conjugated somatostatin receptor-targeting peptide PET in detection of pheochromocytoma and paraganglioma: a systematic review and Metaanalysis. J Nucl Med 2019;60(3):369–76.
31. Barollo S, Bertazza L, Watutantrige-Fernando S, et al. Overexpression of L-type Amino acid transporter 1 (LAT1) and 2 (LAT2): novel markers of neuroendocrine tumors. PLoS One 2016;11(5): e0156044.
32. Bozkurt MF, Virgolini I, Balogova S, et al. Guideline for PET/CT imaging of neuroendocrine neoplasms with (68)Ga-DOTA-conjugated somatostatin receptor targeting peptides and (18)F-DOPA. Eur J Nucl Med Mol Imaging 2017;44(9):1588–601.
33. Feral CC, Tissot FS, Tosello L, et al. 18)F-fluorodihydroxyphenylalanine PET/CT in pheochromocytoma and paraganglioma: relation to genotype and amino

acid transport system L. Eur J Nucl Med Mol Imaging 2017;44(5):812–21.

34. Treglia G, Cocciolillo F, de Waure C, et al. Diagnostic performance of 18F-dihydroxyphenylalanine positron emission tomography in patients with paraganglioma: a meta-analysis. Eur J Nucl Med Mol Imaging 2012;39(7):1144–53.
35. Marzola MC, Chondrogiannis S, Grassetto G, et al. 18F-DOPA PET/CT in the evaluation of hereditary SDH-deficiency paraganglioma-pheochromocytoma syndromes. Clin Nucl Med 2014;39(1): e53–58.
36. King KS, Chen CC, Alexopoulos DK, et al. Functional imaging of SDHx-related head and neck paragangliomas: comparison of 18F-fluorodihydroxyphenylalanine, 18F-fluorodopamine, 18F-fluoro-2-deoxy-D-glucose PET, 123I-metaiodobenzylguanidine scintigraphy, and 111In-pentetreotide scintigraphy. J Clin Endocrinol Metab 2011;96(9):2779–85.
37. Timmers HJ, Chen CC, Carrasquillo JA, et al. Comparison of 18F-fluoro-L-DOPA, 18F-fluoro-deoxyglucose, and 18F-fluorodopamine PET and 123I-MIBG scintigraphy in the localization of pheochromocytoma and paraganglioma. J Clin Endocrinol Metab 2009;94(12):4757–67.
38. Kroiss AS, Uprimny C, Shulkin BL, et al. 68)Ga-DOTATOC PET/CT in the localization of head and neck paraganglioma compared with (18)F-DOPA PET/CT and (123)I-MIBG SPECT/CT. Nucl Med Biol 2019; 71:47–53.
39. Amodru V, Romanet P, Scemama U, et al. Tumor multifocality with vagus nerve involvement as a phenotypic marker of SDHD mutation in patients with head and neck paragangliomas: a (18) F-FDOPA PET/CT study. Head Neck 2019;41(6): 1565–71.
40. Taieb D, Jha A, Guerin C, et al. 18F-FDOPA PET/CT imaging of MAX-related pheochromocytoma. J Clin Endocrinol Metab 2018;103(4):1574–82.
41. Amodru V, Guerin C, Delcourt S, et al. Quantitative (18)F-DOPA PET/CT in pheochromocytoma: the relationship between tumor secretion and its biochemical phenotype. Eur J Nucl Med Mol Imaging 2018;45(2):278–82.
42. Castinetti F, Kroiss A, Kumar R, et al. 15 YEARS OF paraganglioma: imaging and imaging-based treatment of pheochromocytoma and paraganglioma. Endocr Relat Cancer 2015;22(4):T135–45.
43. Kaji P, Carrasquillo JA, Linehan WM, et al. The role of 6-[18F]fluorodopamine positron emission tomography in the localization of adrenal pheochromocytoma associated with von Hippel-Lindau syndrome. Eur J Endocrinol 2007;156(4):483–7.
44. Janssen I, Blanchet EM, Adams K, et al. Superiority of [68Ga]-DOTATATE PET/CT to other functional imaging modalities in the localization of SDHB-associated metastatic pheochromocytoma and paraganglioma. Clin Cancer Res 2015;21(17):3888–95.
45. Zelinka T, Timmers HJ, Kozupa A, et al. Role of positron emission tomography and bone scintigraphy in the evaluation of bone involvement in metastatic pheochromocytoma and paraganglioma: specific implications for succinate dehydrogenase enzyme subunit B gene mutations. Endocr Relat Cancer 2008;15(1):311–23.
46. Janssen I, Chen CC, Millo CM, et al. PET/CT comparing (68)Ga-DOTATATE and other radiopharmaceuticals and in comparison with CT/MRI for the localization of sporadic metastatic pheochromocytoma and paraganglioma. Eur J Nucl Med Mol Imaging 2016;43(10):1784–91.
47. Janssen I, Chen CC, Taieb D, et al. 68Ga-DOTATATE PET/CT in the localization of head and neck paragangliomas compared with other functional imaging modalities and CT/MRI. J Nucl Med 2016;57(2): 186–91.
48. Garcia-Carbonero R, Matute Teresa F, Mercader-Cidoncha E, et al. Multidisciplinary practice guidelines for the diagnosis, genetic counseling and treatment of pheochromocytomas and paragangliomas. Clin Transl Oncol 2021;23(10):1995–2019.
49. Lenders JW, Duh QY, Eisenhofer G, et al. Pheochromocytoma and paraganglioma: an endocrine society clinical practice guideline. J Clin Endocrinol Metab 2014;99(6):1915–42.
50. Niemeijer ND, Alblas G, van Hulsteijn LT, et al. Chemotherapy with cyclophosphamide, vincristine and dacarbazine for malignant paraganglioma and pheochromocytoma: systematic review and meta-analysis. Clin Endocrinol (Oxf) 2014;81(5):642–51.
51. Hadoux J, Favier J, Scoazec JY, et al. SDHB mutations are associated with response to temozolomide in patients with metastatic pheochromocytoma or paraganglioma. Int J Cancer 2014;135(11):2711–20.
52. Tong A, Li M, Cui Y, et al. Temozolomide is a potential therapeutic tool for patients with metastatic pheochromocytoma/paraganglioma-case report and review of the literature. Front Endocrinol (Lausanne) 2020;11:61.
53. Perez K, Jacene H, Hornick JL, et al. SDHx mutations and temozolomide in malignant pheochromocytoma and paraganglioma. Endocr Relat Cancer 2022;29(9):533–44.
54. O'Kane GM, Ezzat S, Joshua AM, et al. A phase 2 trial of sunitinib in patients with progressive paraganglioma or pheochromocytoma: the SNIPP trial. Br J Cancer 2019;120(12):1113–9.
55. Jasim S, Suman VJ, Jimenez C, et al. Phase II trial of pazopanib in advanced/progressive malignant pheochromocytoma and paraganglioma. Endocrine 2017;57(2):220–5.
56. Jimenez C, Fazeli S, Roman-Gonzalez A. Antiangiogenic therapies for pheochromocytoma and paraganglioma. Endocr Relat Cancer 2020;27(7): R239–54.

57. Jimenez C, Subbiah V, Stephen B, et al. Phase II clinical trial of pembrolizumab in patients with progressive metastatic pheochromocytomas and paragangliomas. Cancers (Basel) 2020;12(8):2307.
58. Pryma DA, Chin BB, Noto RB, et al. Efficacy and safety of high-specific-activity (131)I-MIBG therapy in patients with advanced pheochromocytoma or paraganglioma. J Nucl Med 2019;60(5): 623–30.
59. Giammarile F, Chiti A, Lassmann M, et al. EANM procedure guidelines for 131I-meta-iodobenzylguanidine (131I-mIBG) therapy. Eur J Nucl Med Mol Imaging 2008;35(5):1039–47.
60. Carrasquillo JA, Chen CC, Jha A, et al. Systemic Radiopharmaceutical therapy of pheochromocytoma and paraganglioma. J Nucl Med 2021;62(9): 1192–9.
61. Prado-Wohlwend S, Del Olmo-Garcia MI, Bello-Arques P, et al. [(177)Lu]Lu-DOTA-TATE and [(131)I]MIBG phenotypic imaging-based therapy in metastatic/inoperable pheochromocytomas and paragangliomas: comparative results in a single center. Front Endocrinol (Lausanne) 2022;13: 778322.
62. Satapathy S, Mittal BR, Bhansali A. Peptide receptor radionuclide therapy in the management of advanced pheochromocytoma and paraganglioma: a systematic review and meta-analysis. Clin Endocrinol (Oxf) 2019;91(6):718–27.
63. Yadav MP, Ballal S, Sahoo RK, et al. Efficacy and safety of (225)Ac-DOTATATE targeted alpha therapy in metastatic paragangliomas: a pilot study. Eur J Nucl Med Mol Imaging 2022;49(5): 1595–606.
64. Tan TH, Hussein Z, Saad FF, et al. Diagnostic performance of (68)Ga-DOTATATE PET/CT, (18)F-FDG PET/CT and (131)I-MIBG scintigraphy in Mapping metastatic pheochromocytoma and paraganglioma. Nucl Med Mol Imaging 2015;49(2):143–51.
65. Maurice JB, Troke R, Win Z, et al. A comparison of the performance of (6)(8)Ga-DOTATATE PET/CT and (1)(2)(3)I-MIBG SPECT in the diagnosis and follow-up of phaeochromocytoma and paraganglioma. Eur J Nucl Med Mol Imaging 2012;39(8): 1266–70.

Gastro-Entero-Pancreatic Tumors

FDG Positron Emission Tomography/ Computed Tomography

Wajahat Khatri, MD, Ergi Spiro, BS, Amanda Henderson, BS, Steven P. Rowe, MD, PhD, Lilja B. Solnes, MD, MBA*

KEYWORDS

- Gastro-entero-pancreatic neoplasms • ^{18}F-FDG PET/CT • ^{68}Ga-DOTATATE PET/CT
- ^{64}Cu-DOTATATE PET/CT • Well-differentiated neuroendocrine tumors
- Poorly differentiated neuroendocrine tumors • Ki-67 proliferative index

KEY POINTS

- ^{18}F-fluorodeoxyglucose (^{18}F-FDG) PET/CT does not play a significant role in the diagnosis and characterization of well-differentiated gastro-entero-pancreatic neoplasms because the uptake of FDG in these neoplasms is variable but most often minimal.
- However, higher grade/poorly differentiated gastro-entero neuroendocrine neoplasms exhibit significant FDG uptake related to increased tumor-related glycolysis.
- ^{18}F-FDG PET/CT may have a greater utility in the prognostication of patient outcomes, including overall survival, either alone or in combination with more specific molecular imaging radiopharmaceuticals, such as somatostatin analog imaging agents, somatostatin receptor imaging (SSTRI).

Background

Gastro-entero-pancreatic neuroendocrine neoplasms are a class of neoplasms that originate from embryonic neural crest cells. Clinically and biologically diverse, these tumors may histologically range from well differentiated to poorly differentiated. Clinical behavior ranges from indolent, slowly growing to aggressive tumors that spread quickly to other parts of the body; these neoplasms display a broad behavioral spectrum. Neuroendocrine neoplasms (NENs) can seem as sporadic, solitary tumors or as familial tumor syndromes such as in the setting of multiple endocrine neoplasia 1. These tumors can release active peptides, which may have physiologic effects and cause carcinoid syndrome or other symptoms such as hypoglycemia.[1]

Clinically, neuroendocrine neoplasms can be divided into different groups depending on their primary origin, differentiation, Ki67 proliferation index, somatostatin receptor (SSTR) expression, extent of metastatic disease, and secretory status.[2] For larger or functioning tumors, surgical resection is considered the best treatment option with curative intent. However, for carefully selected patients, active surveillance may be an option.[3] In some cases of widespread metastatic disease, surgery may be performed to reduce tumor burden or to treat refractory carcinoid syndrome. For most tumors, initial treatment, if warranted, consists of long-acting somatostatin analogs (SSAs). If patient progresses on first-line therapy, peptide receptor radionuclide therapy (PRRT), chemotherapy, and immunotherapy are all options for patients with advanced disease who do not qualify for surgical resection.[4]

Division of Nuclear Medicine and Molecular Imaging, The Russell H. Morgan Department of Radiology and Radiological Science, Johns Hopkins University School of Medicine, 601 North Caroline Street, JHOC 3, Baltimore, MD 21287, USA
* Corresponding author.
E-mail address: lsolnes1@jhmi.edu

PET Clin 18 (2023) 243–250
https://doi.org/10.1016/j.cpet.2022.11.007

ROLE OF MEDICAL IMAGING IN NEUROENDOCRINE NEOPLASMS

The incidence of neuroendocrine tumors has increased 5-fold in the United States during the past 3 decades.[5] The increasing use of medical imaging for unrelated indications and the resulting detection of asymptomatic, nonfunctioning, neuroendocrine neoplasms is a major factor. In general, molecular imaging is essential for determining the disease extent of neuroendocrine neoplasms, which ultimately determines the optimal clinical management. Computed tomography (CT), MRI, and endoscopic ultrasound (EUS) are examples of conventional anatomical imaging modalities that aid in disease diagnosis and localization. Functional imaging techniques with positron emission tomography (PET) radiotracers, such as ^{68}Ga- or ^{64}Cu-labelled somatostatin analogs (eg, ^{68}Ga-radiolabeled analogue of somatostatin (DOTATOC), ^{68}Ga-radiolabeled analogue of somatostatin (DOTATATE), ^{68}Ga-DOTANOC, and ^{64}Cu-DOTATATE), have largely replaced single-photon emission computed tomography-based imaging with ^{111}In-pentetreotide. These agents play a crucial role in the diagnosis, staging, treatment planning, and prognosis of these tumors.[6] The role of ^{18}F-FDG PET/CT in the evaluation of these tumors is less clear and further prospective studies are needed. ^{18}F-fluorodihydroxyphenylalanine is an emerging radiopharmaceutical that is a valuable diagnostic tool for well-differentiated neuroendocrine neoplasms but is beyond the scope of thisarticle.[7]

CURRENT STATE OF ^{18}F-FDG POSITRON EMISSION TOMOGRAPHY/COMPUTED TOMOGRAPHY IN THE DIAGNOSIS OF GASTRO-ENTERO-PANCREATIC NEOPLASMS

Gastro-entero-pancreatic neuroendocrine tumors (GEP-NETs) comprise the majority of NETs (>75%), with lung NETs comprising an additional approximately 15%.[1] GEP-NETs are characterized by the World Health Organization 2010 classification system based on the Ki-67 index. They are classified as G1 (Ki-67 $\leq$ 2%), G2 (Ki-76 = 3%–20%), or G3 (Ki-67 > 20%), with G1 and G2 characterized as well-differentiated tumors, and G3 tumors characterized as poorly differentiated/dedifferentiated tumors.[8]

The "flip-flop phenomenon" best illustrates the relevance of ^{18}F-FDG PET/CT in the diagnosis and characterization of NENs. In well-differentiated neuroendocrine tumors, a combination of marked SSTR-targeted radiotracer uptake and low ^{18}F-FDG avidity is observed. In contrast, poorly differentiated tumors demonstrate low-SSTR expression and significant ^{18}F-FDG uptake.[8] This phenomenon is explicable by the distinction in proliferation between well-differentiated and poorly differentiated cancers, respectively. Increased SSTR expression in well-differentiated tumors correlates with a low-proliferation index. Similarly, reduced SSTR expression in poorly differentiated tumors suggests a high proliferation index, which results in a high ^{18}F-FDG uptake due to high glycolytic activity.[9]

Moreover, some NETs that undergo dedifferentiation in the later stages of disease may also demonstrate new or increased ^{18}F-FDG uptake relative to previous time periods in the disease course, thus emphasizing the relevance of ^{18}F-FDG PET/CT in advanced, more aggressive, gastro-entero-pancreatic neoplasms. Multiple studies have demonstrated the benefit of ^{18}F-FDG PET/CT in the diagnosis and follow-up of poorly differentiated and advanced NENs; however, its relevance, if any, in the diagnosis and prognosis of well-differentiated neuroendocrine tumors has yet to be determined. Panagiotidis and colleagues[10] demonstrated that ^{18}F-FDG PET/CT has a significant role in the assessment of poorly differentiated neuroendocrine neoplasms, with management planning based solely on ^{18}F-FDG PET/CT (^{68}Ga-DOTATATE and ^{18}F-FDG PET/CT) findings in a subset of patients with more aggressive disease. In addition, Kayani and colleagues[11] concluded in a retrospective analysis that although the sensitivity of ^{18}F-FDG PET/CT in diagnosing well-differentiated neuroendocrine tumors is low, it plays a larger role in diagnosing dedifferentiated neuroendocrine tumors and those with high Ki67 indices. In a prospective study, Binderup and colleagues[12] revealed that higher maximum standardized uptake values (SUVmax) of tumor lesions on ^{18}F-FDG PET/CT were related to lower overall survival. This investigation also confirmed that ^{18}F-FDG avidity was more prevalent among patients with a higher histologic grade. Multiple studies have also recommended dual tracer imaging with ^{18}F-FDG PET/CT and ^{68}Ga-DOTATATE PET/CT as the optimal strategy for the diagnosis of neuroendocrine neoplasms. This method permits tumor localization, accurate staging, and noninvasive whole-body total tumor burden characterization of disease heterogeneity, in addition to potentially providing prognostic information and treatment strategy guidance.[13]

ROLE OF ^{18}F FDG POSITRON EMISSION TOMOGRAPHY/COMPUTED TOMOGRAPHY IN PATIENT SELECTION FOR PEPTIDE RECEPTOR RADIONUCLIDE THERAPY AND ASSESSMENT OF PROGNOSIS

PRRT has been used successfully for the treatment of NETs for several decades, mainly in Europe. Several retrospective studies have shown potential for improving progression-free and overall survival rates.[14] In 2018, the United States Food and Drug Administration approved ^{177}Lu-DOTATATE (PRRT) based on the results of the phase 3 NETTER 1 trial.[15]

The NETTER 1 trial demonstrated increased progression-free survival and quality of life outcomes for patients.[16] The selection and prediction of outcome in patients who will benefit from PRRT is crucial. Currently, patients with SSTR imaging examinations that are positive may be eligible for treatment. Patients with more aggressive disease may be better suited for more aggressive treatments such as chemotherapy or combination therapies in conjunction with PRRT. Studies[17,18] have investigated the role of dual imaging in determining the grade of a patient's tumor. Increased FDG avidity of neuroendocrine tumors has been linked to an increased risk of progression.[19]

Chan and colleagues[19] proposed a grading scheme utilizing dual ^{18}F-FDG and STTR-targeted imaging, "NETPET," for patient risk stratification and possible prognostic implications. The NETPET criteria propose that dividing patients into 3 cohorts: SSTR positive only, SSTR/^{18}F-FDG positive, and SSTR negative/^{18}F-FDG positive correlate with overall survival. This is a more comprehensive imaging approach than a framework that only uses SSTR-targeted PET results, such as the SSTR reporting and data system.[20] However, it also relies on the information from 2 PET scans, increasing the cost and the potential for heterogeneous decision-making associated with NETPET.

^{18}F-FDG PET may predict how patients will respond to ^{177}Lu-based PRRT. A study of patients with Grade 1 and 2, well-differentiated neuroendocrine neoplasms, showed that patients who were

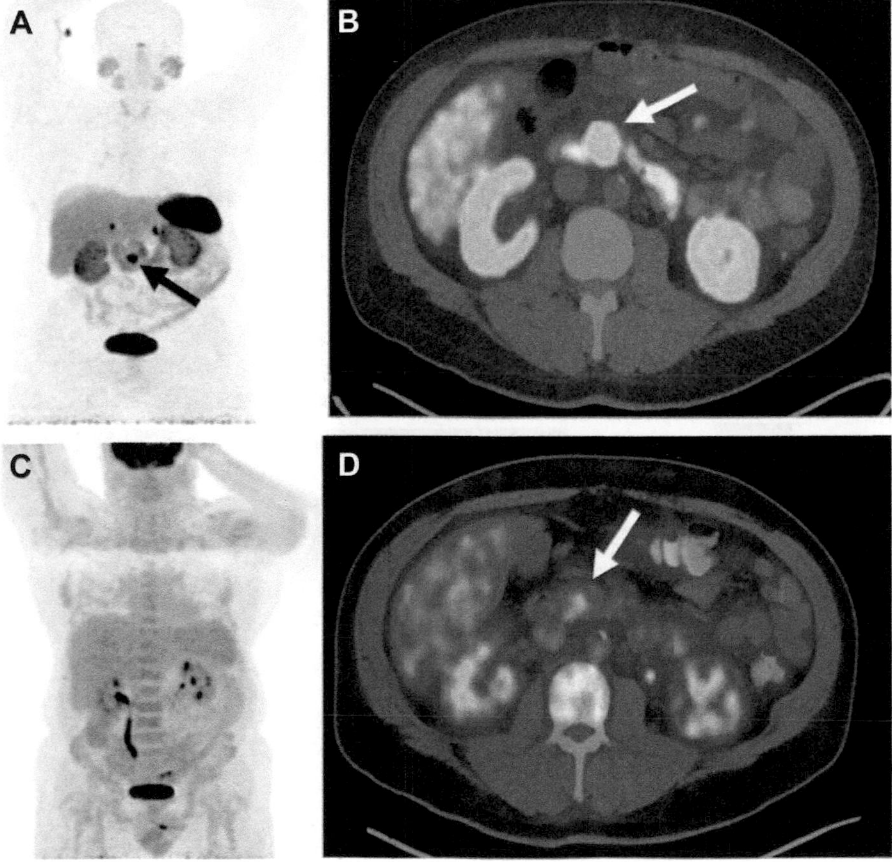

Fig. 1. (*A*) MIP and (*B*) fused axial ^{68}Ga-DOTATATE PET/CT images, (*C*) MIP and (*D*) fused axial ^{18}F-FDG PET/CT images. Note that ^{68}Ga-DOTATATE PET/CT shows intense uptake in the region of the pancreatic head mass in (*A, B*), whereas ^{18}F-FDG PET/CT shows minimal uptake, if any, in the same region in (*C, D*) (*arrows*).

^{18}F-FDG PET/CT negative had better disease control following PRRT than patients with ^{18}F-FDG-avid disease. At the first follow-up assessment following PRRT, none of the ^{18}F-FDG-negative patients had progressed, whereas only 76% of patients with ^{18}F-FDG-avid disease were found to have disease control.[21] Of note, these data suggest that a subset of patients with ^{18}F-FDG-avid disease will still benefit from PRRT and that excluding all patients with ^{18}F-FDG uptake or heterogeneous tumors from therapy would prevent some patients from accessing a beneficial treatment. Going forward, advanced image analysis methods, such as artificial intelligence, may help better select patients for PRRT based on clinical data and multiradiotracer and multimodality imaging findings.

A single course of PRRT in the United States usually consists of 4 infusions 8 weeks apart. Patients who respond positively to PRRT, characterized as sustained disease control, may benefit from additional drug infusions in future cycles.[22,23] A study looked at the role of ^{18}F-FDG PET/CT in patient selection for the second course of therapy and found that ^{18}F-FDG avidity status predicted an overall survival following the second course of PRRT.[24]

In summary, the role of ^{18}F-FDG PET/CT in diagnosing and managing neuroendocrine neoplasms is not well defined. Generally, ^{18}F-FDG PET/CT is thought to have a limited role in low-grade, low Ki67 tumors where SSTR agents are more effective. ^{18}F-FDG PET/CT is helpful in identifying the extent of metastatic disease in more aggressive NET tumors and those that dedifferentiate over time. ^{18}F-FDG PET/CT is likely to play a more prominent role in personalized medicine, tailoring therapeutic regimens to individual patients/tumor profiles. The literature suggests dual imaging with ^{18}F-FDG PET/CT and SSTR agents may offer prognostic information, including prediction of overall survival. Further prospective trials are needed to better understand the role of ^{18}F-FDG PET/CT in the clinical management of neuroendocrine neoplasms.

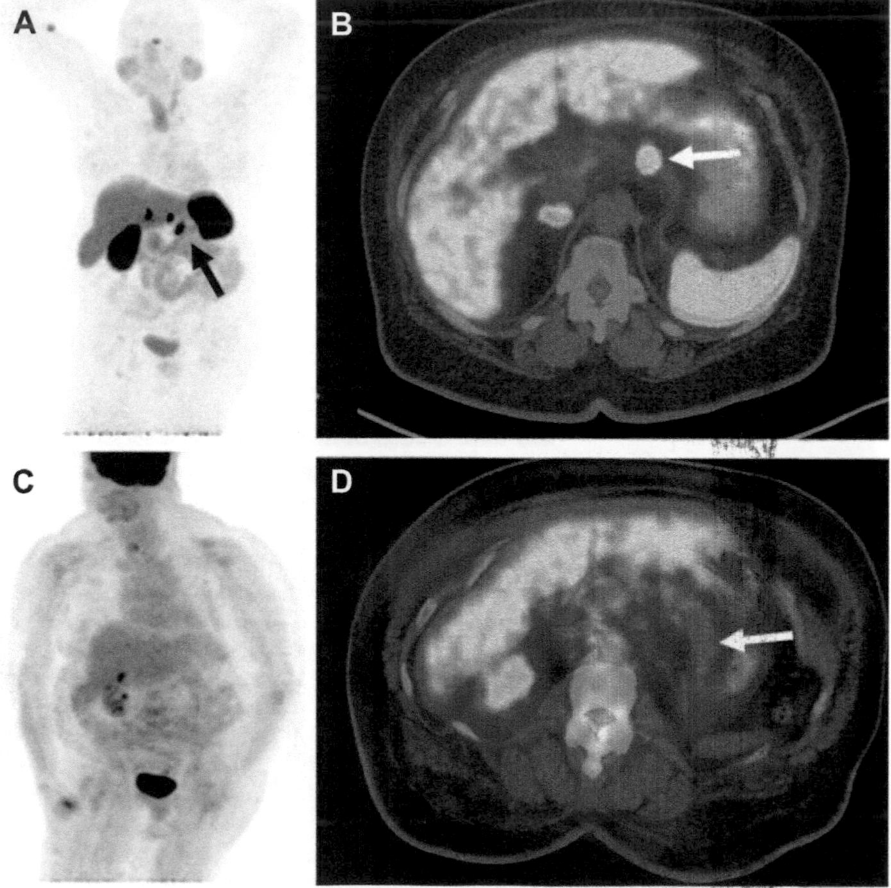

Fig. 2. (*A*) MIP and (*B*) axial fused ^{68}Ga- DOTATATE PET and PET/CT images; (*C*) MIP and (*D*) fused ^{18}F-FDG PET and PET/CT images. Note that ^{68}Ga-DOTATATE PET exhibits intensely avid uptake in the region of the mass in the pancreatic body, in (*A, B*), whereas ^{18}F-FDG PET does not show any uptake in the same region in (*C, D*) (*arrows*).

CASE PRESENTATIONS

Case 1

A 54-year-old patient found to have a pancreatic head mass on cross-sectional imaging. An EUS-guided biopsy revealed a neuroendocrine tumor of the pancreatic head with a Ki67 proliferative index of less than 2% (Grade 1). The patient underwent ^{18}F-FDG PET/CT and ^{68}Ga-DOTATATE PET/CT before surgical resection. ^{68}Ga-DOTATATE PET/CT revealed an intensely radiotracer avid pancreatic head mass corresponding to the patient's primary tumor, whereas ^{18}F-FDG PET/CT did not show significant uptake in the pancreatic head mass. As the tumor was well differentiated and had a low Ki67 proliferation index (grade 1) and the uptake of ^{18}F-FDG was minimal, this patient's clinical picture was concordant with the current evidence suggesting decreased glycolytic activity in well-differentiated neuroendocrine gastro-entero-pancreatic neoplasms. The patient subsequently underwent surgical resection of the tumor with a Whipple procedure (**Fig. 1**).

Case 2

A 68-year-old patient with a well-differentiated neuroendocrine neoplasm of the pancreatic body, initially diagnosed by fine needle aspiration cytology. Patient had dual radiotracer imaging with ^{18}F-FDG PET/CT and ^{68}Ga-DOTATATE PET/CT before surgical resection. Ki67 proliferation index for the tumor was 3% (Grade2). ^{68}Ga-DOTATATE PET/CT revealed an intensely radiotracer-avid pancreatic body mass corresponding to the patient's primary tumor. In contrast, findings on ^{18}F-FDG PET/CT were not convincing owing to the presence of only mild ^{18}F-FDG avidity in the region of the mass because the tumor in the pancreatic body was well-differentiated (grade 2). The patient underwent distal pancreatectomy, splenectomy, and intra-abdominal lymph node dissection (**Fig. 2**).

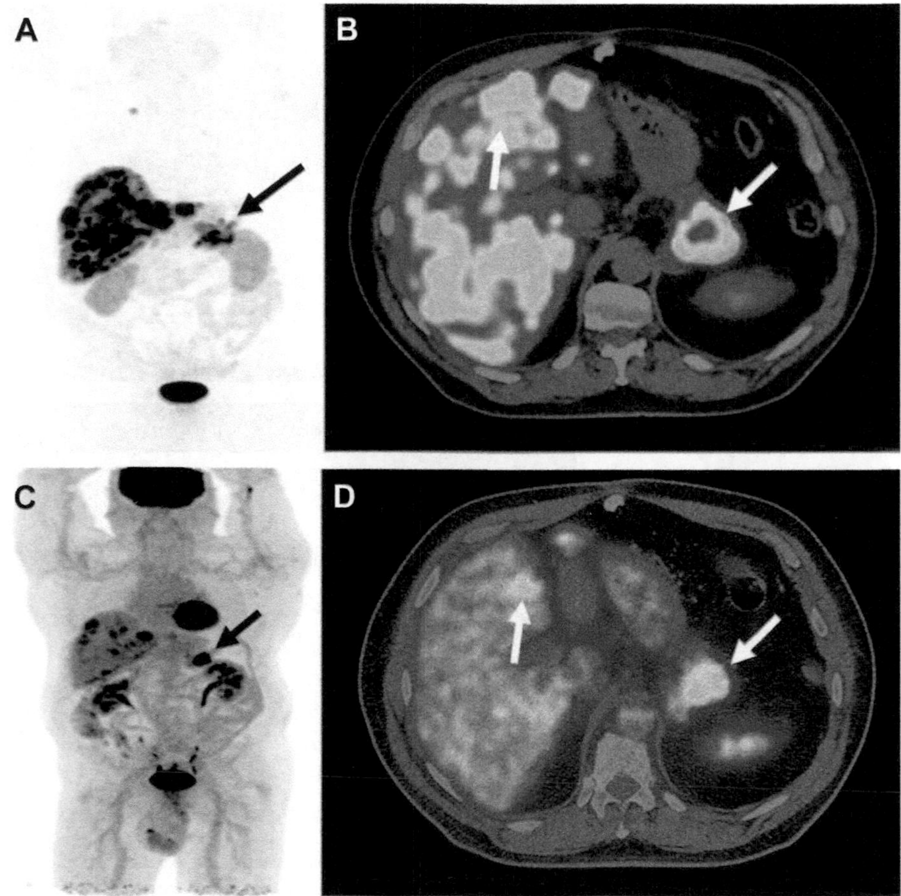

Fig. 3. (*A*) MIP and (*B*) fused ^{64}Cu-DOTATATE PET and PET/CT images, (*C*) MIP and (*D*) fused ^{18}F-FDG PET and PET/CT images. Note that ^{64}Cu-DOTATATE PET/CT exhibits intense avidity in the mass localized to the pancreatic tail and multiple lesions in the liver, in (*A, B*), whereas ^{18}F-FDG PET exhibits mild uptake in the primary lesion and a few lesions in the liver (*arrows*).

Case 3

A 70-year-old patient with neuroendocrine tumor of the pancreatic tail metastatic to the liver. Liver biopsy revealed a low-grade, well-differentiated neuroendocrine tumor with a Ki67 proliferative index of less than 20% (Grade 2). The patient had numerous hepatic lesions consistent with metastases. A ^{64}Cu- DOTATATE PET/CT revealed intense activity in the primary tumor at the tail of the pancreas and in the liver lesions. ^{18}F-FDG PET/CT was also performed within the same time frame and showed mild uptake in the primary tumor, with some ^{18}F-FDG avidity seen in a few hepatic metastatic lesions. Although the tumor was well differentiated, a higher proliferative index could explain the ^{18}F-FDG uptake in some lesions. The patient was treated nonsurgically with chemotherapy and SSAs (**Fig. 3**).

Case 4

A 48-year-old patient with neuroendocrine tumor of the pancreatic tail metastatic to liver, locoregional lymph nodes, and bone. A biopsy of a metastatic lesion in the liver revealed a well-differentiated neuroendocrine tumor with a Ki67 proliferation index of less than 3% (Grade 1). ^{68}Ga-DOTATATE PET/CT revealed intense avidity in the primary tumor in the tail of the pancreas and the liver lesions. ^{18}F-FDG PET/CT was also performed within the same time frame and showed minimal uptake in the primary tumor, with mild

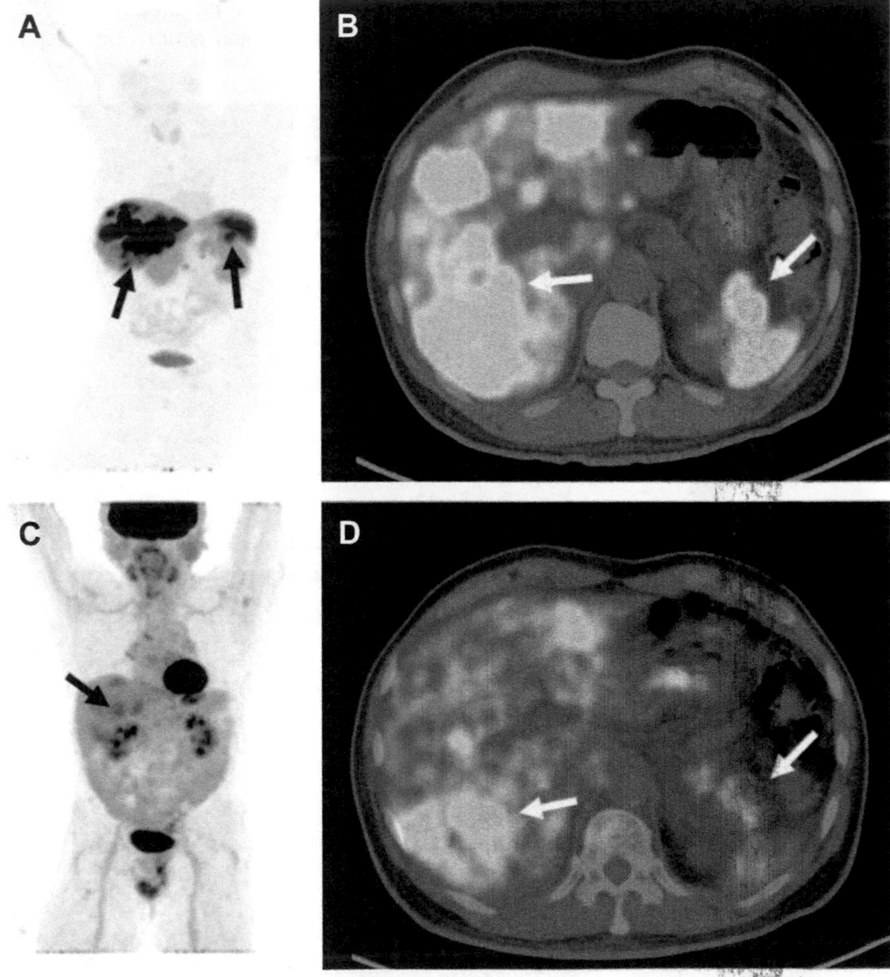

Fig. 4. (*A*) MIP and (*B*) axial fused ^{68}Ga-DOTATATE PET and PET/CT images, (*C*) MIP and (*D*) axial fused ^{18}F-FDG PET and PET/CT images. Note that ^{68}Ga-DOTATATE PET exhibits intense avidity in the mass at the pancreatic tail and multiple lesions in the liver, in (*A, B*), whereas ^{18}F-FDG PET exhibits mild uptake in a few lesions in the liver, with minimal uptake in the pancreatic tail mass (*arrows*). Compared to (*A, B*), the uptake in lesions seen in (*C, D*) is relatively subtle.

^{18}F-FDG avidity seen in a few hepatic metastatic lesions. The patient was treated with chemoembolization of liver lesions and systemic administration of SSAs (**Fig. 4**).

CASE DISCUSSION

All the above cases were diagnosed as well-differentiated neuroendocrine neoplasms, with cases 1 and 2 having disease localized to the pancreas and cases 3 and 4 presenting with systemic metastases, most prominently in the liver. Concerning grading, cases 1 and 4 were grade 1 (Ki67 proliferative index <3%), and cases 2 and 3 were grade 2 (Ki67 proliferative index 3%–20%). However, none of the above cases was poorly differentiated neuroendocrine neoplasm, which corresponds to the minimal-to-mild uptake of ^{18}F-FDG in these neoplasms. In case 3, mild ^{18}F-FDG uptake in the primary tumor and few liver lesions, and in case 4, mild ^{18}F-FDG uptake in a handful of liver lesions, can likely be explained by tumor heterogeneity, with some areas of the tumor and few liver lesions being less well differentiated than other areas and lesions, or having undergone dedifferentiation.[25] Despite the mild uptake, when compared with corresponding ^{68}Ga-DOTATATE PET, the uptake of ^{18}F-FDG in these lesions was subtle and not definitive of a dedifferentiated or high-grade malignant process in the absence of a detailed history and histopathologic confirmation. Overall, the role of ^{18}F-FDG PET/CT in the diagnosis and treatment planning in all the above cases was limited, and ^{68}Ga-DOTATATE PET/CT can be considered to have greater utility in the diagnosis, staging, and treatment planning for these patients.

CLINICS CARE POINTS

- ^{18}F-FDG PET/CT currently does not have any significant role in the diagnosis and prognostication of well and moderately differentiated gastro-entero-pancreatic neoplasms.
- In poorly differentiated gastro-entero-pancreatic neoplasms, ^{18}F-FDG PET/CT does have a role, whether alone or in combination with other imaging modalities such as ^{68}Ga-DOTATATE PET/CT or ^{64}Cu-DOTATATE PET/CT.
- Dual tracer imaging with ^{18}F-FDG PET/CT and ^{68}Ga-DOTATATE PET/CT can be considered a comprehensive strategy for characterizing neuroendocrine neoplasms, especially in cases of tumor heterogeneity.

DISCLOSURE

L.B. Solnes receives research funding from Novartis AG Pharmaceutical Company, Cellectar, Inc., and Precision Molecular, Inc. Consultant for Progenics Pharmaceutical, Inc. Book royalties from Elsevier. S.P. Rowe receives funding from Progenics Pharmaceutical, Inc., Precision Molecular, Inc., and PlenaryAI, Inc. He has consulting agreements with Progenics Pharmaceutical, Inc., Precision Molecular, Inc., and PlenaryAI, Inc. He owns equity in Precision Molecular, Inc. and PlenaryAI, Inc.

REFERENCES

1. Squires MH, Volkan Adsay N, Schuster DM, et al. Octreoscan versus FDG-PET for neuroendocrine tumor staging: a biological approach. Ann Surg Oncol 2015;22(7):2295–301.
2. Alevroudis E, Spei ME, Chatziioannou SN, et al. Clinical utility of 18F-FDG pet in neuroendocrine tumors prior to peptide receptor radionuclide therapy: a systematic review and meta-analysis. Cancers 2021;13(8):1813.
3. Bösch F, Ghadimi M, Angele MK. Personalisierte resektionsverfahren bei neuroendokrinen neoplasien des pankreas [Personalised surgical therapy for neuroendocrine neoplasia of the pancreas]. Zentralblatt für Chirurgie 2022;147(3):264–9.
4. Tsoli M, Chatzellis E, Koumarianou A, et al. Current best practice in the management of neuroendocrine tumors. Ther Adv Endocrinol Metab 2018;10. 204201881880469.
5. Dasari A, Shen C, Halperin D, et al. Trends in the incidence, prevalence, and survival outcomes in patients with neuroendocrine tumors in the United States. JAMA Oncol 2017;3(10):1335–42.
6. Chen SH, Chang YC, Hwang TL, et al. 68Ga-DOTATOC and 18F-FDG PET/CT for identifying the primary lesions of suspected and metastatic neuroendocrine tumors: a prospective study in Taiwan. J Formos Med Assoc 2018;117(6):480–7.
7. Lussey-Lepoutre C, Hindié E, Montravers F, et al. The current role of 18F-FDOPA PET for neuroendocrine tumor imaging. Médecine Nucléaire 2016; 40(1):20–30.
8. Grey N, Silosky M, Lieu CH, et al. Current status and future of targeted peptide receptor radionuclide positron emission tomography imaging and therapy of gastroenteropancreatic-neuroendocrine tumors. World J Gastroenterol 2022;28(17): 1768–80.
9. Hofman MS. Principles and application of molecular imaging for personalized medicine and guiding interventions in neuroendocrine tumors. Diagn Ther Nucl Med Neuroendocrine Tumors 2016;219–38. https://doi.org/10.1007/978-3-319-46038-3_10.

10. Panagiotidis E, Alshammari A, Michopoulou S, et al. Comparison of the impact of 68 Ga-DOTATATE and 18F-FDG PET/CT on clinical management in patients with neuroendocrine tumors. J Nucl Med 2016;58(1): 91–6.
11. Kayani I, Bomanji JB, Groves A, et al. Functional imaging of neuroendocrine tumors with combined PET/CT using 68 Ga-DOTATATE (DOTA-dphe1,tyr3-octreotate) and 18F-FDG. Cancer 2008;112(11): 2447–55.
12. Binderup T, Knigge U, Loft A, et al. 18F-fluorodeoxyglucose positron emission tomography predicts survival of patients with neuroendocrine tumors. Clin Cancer Res 2010;16(3):978–85.
13. Papadakis GZ, Karantanas AH, Marias K, et al. Current status and future prospects of PET-imaging applications in patients with gastro-entero-pancreatic neuroendocrine tumors (GEP-NETs). Eur J Radiol 2021;143:109932.
14. Hicks RJ, Kwekkeboom DJ, Krenning E, et al. ENETS consensus guidelines for the standards of care in neuroendocrine neoplasms: peptide receptor radionuclide therapy with radiolabelled somatostatin analogues. Neuroendocrinology 2017;105(3): 295–309.
15. Strosberg J, El-Haddad G, Wolin E, et al. Phase 3 trial of 177Lu-Dotatate for midgut neuroendocrine tumors. N Engl J Med 2017;376(2):125–35.
16. Strosberg JR, Caplin ME, Kunz PL, et al. 177Lu-Dotatate plus long-acting octreotide versus high-dose long-acting octreotide in patients with midgut neuroendocrine tumours (NETTER-1): final overall survival and long-term safety results from an open-label, randomised, controlled, phase 3 trial. Lancet Oncol 2021;22(12):1752–63.
17. Kayani I, Conry BG, Groves AM, et al. A comparison of 68Ga-DOTATATE and 18F-FDG PET/CT in pulmonary neuroendocrine tumors. J Nucl Med 2009; 50(12):1927–32.
18. Nilica B, Waitz D, Stevanovic V, et al. Direct comparison of 68Ga-DOTA-TOC and 18F-FDG PET/CT in the follow-up of patients with neuroendocrine tumour treated with the first full peptide receptor radionuclide therapy cycle. Eur J Nucl Med Mol Imaging 2016;43(9):1585–92.
19. Chan DL, Pavlakis N, Schembri GP, et al. Dual somatostatin receptor/FDG PET/CT imaging in metastatic neuroendocrine tumours: proposal for a novel grading scheme with prognostic significance. Theranostics 2017;7(5):1149–58.
20. Werner RA, Solnes LB, Javadi MS, et al. SSTR-RADS version 1.0 as a reporting system for SSTR PET imaging and selection of potential PRRT candidates: a proposed standardization framework. J Nucl Med 2018;59(7):1085–91.
21. Severi S, Nanni O, Bodei L, et al. Role of 18FDG PET/CT in patients treated with 177Lu-DOTATATE for advanced differentiated neuroendocrine tumours. Eur J Nucl Med Mol Imaging 2013;40(6): 881–8.
22. Weich A, Werner RA, Serfling SE, et al. Rechallenge with additional doses of 177Lu-DOTATOC after failure of maintenance therapy with cold somatostatin analogs. Clin Nucl Med 2022;47(8):719–20.
23. Kim YI. Salvage peptide receptor radionuclide therapy in patients with progressive neuroendocrine tumors: systematic review and meta-analysis. Nucl Med Commun 2020;42(4):451–8.
24. Rodrigues M, Winkler KK, Svirydenka H, et al. Long-term survival and value of 18F-FDG PET/CT in patients with gastroenteropancreatic neuroendocrine tumors treated with second peptide receptor radionuclide therapy course with 177Lu-DOTATATE. Life 2021;11(3):198.
25. Lapa C, Werner RA, Herrmann K. Visualization of tumor heterogeneity in neuroendocrine tumors by positron emission tomography. Endocrine 2016; 51(3):556–7.

Neuroendocrine Neoplasms

Total-body PET/Computed Tomography

Guobing Liu, MD, PhD[a,b,c,d,1], Chi Qi, PhD[a,b,c,d,1],
Hongcheng Shi, MD, PhD[a,b,c,d,*]

KEYWORDS

• Neuroendocrine neoplasms • Total-body PET/CT • Low dose • Dynamic acquisition

KEY POINTS

- With the high temporospatial resolution, total-body PET/computed tomography (CT) with low-dose gallium-68 (^{68}Ga) DOTATATE or low-dose as well as ultra-low-dose 18F-fluorodeoxyglucose (18F-FDG) with reasonable acquisition time could get qualified imaging to meet the diagnostic request.
- ^{68}Ga DOTATATE PET/CT combined with 18F-FDG PET/CT could effectively diagnose and evaluate the heterogeneity of the neuroendocrine neoplasms.
- Total-body PET/CT dynamic scan could provide more kinetic parameters and time activity curve. It is helpful for understanding tumors' biological characteristics as well as diagnosis and differential diagnosis of neuroendocrine neoplasms.

INTRODUCTION

Neuroendocrine neoplasms (NENs) include neuroendocrine tumor (NET), such as NET Grade 1, Grade 2, and Grade 3, and neuroendocrine carcinoma (NEC) according to the AJCC classification.[1] NENs are a heterogeneous tumor with many different subtypes and the propensity to metastasize. NENs diagnosis may be inaccurate if the results depend on the biopsy performed at a limited range. PET molecular imaging could show NENs characterization as a whole, with well-differentiated sites uptake gallium-68 (^{68}Ga) DOTATATE obviously but poorly differentiated sites accumulation 18F-fluorodeoxyglucose (18F-FDG) mainly. So, ^{68}Ga DOTATATE and 18F-FDG PET/computed tomography (CT) imaging play complementary roles in diagnosis, staging, and evaluation therapy response of NENs. PET molecular imaging-guided biopsy could effectively get target samples and improve the diagnosis accuracy. With the treatment more effective, patients with NENs could live lone time with the disease and may need many times PET scan using different tracers for therapy planning or therapy response evaluation. If the imaging quality could meet the diagnostic request, lower injection activity is more beneficial for the patient.

Long-axial field of view (AFOV) PET/CT is a new trend as it has so many advantages over conventional PET/CT, such as high sensitivity and high imaging quality, as well as long-range dynamic scan with high temporal resolution and so on. It was reported that some of the long AFOV PET has been used in clinical practice or preclinical studies, such as the uExplorer[2] (United Imaging Healthcare), Biograph Vision Quadra[3] (Siemens Healthineers) and the PennPET Explorer[4] (University of Pennsylvania), and so on.

As the first user of the uExplorer total-body PET/CT system with 194 cm AFOV (United Imaging Healthcare, Shanghai, China) in the world,[4] Department of Nuclear Medicine, Zhongshan Hospital,

[a] Department of Nuclear Medicine, Zhongshan Hospital, Fudan University, 180 Fenglin Road, Shanghai, China; [b] Institute of Nuclear Medicine, Fudan University, Shanghai, China; [c] Shanghai Institute of Medical Imaging, Shanghai, China; [d] Cancer Prevention and Treatment Center, Zhongshan Hospital, Fudan University, Shanghai 200032, China

[1] The authors contributed equally to this study.

* Corresponding author.
E-mail address: Shi.hongcheng@zs-hospital.sh.cn

PET Clin 18 (2023) 251–257
https://doi.org/10.1016/j.cpet.2022.11.010

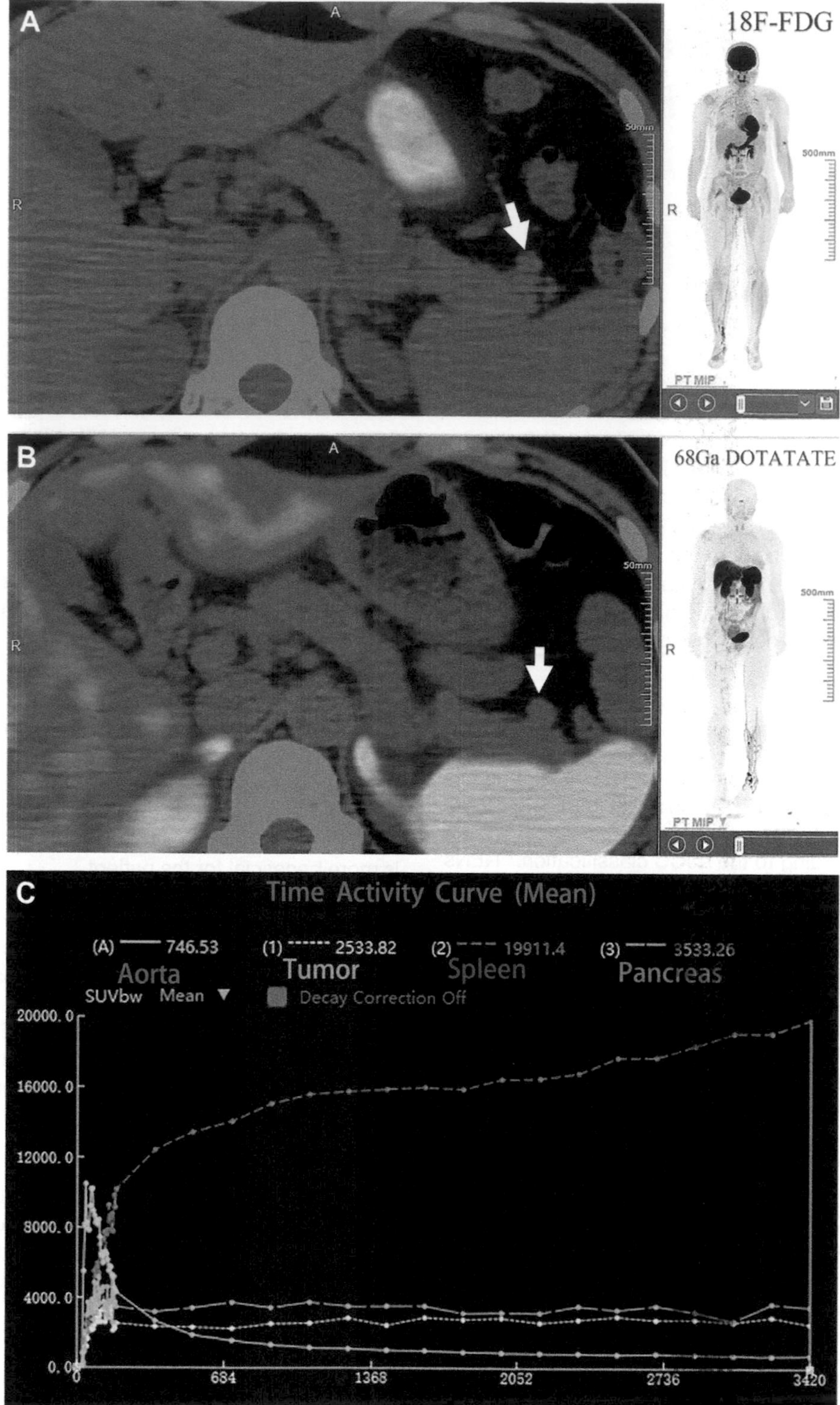

Fig. 1. Pancreatic tail exogenous insulinoma. A 48-year-old woman suffered from hypoglycemia for a month. Blood test results showed that fasting blood glucose level was 2.3 mmol/L (normal range 3.9–5.6 mmol/L) and serum insulin level was 86.3 uU/mL (normal range 2.69–24.9 uU/mL). Enhanced MRI shows a mass in front of the pancreatic tail. 18F-FDG activity of 118.4MBq PET/CT imaging (weight 60 kg, acquisition time 7 min) showed an almost non-FDG avid nodule (SUVmax 1.57) in front of the pancreatic tail (*A*). ^{68}Ga DOTATATE activity of 67.15

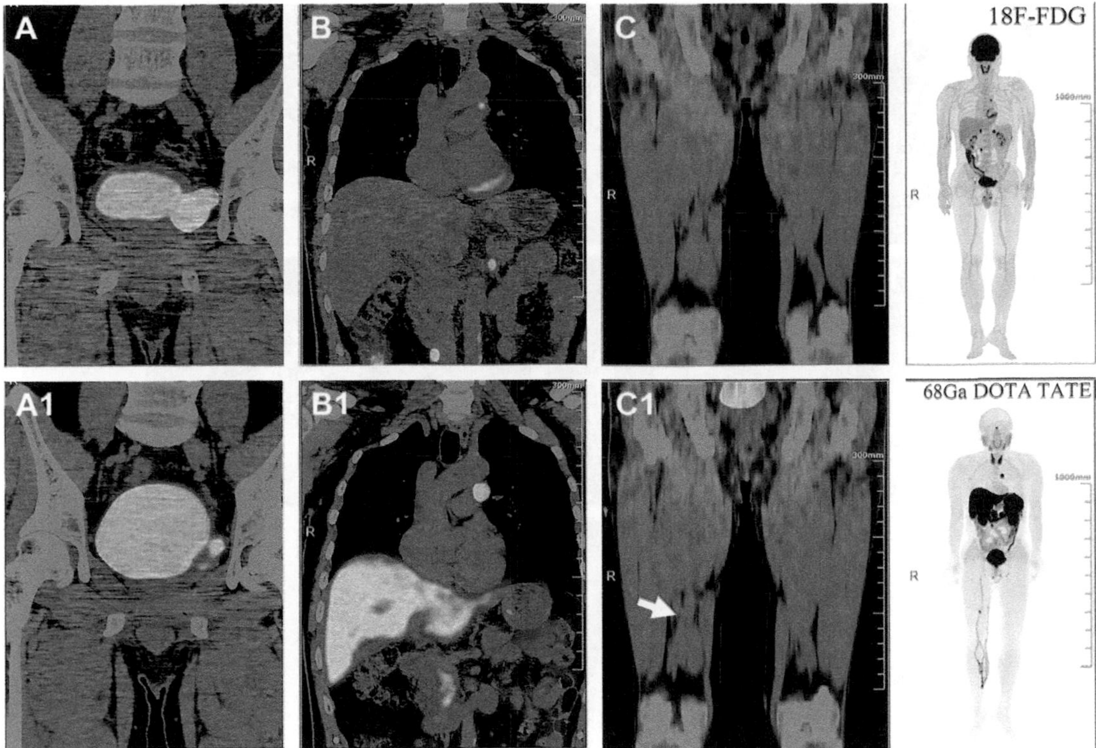

Fig. 2. A patient with paraganglioma and multi metastasis in body. A 49-year-old man with bladder wall paraganglioma diagnosed by biopsy pathology. Total-body 18F-FDG activity of 133.2Mbq (weight 71.1 kg, acquisition time 7 min) and 68 Ga DOTATATE activity of 66.6 MBq (acquisition time 15 min) PET/CT was performed one after another for further evaluation. Total-body PET/CT imaging showed that bladder wall original mass and lymph nodes located by the inferior vena cava and abdominal aorta as well as in mediastinum accumulated 18F-FDG (*A–C*) and ^{68}-Ga DOTATATE (*A1–C1*) at the same time. It reflected the tumor heterogeneity. Another lymph node metastasis was found in the muscle space in the right thigh near the knee in the ^{68}-Ga DOTATATE PET/CT imaging only. It was apt to miss by conventional PET/CT as it located below the middle of the thigh. (*arrows in A, B*) denote the lesion of insulinoma located in front of the pancreatic tail. (arrows in C1) indicate lymph node metastasis in the muscle space of the right thigh near the knee.

Fudan University has examined more than 15000 patients since April 2019, including more than 1500 case 60 min or 75 min dynamic study. From then on, a series of studies have been carried out by our team. We verified that even 30-s fast scans with regular dose (3.7 Mbq/kg),[5–7] half-dose scan (1.85Mbq/kg), or even extra low-dose (0.37 Mbq/kg) scan with one-tenth of regular dose could be used as the qualified selected protocol to meet the different situation request in clinical practice with uExplorer total-body PET/CT system.[8–13] Among the patients, more than 400 patients with or suspected NENs accepted ^{68}Ga DOTATATE PET/CT combined with low or ultra-low-dose 18F-FDG PET/CT examination. Our experience of using total-body PET/CT in a patient with NENs introduced as below.

More Sensitive and Extensive Total-Body Scan in Neuroendocrine Neoplasm Case

With 194 cm AFOV, total-body PET/CT has 40-fold in effective counts rate than a conventional 22 cm AFOV PET/CT scanner.[2] It enhances the ability to find small or radiotracer accumulation slightly lesions based on its high count rate and high sensitivity. In this situation, high-sensitivity PET/CT could play an important role to get more information for the diagnosis of the patient with NENs (**Fig. 1**) or evaluation the status.

MBq PET/CT (acquisition time 10 min) imaging showed the nodule with slightly DOTAT TATE avid (SUVmax 5.25) compared with pancreatic tail (*B*). The shape of time–activity curve of lesion (*yellow*) was different from pancreases (*green*) and spleen (*purple*) (*C*). Pathological diagnosis was insulinoma after the tumor and pancreatic tail resection. (arrows in A, B) denote the lesion of insulinoma located in front of the pancreatic tail.

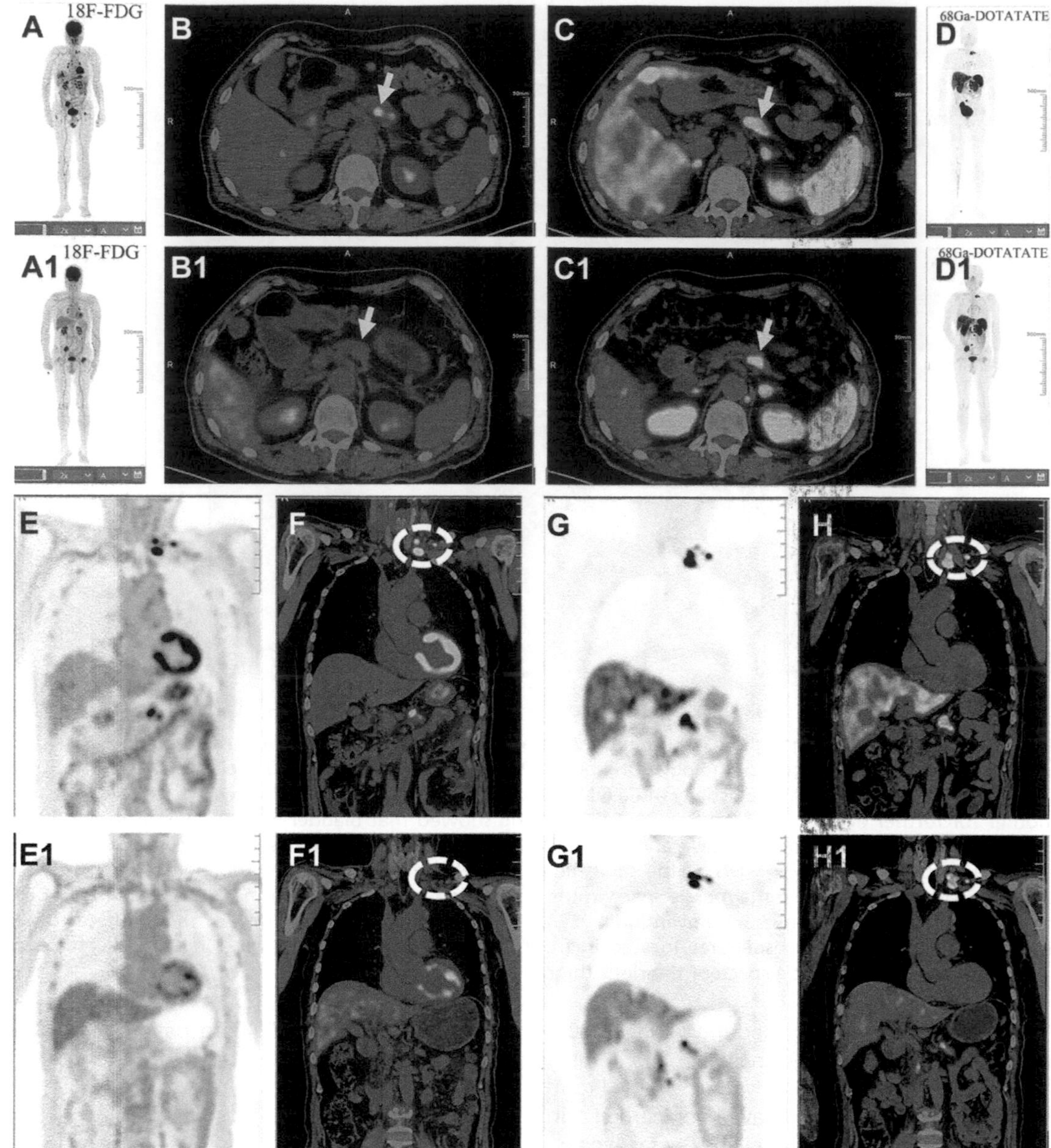

Fig. 3. Therapy response evaluation using low-dose dual-tracer PET/CT. A 66-year-old man was diagnosed pancreases body NET(G2) with liver metastasis by liver biopsy. 18F-FDG activity of 32.19 MBq and ^{68}-Ga DOTATATE activity of 136.9 MBq PET/CT examinations were performed in different day before treatment of staging. The PET/CT imaging showed that pancreas body 18F-FDG avid tumor (*A, B, arrow*) with much more ^{68}-Ga DOTATATE accumulation (*C, D, arrow*). At the same time, left clavicular region multilymph node metastasis shows 18F-FDG (*E, F, circle*) uptake a little less than 68 Ga DOTATATE (*G, H, circle*). After 6 months target therapy, 18F-FDG activity 24.42 MBq and ^{68}-Ga DOTATATE activity of 33.3 MBq PET/CT were performed separately for therapy response evaluation. The PET/CT imaging showed that pancreas body tumor (*A1, B1*) and left clavicular region multilymph node metastasis (*E1, F1*) with no obviously 18F-FDG uptake but obviously ^{68}-Ga DOTATATE accumulation (*C1, D1 and G1, H1*) decreased somewhat than before therapy. It reflects that F-18-FDG combined with ^{68}-Ga DOTATATE PET/CT examination is necessary. (*arrows in C1*) indicate lymph node metastasis in the muscle space of the right thigh near the knee.

It is different from whole-body scan from scalp to middle thigh by multi-bed scan using conventional PET/CT, total-body PET/CT in a single-bed scan could cover scalp to toe. Although it is not common that NENs or its metastasis lesion involves to limb, it is important to detect all the lesions for staging accurately and clinical decision-making (**Fig. 2**).

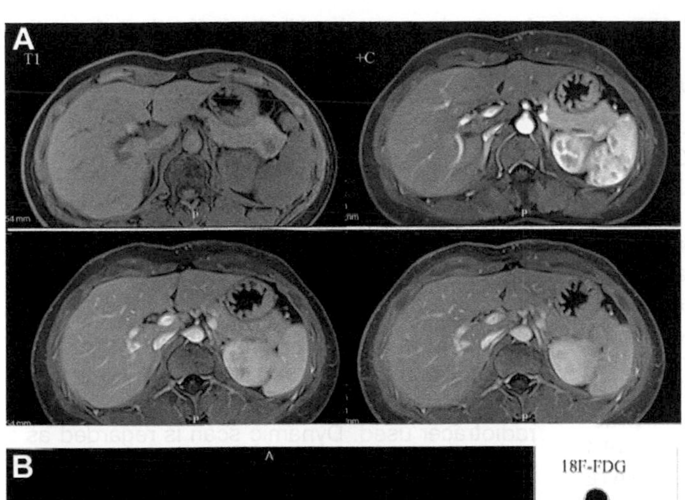

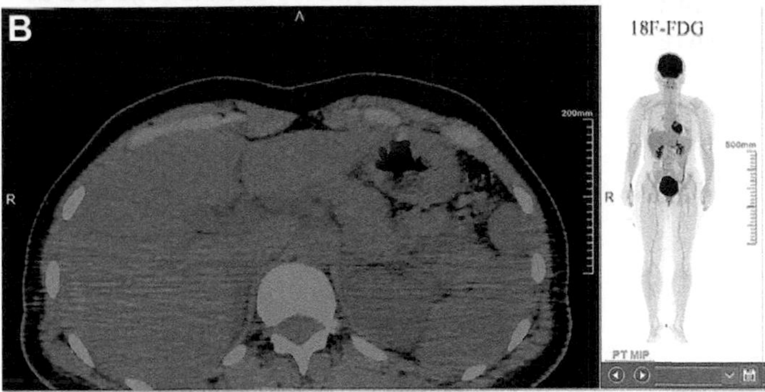

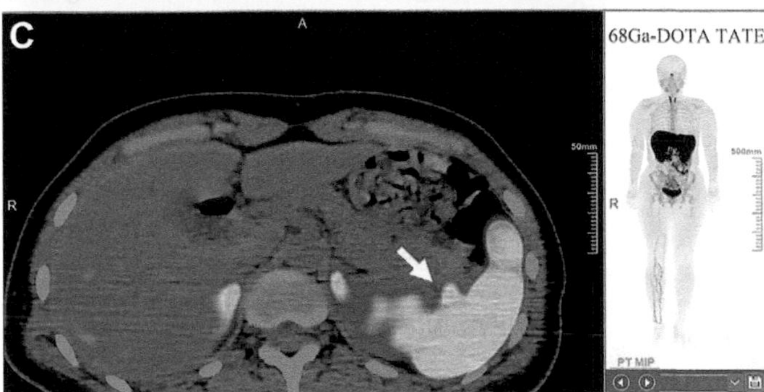

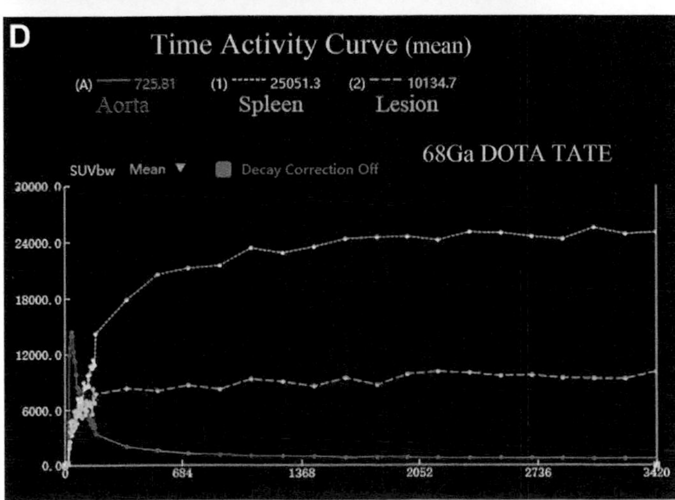

Fig. 4. Accessory spleen in pancreatic tail. A 41-year-old woman suffered from intermittent abdominal pain for a month. Enhanced MRI showed a mass in pancreatic tail and suspected neuroendocrine neoplasms (*A*). Total-body 18F-FDG activity of 24.79 MBq (weight 52.7 kg) and ^{68}-Ga DOTATATE activity of 63.27 MBq dynamic PET/CT was performed one day apart for diagnosis and evaluation. The lesion in pancreatic tail accumulated ^{68}-Ga DOTATATE obviously (SUVmax 16.4) but without FDG in static PET/CT imaging (*B, C, arrow*). The TAC of the lesion almost the same with spleen except for the peak lower (*D*). The lesion TAC was different from the tumor in pancreatic tail (see **Fig. 1C**). Pathological diagnosis of the surgical specimen was accessory spleen.

Low-Dose Gallium-68 DOTATATE and 18F-Fluorodeoxyglucose PET/Computed Tomography Total-Body Static Scan in Neuroendocrine Neoplasm Case

^{68}Ga DOTATATE combined with 18F-FDG PET/CT could evaluate the NENs heterogeneity effectively. It would be meaningful to reduce the radiation exposure for patient accept multi-tracer PET/CT examination and even many times examination during a period of time using low-dose radiotracer (**Fig. 3**). With high sensitivity, total-body PET/CT enables to use low-dose (1.85Mbq/kg) or even extra low-dose (0.37 Mbq/kg) 18F-FDG PET/CT scan to get qualified diagnostic imaging in clinical practice.[8–13] One-third of recommended activity (48.1 to 73.6 MBq) or even lower of ^{68}Ga DOTATATE was used in clinical practice in our center.[14] Low-dose ^{68}Ga DOTATATE PET/CT scan has some advantages; first, it reduces the radiation exposure for patient and staff. It's well known that patients with NENs frequently live with their disease for many years. SSTR-PET/CT combined with 18F-FDG PET/CT examination may play an important role in disease evaluation and/or treatment planning at various times during a patient's disease.[15] As the dual tracer PET/CT scan were performed in our center, not only low-dose radiotracer was given, but also low-dose CT scan was performed for one of the PET/CT examinations to reduce the radiation exposure further if necessary. Second, it was possible to serve more patient when ^{68}Ge/^{68}Ga generator could elute limited radionuclide. Acquisition time for low-dose ^{68}Ga DOTATATE PET/CT is 10 min and 3 to 5 min for low dose(1.85 Mbq/kg) or 7 to 15 min for extra low-dose 18F-FDG PET/CT scan. Patient's feeling was better than or at least equivalent to using conventional PET/CT.

Dynamic Scan in Neuroendocrine Neoplasm Case

Static PET/CT imaging shows the radiotracer distributes at a single time point after the radiotracer is distributed in human body. It reflects a part of biologic and pathologic information of the disease and plays an important role in the disease diagnosis and therapy response evaluation and so on. But static imaging is only a part contents of PET/CT examination, dynamic examination could provide more important characteristics of radiotracer kinetics information, such as tissue delivery, retention, and release back to the blood pool that provide a more comprehensive biologic information in vivo and improve clinical decision making.[16] Limited by the 15 to 30 cm AFOV of conventional PET/CT, dynamic scan could cover short range for a bed scan and get limited effective information to enhance the clinical diagnosis and or evaluation. It was the mainly reason why dynamic scan with conventional PET/CT was not used widely in clinical. With long AFOV, total-body PET/CT could cover long rang or even total-body of the patients and get most or all the organs and tissues dynamic information after a single bed scan. It provides a new opportunity for dynamic scan applications in clinical practice using long AFOV PET/CT.

Sixty minutes or even longer time dynamic scan provide perfusion information at the beginning of the scan and then metabolism or binding to target molecules information according to the different radiotracer used. Dynamic scan is regarded as a promising method for radiopharmaceutical kinetics study. PET kinetic analysis based on the dynamic scan could get many parameters, such as K1, k2, k3, k4, and Ki, that is proposed for understanding the characteristic of the disease.[17] It always takes more time to analyze the PET kinetic parameters and the result has no standard reference in clinical application by now. Time of the activity curve (TAC) is easy to get by drawing the VOI or ROI at the target lesion or tissue. The TAC combined with static PET/CT imaging are also helpful for NENs diagnosis and differential diagnosis (see **Fig. 1**; **Fig. 4**).

SUMMARY

Total-body PET/CT with low-dose ^{68}Ga DOTATATE combined with low-dose 18F-FDG could sensitively detect NENs lesions and objective evaluate its heterogeneity and therapy response. Dynamic scan could provide more tumor biological information to help diagnosis and differential diagnosis.

CLINICS CARE POINTS

- There is evidence showing the effectiveness of somatostatin receptor (SSTR)-targeted imaging for diagnosis, staging, evaluating the possibility of treatment with somatostatin analogs, as well peptide receptor radionuclide therapy (PRRT).
- ^{68}Ga-SSTR, like the ^{68}Ga-DOTATATE, had presented excellent sensitivity and specificity for diagnosing and staging neuroendocrine neoplasms (NENs).
- PET/CT imaging with ^{68}Ga-SSTR complements PET/CT imaging with ^{18}F-FDG toward a personalized therapy in NENs patients.

DISCLOSURE

The authors have nothing to disclose.

FUNDING

This research was supported in part by Science and Technology Committee of Shanghai Municipality (20DZ2201800), Clinical Research Plan of SHDC (No. SHDC2020CR3079B), and Shanghai Municipal Key Clinical Specialty (shslczdzk03401).

REFERENCE

1. Woltering EA, Bergsland EK, Beyer DT. Neuroendocrine tumors of the stomach. American joint committee on cancer 2017. In: Amin MB, editor. AJCC cancer staging manual. Eighth Edition. Springer; 2017. p. 351–9.
2. Badawi RD, Shi H, Hu P, et al. First human imaging studies with the EXPLORER total-body PET scanner. J Nucl Med 2019;60(3):299–303.
3. Alberts I, Hünermund JN, Prenosil G, et al. Clinical performance of long axial field of view PET/CT: a head-to-head intra-individual comparison of the Biograph Vision Quadra with the Biograph Vision PET/CT. Eur J Nucl Med Mol Imaging 2021;48(8):2395–404.
4. Pantel AR, Viswanath V, Daube-Witherspoon ME, et al. PennPET explorer: human imaging on a whole-body imager. J Nucl Med 2020;61(1):144–51.
5. Zhang Y, Hu P, He Y, et al. Ultrafast 30-s total-body PET/CT scan: a preliminary study [published online ahead of print, 2022 May 17]. Eur J Nucl Med Mol Imaging 2022. https://doi.org/10.1007/s00259-022-05838-1.
6. Boellaard R, Delgado-Bolton R, Oyen WJ, et al. FDG PET/CT: EANM procedure guidelines for tumour imaging: version 2.0. Eur J Nucl Med Mol Imaging 2015;42(2):328–54.
7. Sui X, Liu G, Hu P, et al. Total-body PET/computed tomography highlights in clinical practice: experiences from zhongshan hospital, Fudan University. PET Clin 2021;16(1):9–14.
8. Zhang YQ, Hu PC, Wu RZ, et al. The image quality, lesion detectability, and acquisition time of 18F-FDG total-body PET/CT in oncological patients. Eur J Nucl Med Mol Imaging 2020;47(11):2507–15.
9. Hu P, Zhang Y, Yu H, et al. Total-body 18F-FDG PET/CT scan in oncology patients: how fast could it be? Eur J Nucl Med Mol Imaging 2021;48(8):2384–94.
10. Hu Y, Liu G, Yu H, et al. Feasibility of ultra-low 18F-FDG activity acquisitions using total-body PET/CT [published online ahead of print, 2021 Sep 30]. J Nucl Med 2021;121:262038. jnumed.
11. Tan H, Cai D, Sui X, et al. Investigating ultra-low-dose total-body [18F]-FDG PET/CT in colorectal cancer: initial experience. Eur J Nucl Med Mol Imaging 2022;49(3):1002–11.
12. Tan H, Sui X, Yin H, et al. Total-body PET/CT using half-dose FDG and compared with conventional PET/CT using full-dose FDG in lung cancer. Eur J Nucl Med Mol Imaging 2021;48(6):1966–75.
13. Liu G, Hu P, Yu H, et al. Ultra-low-activity total-body dynamic PET imaging allows equal performance to full-activity PET imaging for investigating kinetic metrics of 18F-FDG in healthy volunteers. Eur J Nucl Med Mol Imaging 2021;48(8):2373–83.
14. Bozkurt MF, Virgolini I, Balogova S, et al. Guideline for PET/CT imaging of neuroendocrine neoplasms with (68)Ga-DOTA-conjugated somatostatin receptor targeting peptides and (18)F-DOPA [J]. Eur J Nucl Med Mol Imaging 2017;44(9):1588–601.
15. Hope TA, Bergsland EK, Bozkurt MF, et al. Appropriate use criteria for somatostatin receptor PET imaging in neuroendocrine tumors. J Nucl Med 2018;59(1):66–74.
16. Lammertsma AA. Forward to the past: the case for quantitative PET imaging. J Nucl Med 2017;58(7):1019–24.
17. Pantel AR, Viswanath V, Muzi M, et al. Principles of tracer kinetic analysis in oncology, Part I: principles and overview of methodology. J Nucl Med 2022;63(3):342–52.

Neuroendocrine Tumor Diagnosis: PET/MR Imaging

Heying Duan, MD, Andrei Iagaru, MD*

KEYWORDS

• PET • PET/MRI • MRI • Neuroendocrine tumors • NET • NEN

KEY POINTS

- Functional imaging targeting somatostatin receptors (SSTR) have become indispensable in the management of well-differentiated neuroendocrine tumors (NETs), whereas FDG is used for poorly differentiated NETs and neuroendocrine carcinomas; combined SSTR-targeting and FDG imaging might be advantageous in high-grade well-differentiated NETs.
- Hybrid PET/MR imaging systems acquire PET and MR images simultaneously, offering accurate whole-body staging in a one-stop-shop examination.
- The high soft tissue contrast of MR imaging is particularly superior for evaluation of hepatic metastases, the most frequent site for distant metastases in NETs.
- Continued advancement and improvement of PET/MR imaging protocols allow for shorter image acquisition times at high image quality.
- PET/MR imaging has reduced radiation exposure and is especially advantageous in pediatric patients who require frequent follow-up imaging.

INTRODUCTION

Neuroendocrine tumors (NETs) are rare and sporadic in origin. They can occur in almost every organ; however, the majority are gastroenteropancreatic (GEP) in 61%, bronchial in 25%, and of unknown origin in 14%.[1] GEP NETs occur in the small intestine (33%), rectum (30%), pancreas (13%), stomach (11%), appendix (8%), and colon (5%). The 2022 World Health Organization (WHO) classification categorizes neuroendocrine neoplasia (NEN) into well-differentiated NETs and poorly differentiated neuroendocrine carcinomas (NECs). NETs can be further divided by grading based on their mitotic count and Ki-67 index as markers of cell proliferation: G1 (Ki67 <3%), G2 (Ki67 3%–20%), and well-differentiated G3 (Ki67 >20%), and NECs into small-cell NEC and large-cell NEC.[2] Well-differentiated NETs are most frequent and are slow-growing tumors. Functional tumors secrete hormones, and patients will present with distinct symptoms; however, most patients experience only vague and nonspecific symptoms, making their diagnosis difficult; patients are often misdiagnosed or diagnosed late when the tumor has already metastasized. The unique feature of all well-differentiated NETs is their overexpression of somatostatin receptors (SSTR). Five subclasses of human SSTR have been identified: 1, 2A, 2B, 3, 4, and 5. Subtypes 2 and 5 are the most frequently expressed SSTR in NETs. These SSTR can be targeted with radiolabeled somatostatin analogues. Poorly differentiated NETs and NECs have low or no expression of SSTR. These tumors are imaged with fluorine-18 (^{18}F) fluorodeoxyglucose (FDG). As the tumor biology of NETs is very heterogeneous and the full scope cannot be assessed by a single biopsy, high-grade well-differentiated NETs might benefit from combined imaging of SSTR and FDG-PET, as they might have SSTR-positive and SSTR-negative metastases simultaneously.[3–5]

Department of Radiology, Division of Nuclear Medicine and Molecular Imaging, Stanford University, 300 Pasteur Drive, H2200, Stanford, CA 94305, USA
* Corresponding author.
E-mail address: aiagaru@stanford.edu

PET Clin 18 (2023) 259–266
https://doi.org/10.1016/j.cpet.2022.11.008
1556-8598/23/

Molecular imaging is indispensable in the management of NETs. Hybrid imaging systems, that is, PET combined with computed tomography (CT) or MR imaging, provide functional information with its respective anatomical correlation in a single imaging session. PET/CT systems are widely available nowadays. As the majority of NETs are GEP-NETs and liver metastases are the most common site of metastatic disease, supplemental MR imaging is often necessary. Therefore, PET/MR imaging with its excellent soft tissue contrast may be better suited in patients with GEP-NETs. Simultaneous PET/MR imaging scanners acquire and fuse PET and MR images at the same time and therefore have the potential to provide accurate staging and restaging in a one-stop-shop examination. This article reviews the use of PET/MR imaging for diagnosis of NEN, including advantages and challenges in comparison to PET/CT.

SOMATOSTATIN RECEPTOR-TARGETING PET/MR IMAGING

Accurate diagnostic imaging of NEN is of utmost importance for subsequent treatment stratification. Patients who show distant metastases are not eligible for curative surgical resection. The Food and Drug Administration (FDA) has approved gallium-68 (^{68}Ga) DOTATATE, ^{68}Ga-DOTATOC, and copper-64 (^{64}Cu) DOTATATE for PET imaging. Each of these radiopharmaceuticals have a slightly different affinity profile for the SSTR subtypes, but all bind to SSTR2 and have equally high diagnostic accuracy, sensitivity, and specificity without superiority of one over the other. MR imaging shows superior soft tissue contrast compared with CT and is preferred for imaging of the abdomen, pelvis (**Fig. 1**), bone, and brain in patients with NET.[6] Supplementary MR imaging is also indicated in cases of negative or equivocal SSTR PET/CT.[7] PET/MR imaging combines the best of 2 worlds: the high sensitivity and specificity of SSTR PET and the high soft tissue contrast and functional MR imaging sequences, such as diffusion-weighted imaging (DWI), and offers a convenient one-stop-shop examination for patients with NEN. PET/MR imaging has lower radiation exposure as PET/CT and is particularly beneficial in younger patients in need of continuous imaging. The FDA has cleared several simultaneous PET/MR imaging systems; however, PET/MR imaging is not as widely available as PET/CT and is mostly located in academic centers and used for research. Thus, studies involving NETs at staging were scarce and heterogeneous; most of the below-mentioned studies involved patients at staging and restaging.

The first study demonstrating the feasibility of simultaneous PET/MR imaging in GEP-NETs was published in 2013 and involved a small patient cohort of 8 patients who were imaged with PET/MR imaging and PET/CT using ^{68}Ga-DOTATOC.[8] On a per-patient level, PET/MR imaging accurately identified all 5 patients that had malignant lesions according to the reference standard, whereas PET/CT was false negative in one patient. On a per-lesion level, PET/MR imaging not only visualized all lesions seen on PET/CT, but using a gadolinium contrast-enhanced PET/MR imaging protocol, also visualized lesions that were not seen on triple-phase PET/CT. Particularly, the use of DWI aided in the distinction of malignant and benign hepatic lesions. PET/MR imaging showed limitations in the detection of lung lesions and hypersclerotic bone metastases. In a subsequent study of the same group involving 30 patients with NETs presenting mostly for restaging, PET/MR imaging with gadolinium-enhanced delayed liver-specific phase showed higher accuracy in the detection of NET lesions than dual-phase PET/CT (90.8% vs 86.7%): PET/CT missed subcentimeter hepatic metastases (10/70), whereas PET/MR imaging failed to identify subcentimeter sclerotic bone (3/14) and lung (2/9) metastases, consistent with the findings from their pilot study.[9] However, these missed findings on either hybrid modality did not ultimately alter patient management, as all had advanced, metastatic disease. PET/CT detected more non-NET benign lesions compared with PET/MR imaging (94.5% vs 83.6%). Similar limitations of PET/MR imaging for lung lesions were seen in a cohort of 28 patients with well-differentiated NETs: ^{68}Ga-DOTANOC PET/MR imaging missed all lung and pleural lesions, which were identified by PET/CT.[10] However, overall gadoxetate-enhanced PET/MR imaging with dedicated hepatobiliary phase (HBP) showed a slightly higher sensitivity of 89.8% and accuracy of 97% for NET metastases compared with contrast-enhanced dual-phase PET/CT with 81.6% and 94.6%, respectively; specificity was equally high with 100%.

SOMATOSTATIN RECEPTOR-TARGETING PET/MR IMAGING FOR NEUROENDOCRINE TUMOR LIVER METASTASES

The liver is the most common site of distant metastases in up to 85% of patients with NET.[11,12] As hepatic metastases are the main driver for morbidity and mortality with significantly reduced overall survival, their accurate diagnosis is essential.[13–15] The extent of liver disease directs subsequent treatment management of surgical resection

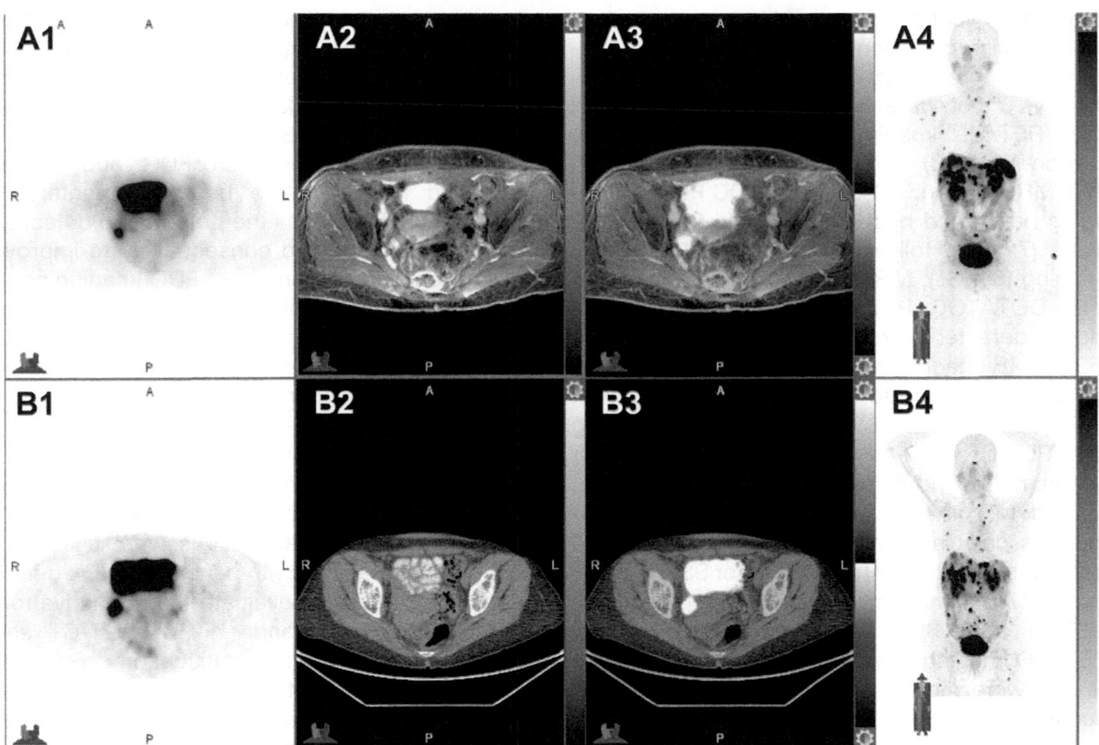

Fig. 1. A 59-year-old woman with a nonfunctional ovarian stromal tumor, Ki-67 8.6%, WHO grade 2, and subsequent diagnosis of metastatic NET, Ki-67 3.2%, WHO grade 2. Primary tumor in the right adnexa and right uterus shows high lesion conspicuity on ^{68}Ga-DOTATATE PET/MR imaging (*A1–A4*, axial PET, MR imaging, fused PET/MR imaging, and maximum intensity projection [MIP] images, respectively). Compared with low-dose ^{64}Cu-DOTATATE PET/CT (*B1–B4*, axial PET, CT, fused PET/MR imaging, and MIP images, respectively), MR imaging offers better tumor delineation and characterization. A T1-weighted LAVA-Flex MR imaging protocol showed enhancement of the lesion in the right posterior uterus relative to the myometrium, demonstrated restricted diffusion and SSTR expression, and was deemed a NET metastasis.

or locoregional or systemic therapy. MR imaging has demonstrated higher sensitivity for liver lesions, which is why patients with suspected or known hepatic lesions will receive additional MR imaging of the abdomen as part of routine imaging.[16] Contrast-enhanced CT and MR imaging are vital, as NET hepatic metastases are hypervascular in the arterial phase.[16–18] Small subcentimeter liver lesions can be masked by partial-volume effect on SSTR PET, as the liver shows high physiologic uptake. The added value of HBP with gadoxetate in simultaneous ^{68}Ga-DOTATOC PET/MR imaging was investigated in 10 patients with known or suspected NET liver metastases.[19] In the whole-body images, all hepatic and nodal lesions seen on PET/CT were also identified on PET/MR imaging. However, additional HBP PET/MR images detected more hepatic lesions (77%) *THAN* PET/CT (63%), which was primarily attributed to MR imaging that identified 99% of all liver lesions. The longer PET/MR imaging acquisition time of 15 minutes for the additional bed position over the liver may have also contributed to better delineation of liver metastases (vs 3 minutes per bed position for PET/CT). A recently published systemic review and meta-analysis evaluated the added value of PET/MR imaging for NET liver metastases and pooled results from studies involving small patient cohorts.[20] In addition to the aforementioned work,[8–10,19] the investigators included 2 more studies, where one compared retrospectively fused PET and MR imaging data with PET/CT.[21] This study is of interest, as it showed that retrospectively fused ^{68}Ga-DOTATOC PET/MR imaging had the highest sensitivity (PET/MR imaging 91.2% vs PET/CT 73.5%), however not significantly higher than MR imaging alone (87.6%), whereas specificity for fused PET/MR imaging (95.6%) did not significantly differ from that of PET/CT (88.2%), however higher than MR imaging alone (86.8%). Overall, fused PET/MR imaging performed better in identifying small, subcentimeter liver lesions, as these may have been below the resolution limit of PET/CT. As PET/MR imaging machines are not ubiquitously available, retrospective software fusion of MR imaging and PET might be a valuable tool.[21,22] However, misalignment or misregistration may limit image interpretation.[23] A more recent study included 11 patients with NET that were evaluated with ^{68}Ga-DOTATOC PET/MR imaging and PET/CT as well as carbon-11 (^{11}C) 5-hydroxy-tryptophan (5-HTP) PET/MR imaging.[24] ^{68}Ga-DOTATOC PET/MR imaging performed best by identifying the most lesions (72.5%), followed by ^{11}C-5-HTP PET/MR imaging (68.2%), MR imaging alone (67.8%), and ^{68}Ga-DOTATOC PET/CT (62.7%), whereas CT alone detected the least amount of lesions (53%). MR imaging performed best regarding liver metastases, followed by PET/MR imaging with ^{68}Ga-DOTATOC and ^{11}C-5-HTP. PET/MR imaging and PET/CT showed equal detection rates for lymph node and bone metastases but outperformed MR imaging and CT alone. The meta-analysis calculated a significantly higher pooled detection rate for liver metastases for SSTR targeting PET/MR imaging at 93.5% compared with PET/CT at 76.8%. The overall added value of PET/MR imaging over PET/CT was 15.3%. These results were mostly attributed to the high lesion conspicuity on HBP MR imaging (**Fig. 2**), especially when combined with DWI.[25] Even without contrast media, whole-body ^{68}Ga-DOTANOC PET/MR imaging with DWI yielded in an equal performance to gadoxetate-enhanced ^{68}Ga-DOTANOC PET/MR imaging for small, subcentimeter lesions in the assessment of abdominal NETs.[26]

FLUORODEOXYGLUCOSE-PET/MR IMAGING

Poorly differentiated NETs and NECs show downregulation of SSTR, whereas glucose transporters are upregulated, known as the *flip-flop phenomenon* (**Fig. 3**). The dedifferentiation progresses on a spectrum with up to 25% of NECs, particularly large-cell NECs, showing SSTR-positive and SSTR-negative lesions simultaneously.[3–5] Imaging with FDG and SSTR-targeting PET therefore is complementary in these patients and has the potential to detect all malignant lesions and consecutively to improve clinical decision making.[27–29] FDG imaging additionally harbors the ability to characterize tumor heterogenicity and predict disease prognosis. A positive FDG-PET is associated with worse outcome with shorter overall survival and progression-free survival.[28] Currently, there are no data available on a direct comparison of PET/MR imaging and PET/CT for FDG and SSTR-targeting imaging. A small number of PET/MR imaging examinations were used in a cohort of 83 patients with pancreatic NEN before surgical resection to evaluate the predictive role of ^{68}Ga-DOTATOC and ^{18}F-FDG-PET/CT and PET/MR imaging for risk stratification.[30] Somatostatin receptor density and total lesion somatostatin receptor density as well as metabolic tumor volume and tumor lesion glycolysis were able to distinguish pT1 and pT2 from pT3 and pT4 tumors. ^{68}Ga-DOTATOC maximal standardized uptake value (SUV) was a predictor for distant metastases, whereas metabolic tumor volume and tumor lesion glycolysis were predictors for angioinvasion. Dual-tracer imaging in patients with high-grade NENs and NECs provides relevant clinical information regarding tumor spread and aggressiveness, which impacts subsequent patient management.

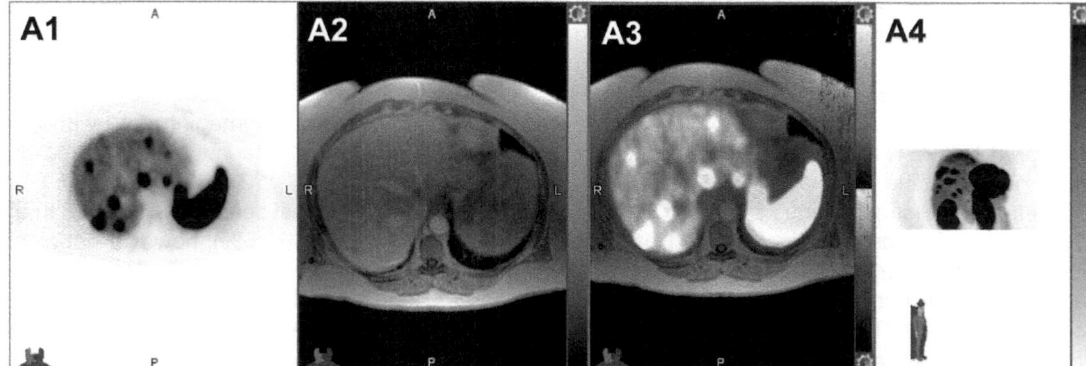

Fig. 2. A 68-year-old woman with NET (atypical carcinoid) of the lung. ^{68}Ga-DOTATATE PET/MR imaging (*A1–A4*, axial PET, MR imaging, fused PET/MR imaging, and MIP images, respectively) shows multiple hepatic lesions, which are generally mildly T2 and DWI hyperintense and hypointense on the HBP on MR imaging, whereas all demonstrate SSTR expression on PET. As this patient has a history of several liver-directed treatments (transarterial chemoembolization), PET/MR imaging follow-up imaging was chosen as the appropriate single-examination modality.

CHALLENGES

Attenuation Correction

Annihilation PET photons that arise from deep tissues have a higher tissue attenuation until they arrive at the detectors (eg, signal reduction) compared with PET photons arising from surface structures. Attenuation correction (AC) accounts for these photons that are more attenuated by adjusting the quantitative measure of tracer uptake, that is, SUV, to their corresponding tissue density. This enables quantitative accuracy of lesion comparison within and between imaging studies. PET/CT has the unique advantage that the CT transmission data can be used to create a CT energy photon attenuation map, which consecutively can be converted to a PET attenuation map for AC.[31] Conversely, MR images lack transmission sources owing to the high magnetic field and cannot be used for AC. Multiple alternate approaches to MR imaging–based attenuation correction (MRAC) for PET/MR imaging have been proposed.[32] The biggest challenge is to distinguish bone and lung (air) from other tissues, as both have near-zero signal in conventional MR imaging. The 2 major categories of MRAC are the atlas- and the direct imaging–based methods. In short, atlas-based method uses population data to generate an MR imaging/CT atlas that is aligned with MR images to create a pseudo-CT that is used for MRAC. This method relies on normal anatomy and tissue density; thus, any abnormalities, even in bone density, that divert from the population average may lead to large AC errors.[33] It has been well explored in neuroimaging but is not used for whole-body imaging. The direct imaging–based methods generate attenuation maps using the patient's MR imaging sequences, such as Dixon, ultrashort echo time (UTE), or zero echo time (ZTE), to characterize tissue qualities for MRAC. It is most accurate when used in conjunction with the segmentation method and MR/CT conversion. Particularly, UTE and ZTE sequences are used to assess osseous and air-filled structures (lung and bowel) in order to improve segmentation.[34,35] Machine learning has been used to derive a relationship between

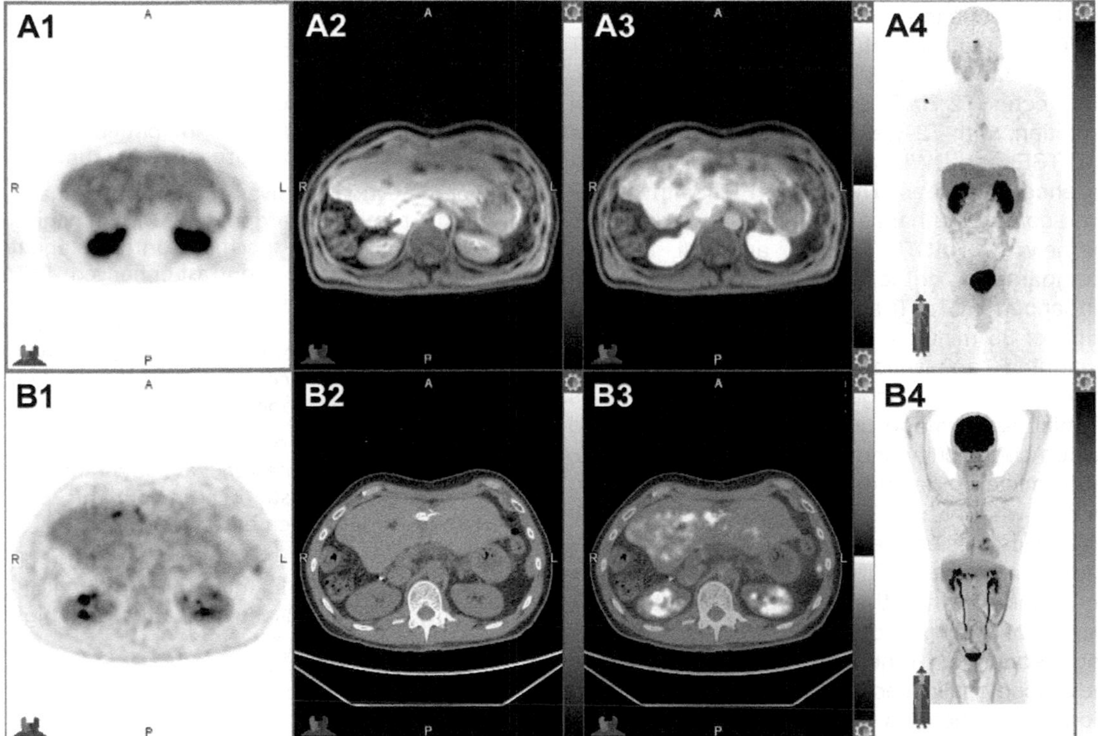

Fig. 3. A 50-year-old man with well-differentiated, Ki-67 10.5%, WHO grade 2 pancreatic NET and status post multiple hepatic resections. ^{68}Ga-DOTATATE PET/MR imaging (*A1–A4*, axial PET, MR imaging, fused PET/MR imaging, and MIP images, respectively) shows a 1.4-cm T2 hyperintense, DWI hyperintense, HBP hypointense lesion in segment IVb as well as a small hypoenhancing focus in segment 2. As no SSTR expression is seen, an ^{18}F-FDG-PET/CT (*B1–B4*, axial PET, CT, fused PET/MR imaging, and MIP images, respectively) was performed that shows hypermetabolic activity of the suspected hepatic lesions, which are, however, better delineated anatomically on MR imaging.

CT Hounsfield unit and MR imaging signal or to automatically segment bone tissues that can be used to generate a pseudo-CT for MRAC.[36–38] Inaccurate segmentation of bone tissues results in errors in SUV, whereas the area within or adjacent to cortical bone is the most affected. The resulting deviations in SUV of 10% to 20% were not clinically significant, even for the detection of bone metastases; however, the MRAC map should be reviewed for accuracy in bone tissue delineation when interpreting PET/MR imaging studies.[39–43]

IMAGING PROTOCOLS

The long acquisition time of multiple MR imaging sequences is challenging, not only for the clinical workflow but also for the patients, as the PET/MR imaging gantry is longer and narrower. Efforts were made to shorten MR imaging sequences to reduce overall imaging time. In a retrospective study including 29 patients with well-differentiated, metastasized NETs, fast non-contrast-enhanced PET/MR imaging examination protocols were compared with multiphase contrast-enhanced PET/CT.[44] Specifically, 4 PET/MR imaging setups were compared: PET and T2 half Fourier acquisition single shot turbo spin echo (T2 HASTE) acquisition alone, and in addition, with T2-weighted spin-echo sequence (T2 TSE) and DWI, respectively, and last, all sequences together. The latter, PET with only 3 non-contrast-enhanced MR imaging sequences, namely T2 HASTE, T2 TSE, and DWI, showed comparable detection rates to contrast-enhanced PET/CT at a reduced total imaging time of 35 minutes. Another fast dual-echo T2-weighted acquisition technique allowed for whole-body MR image acquisition in as little as 7 minutes.[45] Image quality was high with good lesion conspicuity and high signal-to-noise ratio, and minimal geometric distortion. Compared with whole-body PET/MR imaging DWI sequence, lesion detection of metastatic renal cancer was better. This fast technique allows for a quick scan of the whole body with the possibility of adding dedicated functional MR imaging sequences if needed. With the continued advancement in shortening MR image acquisition time, there is an increasing demand to match PET acquisition times. A reduced PET image acquisition time of 3 minutes per bed position has been shown to not impact image quality.[46] Efforts are also being made in improving lung sequences such as breath-hold techniques[47,48] or iterative motion-compensation reconstruction.[49]

SUMMARY

SSTR-targeted functional imaging using simultaneous PET/MR imaging has been shown to be valuable at staging and restaging of patients with well-differentiated NETs. The sensitivity and specificity were equally high compared with the current gold-standard PET/CT. Particularly in patients with liver metastases, PET/MR imaging with hepatocyte-specific contrast media outperformed PET/CT in diagnostic accuracy. PET/MR imaging offers the possibility of a one-stop-shop examination, streamlining the workflow for the clinician and offering the convenience of a single scan to the patient. PET/MR imaging protocols are advancing, providing faster sequences that are faster or on par with PET/CT acquisition times, and better lesion conspicuity in the lungs. With increasing availability and clinical adoption of PET/MR imaging systems, SSTR targeting PET/MR imaging has enormous potential to become standard of care in imaging of patients with NETs.

CLINICS CARE POINTS

- Somatostatin receptors targeting PET/MR imaging showed equally high sensitivity, specificity, and diagnostic accuracy with PET/computed tomography in patients with well-differentiated neuroendocrine tumors.
- For detection of liver metastases, somatostatin receptors targeting PET/MR imaging with hepatocyte-specific contrast agent were superior to contrast-enhanced PET/computed tomography; non-contrast-enhanced PET/MR imaging in combination with diffusion-weighted imaging showed equal performance to contrast-enhanced PET/computed tomography.
- PET/MR imaging offers a convenient one-stop-shop examination at low-radiation exposure that mostly benefits patients with liver-dominant disease.
- Limitations of ^{68}Ga-DOTA-somatostatin analogue PET/MR imaging include the availability only in academic centers and high costs.

DISCLOSURE

The authors have nothing to disclose.

REFERENCES

1. Fernandez CJ, Agarwal M, Pottakkat B, et al. Gastroenteropancreatic neuroendocrine neoplasms: a

clinical snapshot. World J Gastrointest Surg 2021; 13(3):231–55.
2. Rindi G, Mete O, Uccella S, et al. Overview of the 2022 WHO classification of neuroendocrine neoplasms. Endocr Pathol 2022;33(1):115–54.
3. Panagiotidis E, Alshammari A, Michopoulou S, et al. Comparison of the impact of 68Ga-DOTATATE and 18F-FDG PET/CT on clinical management in patients with neuroendocrine tumors. J Nucl Med 2017;58(1): 91–6.
4. Rindi G, Wiedenmann B. Neuroendocrine neoplasia of the gastrointestinal tract revisited: towards precision medicine. Nat Rev Endocrinol 2020;16(10): 590–607.
5. Konukiewitz B, Schlitter AM, Jesinghaus M, et al. Somatostatin receptor expression related to TP53 and RB1 alterations in pancreatic and extrapancreatic neuroendocrine neoplasms with a Ki67-index above 20. Mod Pathol 2017;30(4):587–98.
6. Sundin A, Arnold R, Baudin E, et al. ENETS consensus guidelines for the standards of care in neuroendocrine tumors: radiological, nuclear medicine & hybrid imaging. Neuroendocrinology 2017; 105(3):212–44.
7. Blanchet EM, Millo C, Martucci V, et al. Integrated whole-body PET/MRI with 18F-FDG, 18F-FDOPA, and 18F-FDA in paragangliomas in comparison with PET/CT: NIH first clinical experience with a single-injection, dual-modality imaging protocol. Clin Nucl Med 2014;39(3):243–50.
8. Beiderwellen KJ, Poeppel TD, Hartung-Knemeyer V, et al. Simultaneous 68Ga-DOTATOC PET/MRI in patients with gastroenteropancreatic neuroendocrine tumors: initial results. Invest Radiol 2013;48(5):273–9.
9. Sawicki LM, Deuschl C, Beiderwellen K, et al. Evaluation of (68)Ga-DOTATOC PET/MRI for whole-body staging of neuroendocrine tumours in comparison with (68)Ga-DOTATOC PET/CT. Eur Radiol 2017;27(10):4091–9.
10. Berzaczy D, Giraudo C, Haug AR, et al. Whole-body 68Ga-DOTANOC PET/MRI versus 68Ga-DOTANOC PET/CT in patients with neuroendocrine tumors: a prospective study in 28 patients. Clin Nucl Med 2017;42(9):669–74.
11. Modlin IM, Lye KD, Kidd M. A 5-decade analysis of 13,715 carcinoid tumors. Cancer 2003;97(4): 934–59.
12. Oberg K, Eriksson B. Endocrine tumours of the pancreas. Best Pract Res Clin Gastroenterol 2005; 19(5):753–81.
13. Frilling A, Li J, Malamutmann E, et al. Treatment of liver metastases from neuroendocrine tumours in relation to the extent of hepatic disease. Br J Surg 2009;96(2):175–84.
14. Madeira I, Terris B, Voss M, et al. Prognostic factors in patients with endocrine tumours of the duodenopancreatic area. Gut 1998;43(3):422–7.
15. Tomassetti P, Campana D, Piscitelli L, et al. Endocrine pancreatic tumors: factors correlated with survival. Ann Oncol 2005;16(11):1806–10.
16. Dromain C, de Baere T, Lumbroso J, et al. Detection of liver metastases from endocrine tumors: a prospective comparison of somatostatin receptor scintigraphy, computed tomography, and magnetic resonance imaging. J Clin Oncol 2005;23(1):70–8.
17. Sahani DV, Bonaffini PA, Fernandez-Del Castillo C, et al. Gastroenteropancreatic neuroendocrine tumors: role of imaging in diagnosis and management. Radiology 2013;266(1):38–61.
18. Ronot M, Cuccioli F, Dioguardi Burgio M, et al. Neuroendocrine liver metastases: vascular patterns on triple-phase MDCT are indicative of primary tumour location. Eur J Radiol 2017;89:156–62.
19. Hope TA, Pampaloni MH, Nakakura E, et al. Simultaneous (68)Ga-DOTA-TOC PET/MRI with gadoxetate disodium in patients with neuroendocrine tumor. Abdom Imaging 2015;40(6):1432–40.
20. Raj N, Coffman K, Le T, et al. Treatment response and clinical outcomes of well-differentiated high-grade neuroendocrine tumors to lutetium-177-DOTATATE. Neuroendocrinology 2022. https://doi.org/10.1159/000525216.
21. Schreiter NF, Nogami M, Steffen I, et al. Evaluation of the potential of PET-MRI fusion for detection of liver metastases in patients with neuroendocrine tumours. Eur Radiol 2012;22(2):458–67.
22. Donati OF, Hany TF, Reiner CS, et al. Value of retrospective fusion of PET and MR images in detection of hepatic metastases: comparison with 18F-FDG PET/CT and Gd-EOB-DTPA-enhanced MRI. J Nucl Med 2010;51(5):692–9.
23. Monti S, Cavaliere C, Covello M, et al. An evaluation of the benefits of simultaneous acquisition on PET/MR coregistration in head/neck imaging. J Healthc Eng 2017;2017:2634389.
24. Jawlakh H, Velikyan I, Welin S, et al. 68) Ga-DOTATOC-PET/MRI and (11) C-5-HTP-PET/MRI are superior to (68) Ga-DOTATOC-PET/CT for neuroendocrine tumour imaging. J Neuroendocrinol 2021; 33(6):e12981.
25. Hayoz R, Vietti-Violi N, Duran R, et al. The combination of hepatobiliary phase with Gd-EOB-DTPA and DWI is highly accurate for the detection and characterization of liver metastases from neuroendocrine tumor. Eur Radiol 2020;30(12):6593–602.
26. Mayerhoefer ME, Ba-Ssalamah A, Weber M, et al. Gadoxetate-enhanced versus diffusion-weighted MRI for fused Ga-68-DOTANOC PET/MRI in patients with neuroendocrine tumours of the upper abdomen. Eur Radiol 2013;23(7):1978–85.
27. Reubi JC. Peptide receptor expression in GEP-NET. Virchows Arch 2007;451(Suppl 1):S47–50.
28. Binderup T, Knigge U, Johnbeck CB, et al. (18)F-FDG-PET is superior to who grading as a prognostic

tool in neuroendocrine neoplasms and useful in guiding PRRT: a prospective 10-year follow-up study. J Nucl Med 2021;62(6):808–15.

29. Naswa N, Sharma P, Gupta SK, et al. Dual tracer functional imaging of gastroenteropancreatic neuroendocrine tumors using 68Ga-DOTA-NOC PET-CT and 18F-FDG PET-CT: competitive or complimentary? Clin Nucl Med 2014;39(1):e27–34.
30. Mapelli P, Partelli S, Salgarello M, et al. Dual tracer 68Ga-DOTATOC and 18F-FDG PET improve preoperative evaluation of aggressiveness in resectable pancreatic neuroendocrine neoplasms. Diagnostics (Basel) 2021;11(2). https://doi.org/10.3390/diagnostics11020192.
31. Kinahan PE, Hasegawa BH, Beyer T. X-ray-based attenuation correction for positron emission tomography/computed tomography scanners. Semin Nucl Med 2003;33(3):166–79.
32. Chen Y, An H. Attenuation correction of PET/MR imaging. Magn Reson Imaging Clin N Am 2017;25(2):245–55.
33. Akbarzadeh A, Ay MR, Ahmadian A, et al. MRI-guided attenuation correction in whole-body PET/MR: assessment of the effect of bone attenuation. Ann Nucl Med 2013;27(2):152–62.
34. Delso G, Wiesinger F, Sacolick LI, et al. Clinical evaluation of zero-echo-time MR imaging for the segmentation of the skull. J Nucl Med 2015;56(3):417–22.
35. Delso G, Carl M, Wiesinger F, et al. Anatomic evaluation of 3-dimensional ultrashort-echo-time bone maps for PET/MR attenuation correction. J Nucl Med 2014;55(5):780–5.
36. Hwang D, Kang SK, Kim KY, et al. Generation of PET attenuation map for whole-body time-of-flight (18)F-FDG PET/MRI using a deep neural network trained with simultaneously reconstructed activity and attenuation maps. J Nucl Med 2019;60(8):1183–9.
37. Leynes AP, Yang J, Wiesinger F, et al. Zero-Echo-Time and Dixon Deep Pseudo-CT (ZeDD CT): direct generation of pseudo-CT images for pelvic PET/MRI attenuation correction using deep convolutional neural networks with multiparametric MRI. J Nucl Med 2018;59(5):852–8.
38. Zaharchuk G, Davidzon G. Artificial intelligence for optimization and interpretation of PET/CT and PET/MR images. Semin Nucl Med 2021;51(2):134–42.
39. Seith F, Gatidis S, Schmidt H, et al. Comparison of positron emission tomography quantification using magnetic resonance- and computed tomography-based attenuation correction in physiological tissues and lesions: a whole-body positron emission tomography/magnetic resonance study in 66 patients. Invest Radiol 2016;51(1):66–71.
40. Liu G, Cao T, Hu L, et al. Validation of MR-based attenuation correction of a newly released whole-body simultaneous PET/MR system. Biomed Res Int 2019;2019:8213215.
41. Fraum TJ, Fowler KJ, McConathy J. Conspicuity of FDG-Avid osseous lesions on PET/MRI versus PET/CT: a quantitative and visual analysis. Nucl Med Mol Imaging 2016;50(3):228–39.
42. Moradi F, Iagaru A, McConathy J. Clinical applications of PET/MR imaging. Radiol Clin North Am 2021;59(5):853–74.
43. Samarin A, Burger C, Wollenweber SD, et al. PET/MR imaging of bone lesions–implications for PET quantification from imperfect attenuation correction. Eur J Nucl Med Mol Imaging 2012;39(7):1154–60.
44. Seith F, Schraml C, Reischl G, et al. Fast non-enhanced abdominal examination protocols in PET/MRI for patients with neuroendocrine tumors (NET): comparison to multiphase contrast-enhanced PET/CT. Radiol Med 2018;123(11):860–70.
45. Wang X, Pirasteh A, Brugarolas J, et al. Whole-body MRI for metastatic cancer detection using T2-weighted imaging with fat and fluid suppression. Magn Reson Med 2018;80(4):1402–15.
46. Duan H, Baratto L, Hatami N, et al. Reduced acquisition time per bed position for PET/MRI using (68)Ga-RM2 or (68)Ga-PSMA-11 in patients with prostate cancer: a retrospective analysis. AJR Am J Roentgenol 2022;218(2):333–40.
47. Crimi F, Varotto A, Orsatti G, et al. Lung visualisation on PET/MRI: implementing a protocol with a short echo-time and low flip-angle volumetric interpolated breath-hold examination sequence. Clin Radiol 2020;75(3):239.e15–21.
48. Chassagnon G, Martin C, Ben Hassen W, et al. High-resolution lung MRI with ultrashort-TE: 1.5 or 3 Tesla? Magn Reson Imaging Sep 2019;61:97–103.
49. Zhu X, Chan M, Lustig M, et al. Iterative motion-compensation reconstruction ultra-short TE (iMoCo UTE) for high-resolution free-breathing pulmonary MRI. Magn Reson Med 2020;83(4):1208–21.

Neuroendocrine Tumor Therapy Response Assessment

Vetri Sudar Jayaprakasam, MBBS, FRCR, FEBNM[a], Lisa Bodei, MD, PhD[a,*]

KEYWORDS

• Neuroendocrine neoplasms • Peptide receptor radionucleotide therapies • DOTA-Tyr^3-octreotate • Response • NETest • PPQ

KEY POINTS

- Response assessment of NENs is challenging due to their diverse morphologic and functional characteristics.
- Anatomic and functional imaging are synergistic in NEN management. ^{68}Ga-DOTA-SSA-peptides plays an integral role in diagnosis, response assessment, and follow-up of patients with NENs.
- SSR PET/MRI, artificial intelligence/machine learning, radiomics and multigenomic assays, like NETest and PPQ, will likely play a major role in NEN management and response assessment.

INTRODUCTION

Current nonsurgical treatment options available for the management of neuroendocrine neoplasms (NEN) include somatostatin analogues, targeted therapies, chemotherapy, and peptide receptor radionuclide therapies (PRRT). In the last decade, PRRT has reshaped the treatment paradigm of metastatic or inoperable NENs.[1,2] First described in the 1990s, radiolabeled somatostatin analogues using ^{111}In–DTPA–octreotide paved the way for a targeted form of diagnosis and systemic radiotherapy, allowing the delivery of radionuclides directly to the tumor cells.[3] More recently, β-emitting radionuclides (lutetium-177 [^{177}Lu] or yttrium-90 [^{90}Y]) chelated to oligopeptides, such as DOTATATE (DOTA-Tyr^3-octreotate) or DOTATOC (DOTA-D-Phe^1,Tyr^3-octreotide), target the somatostatin receptors, overexpressed on the cell surface of the NENs, delivering highly specific cytotoxic radiation therapy to the tumor cells.[4]

Several clinical trials have proven the efficacy and tolerability of the PRRT either on its own or in combination with other treatment modalities. Some of the earliest studies at the turn of the-century investigated PRRT with ^{90}Y, demonstrating an objective response rate of 26% and an overall clinical benefit in 76% of patients.[5] ^{177}Lu, with its ability of partial decay into γ-photons, proved useful for dosimetry and immediate response assessment, and replaced ^{90}Y in the treatment of NEN.[6,7] The landmark NETTER – 1 study showed a greater median overall survival (OS) of around 12 months in patients treated with ^{177}Lu-DOTATATE when compared with those receiving high-dose long-acting octreotide alone.[2] Significant improvement was seen in the quality of life, including global health status, physical functioning, and clinical symptom relief such as fatigue, pain, and diarrhea.[8] Prolongation in progression-free survival (PFS) was noted regardless of baseline liver tumor burden, target lesion size, or alkaline phosphatase levels.[9] In patients with advanced bronco-pulmonary carcinoid, treatment with ^{177}Lu-DOTATATE resulted in higher OS (61.4%) and greater morphologic responses (29.2%) compared to patients treated with ^{90}Y- DOTATATE alone (31.6% and 18.2% respectively).[10] The currently ongoing COMPETE trial aims to evaluate the efficacy and safety of

The authors have no conflic of interest related to the present work.

[a] Molecular Imaging and Therapy Service, Memorial Sloan Kettering Cancer Center, New York, NY, USA
* Corresponding author.
E-mail address: bodeil@mskcc.org

PET Clin 18 (2023) 267–286
https://doi.org/10.1016/j.cpet.2022.11.009
1556-8598/23/

^{177}Lu-DOTATOC (edotreotide) PRRT compared with everolimus in patients with inoperable, progressive, gastro-entero-pancreatic-NET.[11] Other clinical trials currently underway are investigating different treatment strategies and newer options, such as

- COMPOSE trial assessing efficacy of ^{177}Lu-edotreotide compared with best standard of care in well-differentiated Grade 2 and 3 GEP-NET
- SEQTOR trial evaluating the efficacy and safety of everolimus and STZ-5FU in advanced pancreatic NET
- AXINET trial comparing combination therapy of sandostatin LAR and axitinib to placebo in patients with well-differentiated nonpancreatic NEC[12,13]

Recently, treatment with alpha-emitting radioisotopes with high linear energy transfer, such as actinium-225 (^{225}Ac) and bismuth-213 (^{213}Bi) has gained interest, although clinical validation is still required.[14,15] Locoregional treatments such as transarterial embolization (TAE), transarterial chemoembolization (TACE), or radioembolization are now offered routinely in select tertiary centers, not only for high tumor burden or disease progression, but also for symptom control and treatment of disease complications.[16]

Overall, PRRT has a favorable safety profile with mild-to-moderate reversible toxicities, even in extensively pretreated metastatic NEN patients when standard protocols are followed.[17] The critical organs at risk are the kidneys and bone marrow. ^{177}Lu-DOTATATE treatment was found to be associated with lower rates of nephrotoxicity compared with ^{90}Y- DOTATATE therapy, 26% versus 44%, none of which were severe.[18] Most patients treated with ^{177}Lu-DOTATATE showed mild and reversible hematological toxicity.[2,18] Approximately 2% of patients treated with ^{177}Lu-DOTATATE develop myelodysplastic syndrome, and a smaller proportion progress to acute leukemia, although risk factors such as previous chemotherapy and platelet toxicity during PRRT do not always correlate with this untoward event.[18,19] In patients with bronchopulmonary carcinoid, combination ^{177}Lu-DOTATATE and ^{90}Y-DOTATOC therapy protocol demonstrated the highest association with hematological toxicities and resulted in decreased survival.[10] It should also be noted that approximately 15% to 20% of patients develop disease progression either during therapy or within 6 months to 1 year of completion of PRRT.[1,20]

The multiple treatment options highlight the varied treatment strategies available for the management of NEN, which is therefore multidisciplinary. Because of their generally slow-growing nature and the long development of the response to treatments such as radionuclide therapies or biotherapies, response assessment, particularly a timely appraisal of the disease trajectory, is a challenging task. Understanding the distinct biochemical, morphologic, and functional changes occurring in the tumor secondary to treatment is essential in management of patients with NEN.

Response Assessment

Inherent tumor characteristics of the NEN and different mechanisms of action of the treating agents present unique challenges in the response assessment. Traditional approaches to response assessment with computed tomography (CT) or MRI may not uncover the true extent or nature of response in these heterogenous groups of neoplasms. Currently, various prognostic and predictive clinical, biochemical, morphologic, and functional biomarkers are available in the management of patients with NEN. Overall response assessment should be based on the awareness of the strength and weakness of these individual modalities and inclusive of the newly developing biological, metabolic, and functional techniques.

Clinical Biomarkers–Patient Reported Outcome Measures

Clinically symptomatic NEN secondary to the functions of the secreted hormones can severely impact patient quality of life (QoL).[21] These symptoms can be diverse and nonspecific including diarrhea, flushing, pain, cramps, bronchospasm, palpitations, and weight loss. Carcinoid syndrome, associated with triad of flushing, diarrhea, and abdominal pain, is seen in approximately 20% of patients with NEN.[22] Symptoms may also be nonspecific and relate purely to overall tumor burden. In a large, global survey of 1928 patients with NENs, a considerable proportion of patients reported significant impact of the disease on their personal and professional lives, with complaints of poor to fair health (37%), fatigue/weakness (56%), and negative impact of finances (50%) and emotional health (60%).[21] The patient-reported outcome measures (PROM) constitute an important aspect of response assessment for patients undergoing treatment for NEN.[23] Health-related QoL (HR-QoL), a subset of PROM, is a subjective assessment of patient wellbeing, including the physical, psychological, and social aspects, that can be influenced by the disease and treatment.[24] HR-QoL related measurement tools allow for a better communication of the patient's own assessment of the disease symptoms and the effect of the treatment to the clinical team.[25]

In the recent years, there has been an increasing trend in utilization of the HR-QoL measurements in clinical trials. Some of these tools are generic and some specific to NEN. These can be administered using Likert scales, either on paper copies, online, or via a mobile application. The Karnofsky Performance Status Scale (KPSS), originally developed in 1948, measures the ability of patients to perform ordinary daily tasks and can be used to compare the effectiveness of different treatment modalities and assess prognosis.[26] The Eastern Cooperative Oncology Group (ECOG) performance criteria measure functional status, with a score ranging from "0" (fully active) to "5" (dead) and have been adopted by World Health Organization.[27] European Organization for Research and Treatment of Cancer (EORTC) QoL questionnaire (QLQ C-30) consists of 30 validated questions covering functional, symptom, global health, and QoL scales and converts the reported data into a score between 1 and 100.[28] Functional Assessment of Cancer Therapy - General (FACT-G) is a generic cancer self-report instrument to measure QoL incorporating physical, functional, social, and emotional subscales.[29]

Based on EORTC guidelines, NEN disease-specific questionnaire QLQ-GINET-21 was developed for assessing QoL in patients with gastrointestinal (GI) NEN.[30] This contains a total of 21 items, including assessment of muscle/bone pain, body image, sexual functioning, endocrine and GI symptoms, disease- and treatment-related worries. Norfolk QoL-NET is another NEN disease-specific 7-domain tool that incorporates respiratory, cardiovascular, and flushing scales in addition to the physical and mental assessment.[31] HR-QoL scores at baseline and during treatments can be used to assess changes in patient health status and compare between patient groups. A brief overview of the different components of the various HR-QoL questionnaire is presented in **Fig. 1**.

In a retrospective study of 504 patients with GEP-NETS undergoing treatment with ^{177}Lu-octreotate, Kwekkeboom and colleagues[32] reported a significant prognostic correlation of tumor remission prediction with a KPSS score of greater than 70 (P>.05). In the NETTER-1 trial, HR-QoL was assessed based on QLQ C-30 and GINET-21 questionnaires.[8] The study demonstrated significantly longer time to deteriorate (TTD) in the ^{177}Lu- DOTATATE arm in several health domains such as global health status (hazard ratio, HR, 0.41), physical functioning (HR, 0.52), diarrhea (HR, 0.47) and disease-related worries (HR, 0.57). Similar improvements in HR-QoL assessed by EORTC QLQ-C30 were reported by Marinova and colleagues[33] in patients with pancreatic NEN following PRRT. There was improvement in the global health status (P=.008) and social functioning (P=.049) at the end of the treatment and significant alleviation of symptoms such as fatigue, nausea, vomiting, and dyspnea. In patients with inoperable or metastasized GEP or bronchial NEN treated with ^{177}Lu- DOTATATE, Khan and colleagues[34] noticed a significant decrease in the EORTC global health status QoL and KPSS with disease progression after an initial response to treatment (ANOVA, $P \leq .01$).

One of the major limitations of the PROM/HR-QoL assessment tools is the reliance on patient understanding of the process and accurate communication. Although tools have been created to overcome the language and cultural barriers, they are still not perfect. Technical issues with data entry, lengthy questionnaires, or lack of easy accessibility to instruments can deter patient involvement. Easy-to-use, reliable, accessible and validated PROM/HR-QoL instruments, and patient education and awareness are the cornerstones in establishing accurate clinical response assessment.

Serum Biomarkers

Neoplastic cells secrete various peptides, amines or other molecules into the blood that can be measured and used as a diagnostic or prognostic biochemical biomarker. Several circulating serum biomarkers are used in the management of patients with NEN. These can be grouped as general biomarkers, seen in various NENs, or specific biomarkers associated with a particular type of NEN (**Fig. 2**). General circulating serum biomarkers include biomarkers such as chromogranin A (CgA), neuron-specific enolase (NSE), progastrin-releasing peptide, and inflammation-based index, derived from C-reactive protein and albumin (IBI).[35] CgA, a secretory granin protein present in the nervous, endocrine, and immune system, is considered as the default serum biomarker, despite its low accuracy.[36,37] Although still used routinely in clinical practice as a surrogate for tumor burden, it neither measures tumor behavior nor assesses response to treatment.[38] In a study by Brabander and colleagues,[39] the authors reported a 20% increase in the CgA levels after first cycle of PRRT in approximately 29% of patients, without a significant correlation between different response groups. It is also nonspecific, seen in benign conditions such as inflammatory bowel

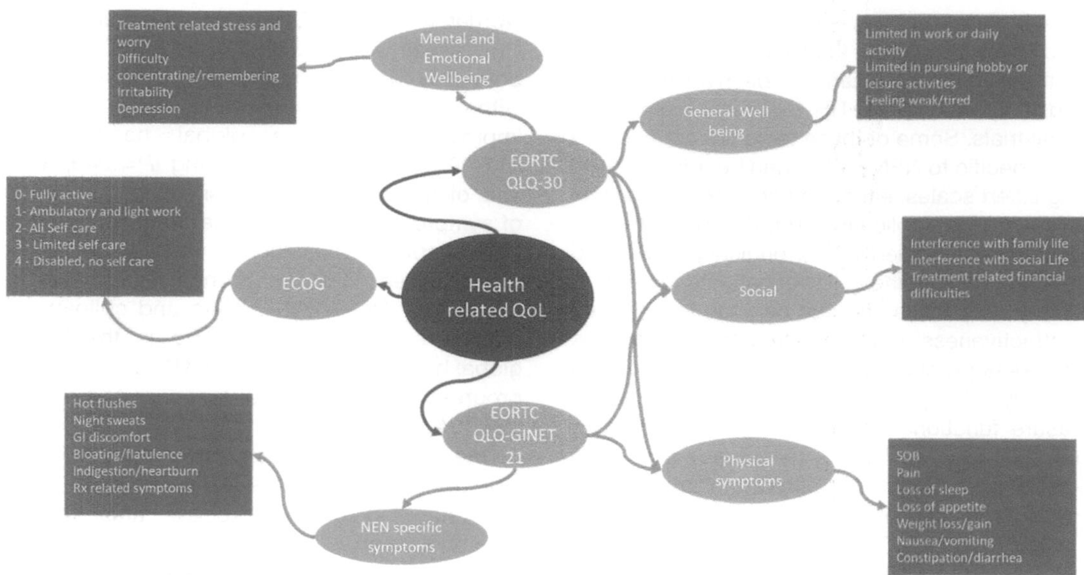

Fig. 1. Brief illustration of the HR-QoL assessment questionnaires relating to various domains.

disease, and in non-neuroendocrine malignancies such as hepatocellular carcinoma and prostate and thyroid cancers.[40–42] In addition, some NENs such as insulinoma, bronchopulmonary and poorly differentiated NENs are known to have low CgA expressions.[43] NSE is a glycolytic enzyme present in neurons and neuroendocrine cells. It is frequently elevated in patients with NEN, particularly those with small cell lung cancer and Merkel cell carcinoma.[44–46] However, it has a low specificity, with elevated levels seen in 46% of patients with peripheral NENS compared with 35% of non-NEN patients.[47]

Specific circulating serum biomarkers are associated with clinical syndromes such as serotonin and its metabolite 5-hydroxyindolacetic acid (5-

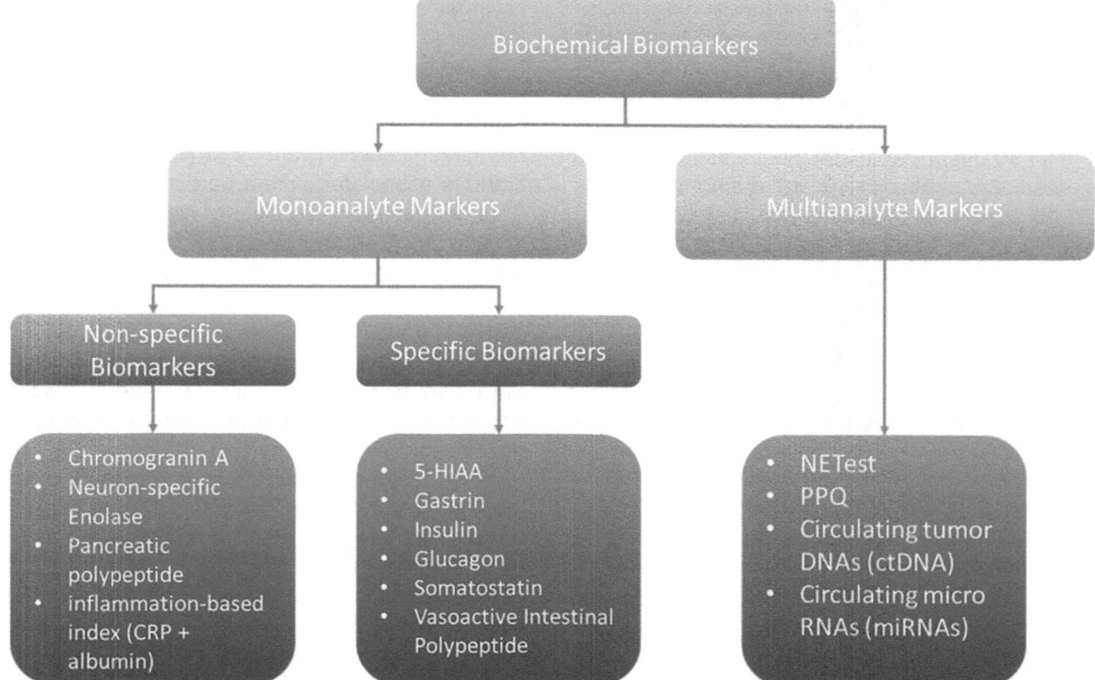

Fig. 2. Various biochemical biomarkers used in the detection and assessment of neuroendocrine neoplasms.

HIAA), insulin, gastrin, and vasoactive intestinal peptide (VIP). One of the commonly used specific biomarker is the 5-HIAA, which is the metabolite of serotonin and is secreted in the urine.[48] Serotonin is overexcreted in patients with small bowel NEN and is main cause for serotonin syndrome, particularly in setting of liver metastases, where the excess serotonin escapes liver metabolism.[49] The serum and plasma 5-HIAA have been shown to act as a surrogate for the 24-hour urinary 5-HIAA in patients with adequate renal function; however, larger studies are needed for validation.[50] Although the urinary 5-HIAA has an overall sensitivity and specificity of 70% and 90%, respectively, in the presence of carcinoid syndrome, existing data do not support its use as a reliable prognostic marker.[51,52] In the post-treatment setting, there may be a reduction in the levels of these specific biomarkers; however, neither the degree of reduction nor the absolute levels indicate the extent of response to treatment. Several clinical trials, including NETTER-1, have shown that these single-analyte biochemical biomarkers do not correlate with response to PRRT or survival outcome.[53]

In order to address the limitations of these monoanalyte biomarkers, there has been an increasing interest in developing multianalyte algorithmic assay (MAAA) which comprises circulating tumor DNA (ctDNA), circulating tumor cells (CTC), and micro RNAs (miRNAs).[54] These so-called liquid biopsies capture multidimensional information of tumor behavior and assess real-time treatment response. The technique has been used in other malignant and non-malignant conditions, such as ovarian cancers and liver disease.[55,56] Although ctDNA and miRNAs have shown promises in other malignancies, the role of these biomarkers has been limited in the response assessment of NEN. NETest is a polymerase chain reaction (PCR)-based multigene expression assay of 51 circulating NEN specific mRNAs, functioning as a liquid biopsy to identify NEN and monitor response to PRRT.[57,58] The 2-step protocol test involves mRNA isolation, cDNA production, and PCR from the collected blood samples, followed by normalization and quantification of the 51 marker-gene expressions.[58] It has been shown to be useful in detection, clinical monitoring, and prediction of PFS in NENs. It also correlates well with imaging assessment with CT/MR and RECIST measurements. In a validation study by Modlin and colleagues,[59] the NETest demonstrated a high sensitivity (85%–98%) and specificity (93%–97%) in differentiating of GEP-NETS from controls. Liu and colleagues[60] reported similar results in a mixed cohort of NEN patients. The NETest has a better sensitivity in detecting GEP-NETS when compared with CgA (85% vs 32%).[59] Malczewska and colleagues[61] demonstrated a significantly elevated of NETest score in patients with bronchopulmonary carcinoids when compared with controls (45 ± 25 vs 9 ± 8; $P<.0001$). The authors found significantly lower levels of NETest in the patients with non-NEN lung malignancies and benign lung disease when compared to patients with NEN ($P<.001$). NETest was also concordant with RECIST-based assessment of disease status and prognostic for PFS (odds ratio, 6.1; $P<.0001$).[60] In patients with advanced and inoperable GEP- and bronchopulmonary NEN undergoing PRRT, RECIST responders showed decreased levels of NETest compared with RECIST nonresponders ($-47 \pm 3\%$, $P<.0001$ vs $+ 79 \pm 19\%$, $P<.0005$).[57] NETest demonstrated increased accuracy in differentiating progressive versus stable disease (61 ± 26 vs 35.5 ± 18; $P<.0001$), and detection of patients with metastatic disease.[61]

PRRT Predictive Quotient (PPQ) is an algorithm that integrates NEN-specific gene transcripts (growth factor signaling and metabolism) with Ki-67 values to predict efficacy of the ^{177}Lu-DOTATATE PRRT and differentiate between PRRT responders and nonresponders.[62] In a set of 2 validation cohorts containing 44 and 42 patients each, PPQ accurately predicted response to PRRT in patients at baseline and follow-up, with a sensitivity of 94% to 97% and negative predictive value (NPV) of 93% to 95%.[62] There was significant difference in the median PFS between the PPQ + responders (not reached) and PPQ-nonresponders (10–14 months; HR 18–92, $P<.0001$). It was also demonstrated to be highly specific for PRRT, having no significant difference in prediction for median PFS in patients undergoing treatment with SSA alone. There was a positive correlation between the NETest levels and PPQ, with high levels of pretreatment NETest followed by significant decrease after treatment in PPQ + patients, namely responders and, vice-versa, increase in PPQ- or nonresponding patients.[57]

Imaging Biomarkers

In addition to the clinical and biochemical assessments, imaging biomarkers comprise an essential cornerstone in the management of the patients with NEN. Both anatomic and functional imaging play a key role in the staging, response assessment, and recurrent disease evaluation, and as such these should be used in conjunction to each other. Contrast-enhanced CT is one of the most commonly performed imaging modalities, and the accuracy of the study depends upon technique of acquisition.[63] NENs tend to be hypervascular, and hence, the CT is typically performed as a multiphase contrast-enhanced scan, including the arterial and portal-venous phase. MRI can be performed with either extracellular or hepatocyte-specific contrast agents. Diffusion weighted imaging (DWI) and apparent diffusion coefficient (ADC) maps are routinely included in the MRI protocol. Somatostatin receptor imaging (SSR) is performed with gallium-68 (^{68}Ga)-labeled SSA such as DOTATATE or DOTATOC in combination with CT or MRI, with or without intravenous contrast. ^{68}Ga-DOTA-SSA positron emission tomography (PET)/CT has now replaced ^{111}In-pentetreotide scintigraphy. ^{18}F-fluorodeoxyglucose (FDG) PET/CT can play an important role in poorly differentiated NENs or those with low or heterogeneous SSR expression. Imaging based response assessment in NEN can be challenging because of heterogenous tumor biology, variable growth kinetics, and the atypical effect of the therapy agents currently used in clinical practice and research settings.

NENs tend to be slow-growing tumors with delay in substantial increase or decrease in tumor size despite clinically benefitting from the treatment. Even in the setting of metastatic disease, patients with NET have prolonged survival. Several response criteria have been tried in the response assessment of NENs (**Fig. 3**). In most clinical trials, the objective tumor response is based on RECIST 1.1 criteria, developed mainly to evaluate response to cytotoxic chemotherapies. Based on RECIST 1.1, a 30% decrease in the sum of diameters of the target lesions signifies partial response, whereas a 20% increase is defined as progression.[64] Aside from the occurrence of unequivocal progression (markedly increased size or appearance of new lesions), or instances where there has been no significant interval change, the assessment of response is challenging (**Figs. 4** and **5**). Several studies have shown discordance between survival outcomes and the RECIST-based response assessments.[65] In a study of patients with advanced GEP-NET undergoing treatment with sunitinib, the time to tumor progression (TTP) was significantly different between the PR versus PD and SD versus PD groups categorized by RECIST 1.1 (P=.007 and P<.001 respectively). However, there was no significant difference in TTP between the PD and the SD groups (P=.131).[66] In patients with pancreatic NET treated with sunitinib who were deemed SD or PR based on RECIST, there was no statistically significant association between RECIST-based tumor response assessment and PFS in patients deemed SD or PR (Mantel–Byar test, P=.4).[67] In patients with progressive GEP NET undergoing PRRT with ^{177}Lu-DOTATATE, changes in 2-dimensional size based on REICST 1.1 criteria did not predict disease progression after 2 cycles of PRRT.[68]

Anatomic assessment alone of disease in some locations or under certain conditions may not always be accurate or feasible. Cardiac metastases are usually occult on CT[69] (**Fig. 6**). Osseous or peritoneal metastases on CT are considered unmeasurable based on RECIST 1.1 unless they

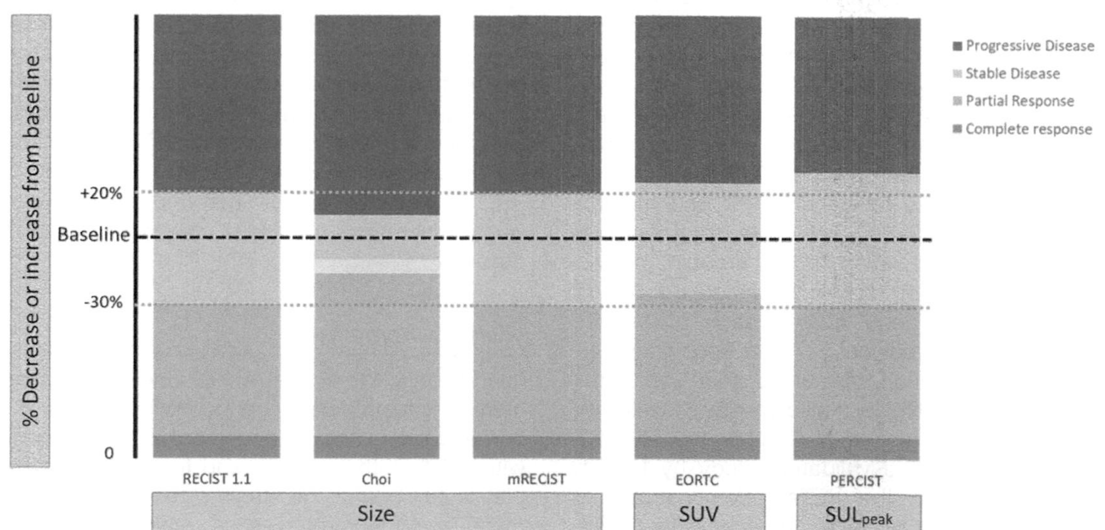

Fig. 3. Response assessment criteria used in neuroendocrine neoplasms. RECIST 1.1, CHOI, and mRECIST use size measurements for response assessment. CHOI criteria also use decrease in density for assessing partial response (*light yellow bar*). EORTC and PERCIST use changes in SUV and SULpeak for response assessment respectively.

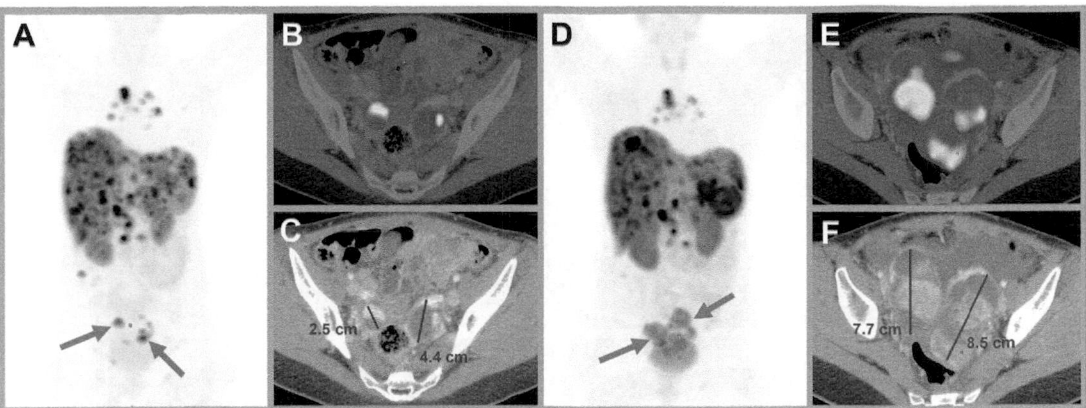

Fig. 4. 29-year-old woman with well-differentiated, high-grade pancreatic neuroendocrine tumor metastatic to the peritoneum, ovaries, omentum, lymph nodes, and liver, 1 year after diagnosis. Baseline ^{68}Ga-DOTATATE maximum intensity projection (MIP) (*A*) fused axial PET/CT (*B*) and contrast-enhanced CT (*C*) images before ^{177}Lu-DOTATATE therapy show intensely avid SSR-positive bilateral adnexal masses (*blue arrows*) and lung, liver, and nodal metastases. Following 4 cycles of ^{177}Lu-DOTATATE therapy, 68Ga-DOTATATE MIP (*D*), fused axial PET/CT (*E*), and contrast-enhanced CT (*F*) images show markedly increased bilateral adnexal masses, consistent with progression. Palliative resection of the adnexal masses was planned; however, the patient deteriorated clinically and passed away 5 months after completion of therapy.

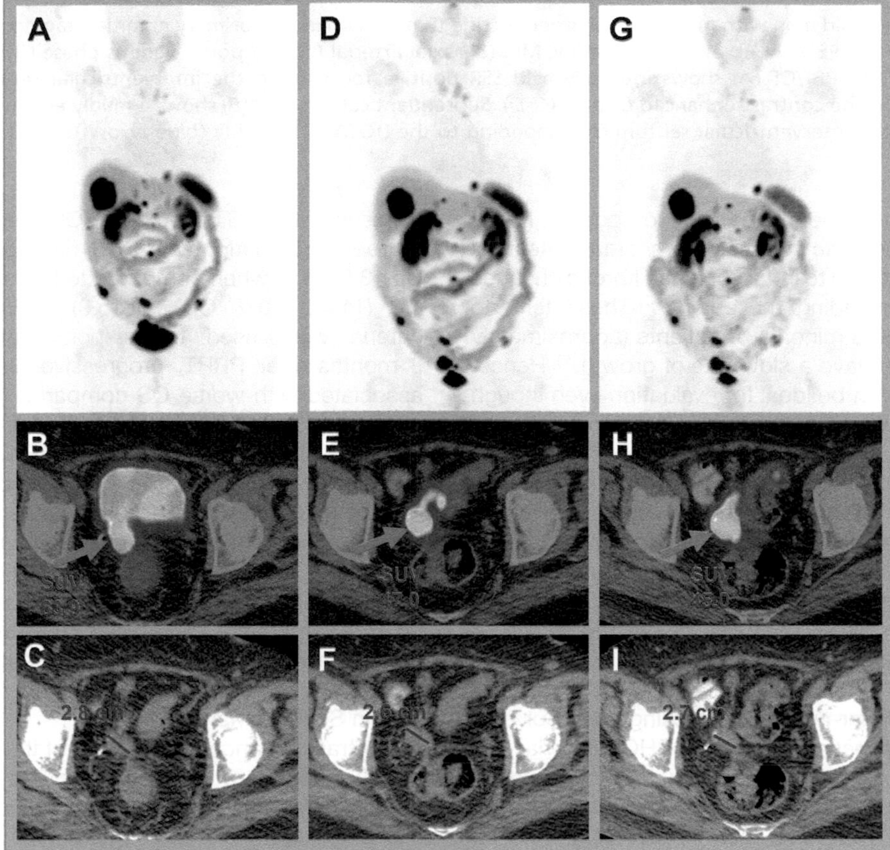

Fig. 5. 81-year-old woman with metastatic small bowel neuroendocrine tumor to liver, lymph nodes and peritoneum, 14 years after diagnosis. MIP (*A, D* and *G*), fused axial ^{68}Ga-DOTATATE PET/CT (*B, E,* and *H*), and low-dose companion CT (*C, F,* and *I*) images from baseline (*A–C*), immediately after (*D, F* and *G*) and post 1-year (*G–I*) following 4 cycles of ^{177}Lu-DOTATATE therapy, showing stable disease within the pelvic peritoneal nodule (*blue arrows*).

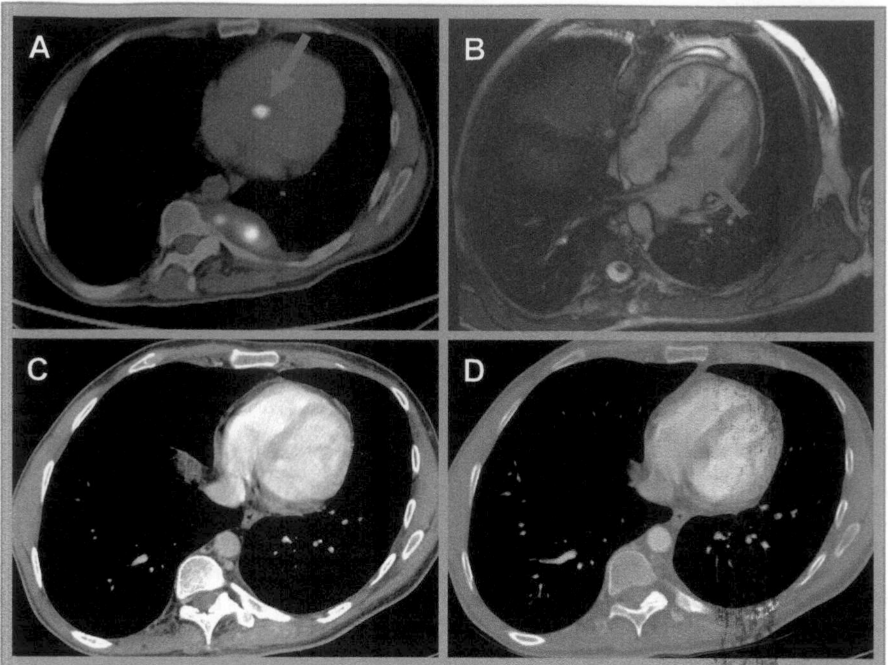

Fig. 6. 41-year-old man with metastatic neuroendocrine tumor of unknown primary at initial staging. Fused axial ^{68}Ga-DOTATATE PET/CT (*A*), axial T2W cardiac MRI (*B*), axial arterial (*C*) and portal venous phase CT (*D*) images. ^{68}Ga-DOTATATE PET/CT (*A*) shows intensely avid SSR positive focus along the interventricular septum, which was occult on the contrast-enhanced CT scan (*C, D*). Subsequent cardiac MRI (*B*) shows a mildly enhancing metastasis along the interventricular septum corresponding to the DOTATATE avidity (*blue arrows*).

have a well-defined soft tissue component. Metastatic mesenteric masses from small intestinal NETs are known to induce intense fibrotic changes in the surrounding mesentery.[70] These tend to grow only in a minority of patients (approximately 13.5%) and have a slow rate of growth.[71] Hence, these may not be ideal for evaluation even though they may be considered measurable lesion based on RECIST 1.1.

Since the introduction of targeted therapies in oncological treatments, it has been understood that anatomic information alone is not enough for response assessment. Response to targeted therapies may occur via decrease in tumor vascularity, increase in tumor necrosis, or cavitation with or without significant change in size.[72,73] Tumor necrosis can make a lesion more conspicuous or make it appear as new, mimicking stable or progressive disease[74] (**Fig. 7**). CHOI criteria use both tumor size and density in the response assessment. Partial response is described as a more than 10% decrease in size or more than 15% decrease in tumor density.[75] Huizing and colleagues[53] compared RECIST 1.1 and CHOI criteria for early response assessment and prediction of survival in patients undergoing PRRT. In 107 patients with pancreatic NET undergoing treatment with sunitinib, PFS based on CHOI criteria showed a greater correlation with OS (15.8 months; 95% CI, 13.9–25.7) when compared to PFS by RECIST 1.1 (11.42; 95% CI, 9.7–15.9).[67] When CHOI criteria were used for response assessment 9 months after PRRT, progressive disease was associated with worse OS compared with stable disease (HR 6.10; 95% confidence interval [CI] 1.38–27.05) and partial response (HR 22.66; 95% CI 2.33–219.99). Progressive disease on RECIST 1.1 showed worse prognosis compared with stable disease but not compared with partial response. Given the limitation of the morphologic assessments, determination of response based on RECIST criteria (82%), and Hounsfield Units (CHOI criteria) (76%) received a negative assessment in a multidisciplinary meeting of experts held in Spain in March 2015.[76]

Contrast enhancement pattern of the NEN seen on CT correlates with vascularity of the tumor and poorly differentiated NENs are generally less vascular than the well-differentiated NENs[77] (**Fig. 8**). NENs with decreased vascularity are associated with decreased OS. Arai and colleagues[78] evaluated the CT-based contrast enhancement ratio (CER) of pancreatic NEN to predict disease recurrence after resection. The

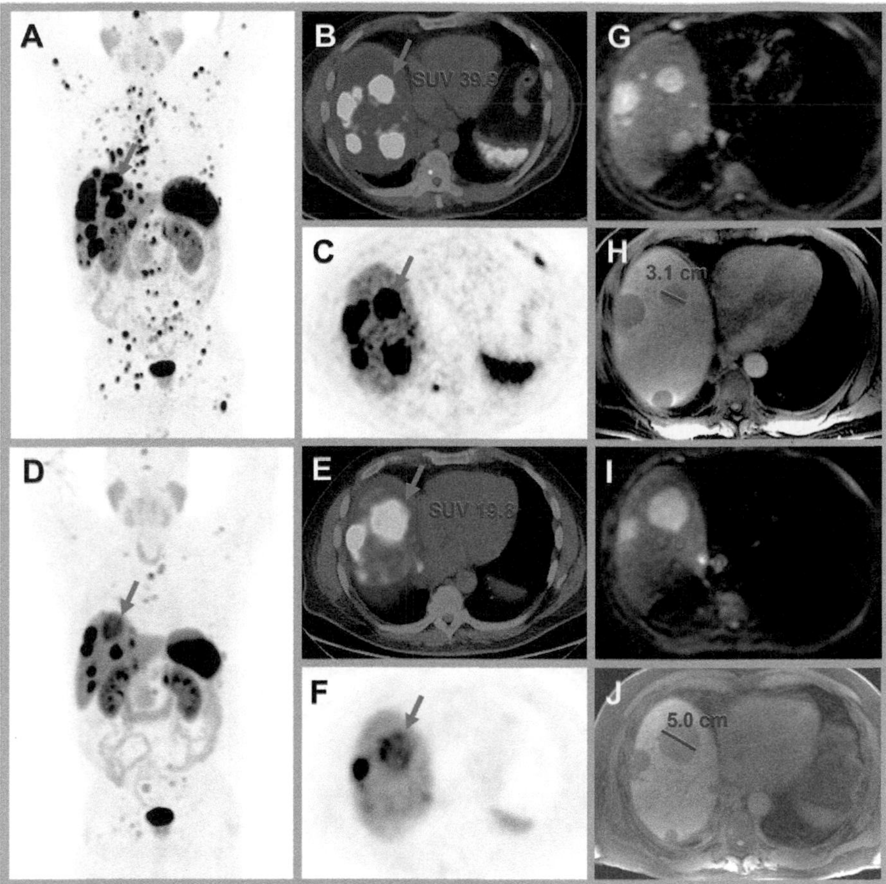

Fig. 7. 60-year-old man with metastatic bronchial carcinoid 6 years after diagnosis. Baseline ^{68}Ga-DOTATATE MIP (*A*), fused axial PET/CT (*B*), and PET (*C*) images before ^{177}Lu-DOTATATE therapy show intensely avid somatostatin receptor-positive hepatic and osseous metastases. Pretreatment axial DWI (*G*) and delayed contrast-enhanced (*H*) MRI demonstrate diffusion-restricting and hypo-enhancing liver metastases. Following 4 cycles of 177Lu-DOTATATE therapy, ^{68}Ga-DOTATATE MIP (*D*), fused axial PET/CT (*E*), and PET (*F*) images show decreased hepatic and osseous metastases, including decreased uptake within a superior segment 4 metastasis (*blue arrows*). Post-treatment axial DWI (*I*) and delayed contrast (*J*) MRI show increased size of the segment 4 metastasis from 3.1 cm to 5.0 cm, consistent with pseudoprogression. Sustained durable response was seen at 18 months following completion of PRRT (images not shown).

CER was calculated by dividing the CT Hounsfield unit (HU) at maximum enhanced phase by the HU of the precontrast scan. The authors reported a significantly lower median CER value for patients with recurrence compared to those without recurrence (2.9 vs 4.3, *P*=.013). Changes in tumor contrast enhancement patterns in patients with metastatic pancreatic NEN undergoing PRRT were evaluated by Pettersson and colleagues.[79] In this study of 37 patients, the authors found that there was an increase in the contrast enhancement of the metastases early on in the treatment (baseline to mid-treatment), followed by decreased contrast enhancement at later time points of therapy, and the early increased contrast enhancement had a moderate correlation with PFS. Changes in perfusion CT parameters such as tumor blood flow, blood volume, and mean transit time in patients with NEN undergoing treatment with bevacizumab has been tried in few studies, with decrease in perfusion parameters considered a sign of response assessment.[80,81] However, larger studies are needed to validate these hypotheses.

Multiparametric imaging with MRI (mpMRI) using with DWI and dynamic contrast-enhanced (DCE) sequences can be helpful in further assessment of response to treatment, although no standardized criteria exist (**Fig. 9**). DWI and DCE MRI images were evaluated for the early prediction of response in patients with NEN-related hepatic metastases undergoing therapy with ^{90}Y-

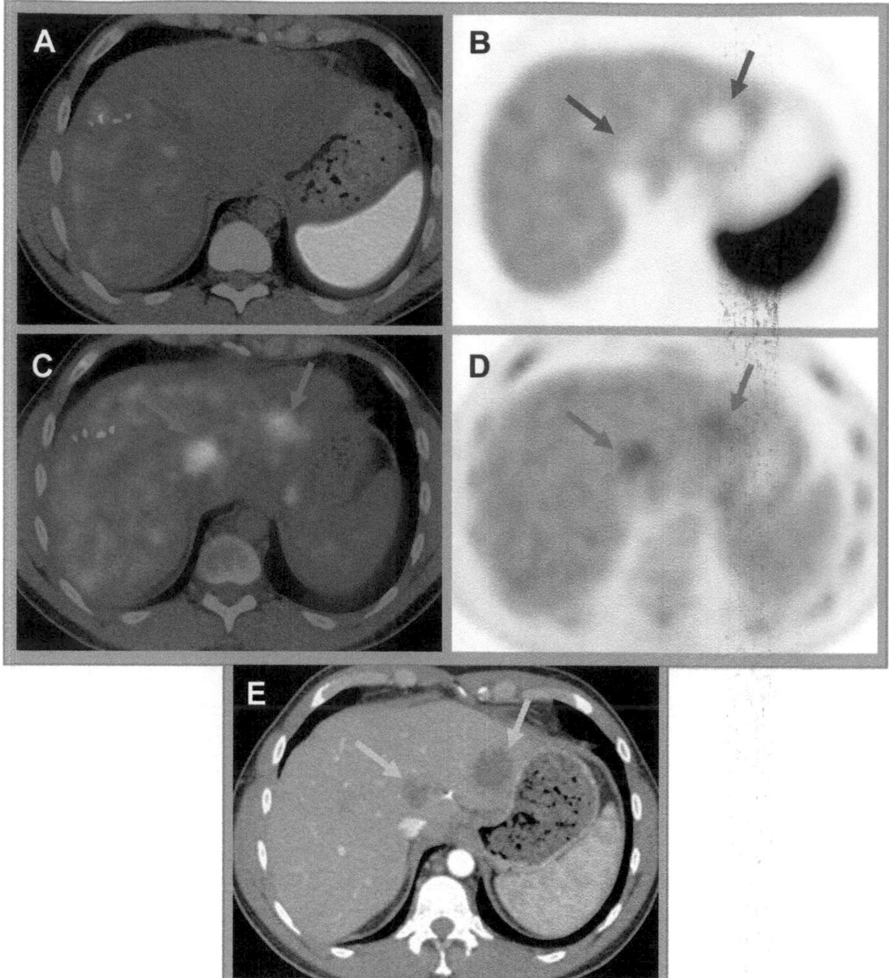

Fig. 8. 39-year-old man with poorly differentiated rectal neuroendocrine tumor metastatic to liver and nodes with Ki-67 of 80% at 15 months after diagnosis. ^{68}Ga-DOTATATE fused axial PET/CT (*A*) and PET (*B*) images show no SSR-positive focus within the liver metastases (*red arrows*). ^{18}F-FDG fused axial PET/CT (*C*) and PET (*D*) show moderately avid FDG uptake within the liver metastases (*blue arrows*), and arterial contrast-enhanced CT (E) shows poor vascularization within the metastases (*yellow arrows*), consistent with poor differentiation. Patient was treated with systemic chemotherapy.

DOTATOC[82] before and 48 hours after ^{90}Y-DOTATOC mpMRI was performed in 20 patients. Statically significant decreased restriction with higher ADC values were seen in the regressive liver lesions (*P*=.026). Miyazaki and colleagues[83] reported a better response to treatment in metastatic NEN with lower pretreatment distribution volume and high arterial flow fraction.

Somatostatin Receptor Imaging

SSR imaging using ^{68}Ga-DOTA-SSA-peptides plays an integral role in diagnosis, response assessment, and follow-up of patients with NENs. Standardized reporting system analogous to the PSMA-RADS has been proposed to help identify potential pitfalls, measure readers confidence in the presence of SSR expression tumor, and to guide the clinical team in selecting patients for PRRT.[84] Modified Krenning score, extrapolated from the one used in ^{111}In-Octreoscan, assigns a grade from a 5-point scale on the basis of qualitative assessment of uptake relative to blood pool and hepatic activity.[85] Patients with lesions larger than 2 cm and score of 3 or 4 should be considered for PRRT.

Several prognostic parameters have been evaluated based on the tumor SSTR expression as indicated by baseline ^{68}Ga-DOTA-SSA-peptides PET/CT. In patients with G1 and G2 pancreatic

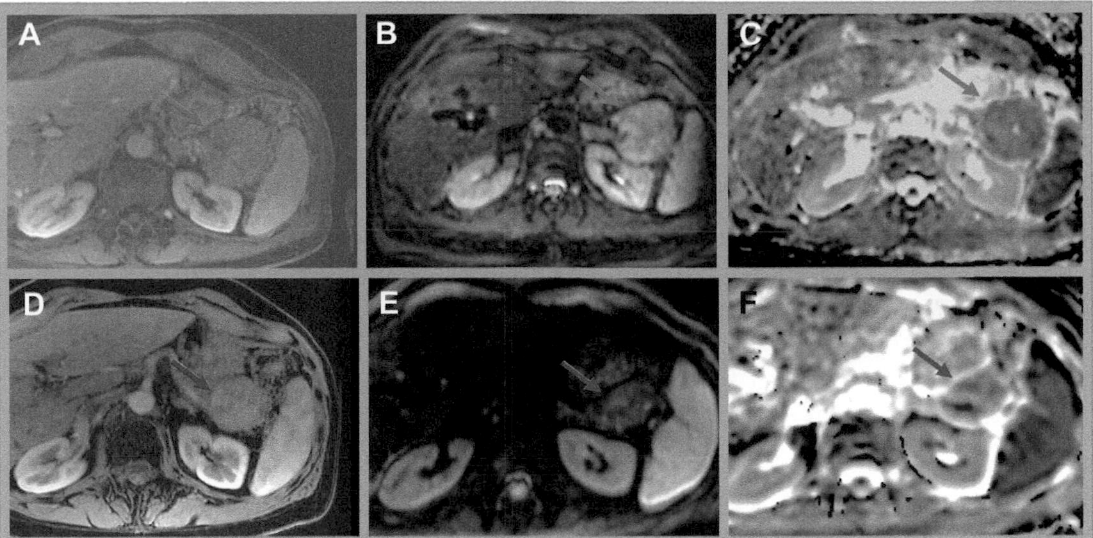

Fig. 9. 64-year-old man with pancreatic neuroendocrine tumor. Axial delayed contrast-enhanced MRI (*A, D*), diffusion-weighted images (*B, E*), and ADC maps (*C, F*) at baseline (*A–C*) and following 4 cycles of ^{177}Lu-DOTATATE therapy (*D–F*). Pretreatment images show enhancing pancreatic tail mass with restricted diffusion (*blue arrows*). Following PRRT, there is decrease in size with loss of restricted diffusion (*red arrows*), consistent with response to treatment.

NET, lower lesion maximum standardized uptake value (SUVmax) measured on ^{68}Ga-DOTANOC PET/CT was found to be associated with worse outcome (SUVmax ≤37.8; HR, 3.09; *P*=.003) and shorter PFS (SUVmax <37.8 vs >38.0; 16.0 vs 27.0 months; *P*=.002).[86] For response prediction to PRRT, Kratochwil and colleagues[87] proposed a SUVmax cut off of greater than 16.4 on ^{68}Ga-DOTATOC PET/CT for PRRT patient selection and a tumor-to-liver (T/L) ratio of greater than 2.2. Durmo and colleagues[88] found a high baseline whole-body tumor volume to be a predictor of unfavorable response to PRRT and decreased OS (HR 12.76, 95%CI 1.53–107, *P*=.01). For objective response prediction to PRRT, Sharma and colleagues[89] suggested single-lesion SUVmax and SUVmax-av (using up to 5 target lesions in multiple organ sites). Ortega and colleagues[90] demonstrated various baseline PET parameters such as higher mean SUVmax, ratio of lesion to liver SUVmax to predict response. However, none of these parameters have been validated for routine clinical assessment and, most importantly, cannot predict the response in a single patient.

In patients undergoing PRRT, post-therapy ^{177}Lu-DOTATATE whole-body planar imaging can be performed for dosimetry calculations and/or visual analysis of tracer distribution (**Fig. 10**). In a study of 16 patients undergoing PRRT, analysis of 53 post-therapy whole-body scans was found to be effective in the immediate validation of successful treatment and preliminary monitoring of the disease.[91] Development of ascites on the post-PRRT single-photon emission CT (SPECT)/CT suggested poor outcome, with decrease in OS compared to those who did not (13.2 months vs 37.9 months; *P*<.001).[92]

PRRT is usually offered for 4 cycles over a period of 8 months. During this time, the patients are followed by clinical and biochemical parameters. Imaging is performed only if clinically indicated. There is no definite role for interim ^{68}Ga-DOTA-SSA imaging. In the study by Durmo and colleagues,[88] an interim PET after 2 cycles of PRRT did not provide any useful information on response prediction or survival outcome. There may be an increase in size of the lesions on the post-PRRT scan caused by radiation-induced inflammation rather than true progression, known as pseudoprogression.[39] Hence, a delay of 2 to 3 months in performing the SSA PET/CT following completion of PRRT is advised. There is no unified consensus on the choice of imaging technique or the timing for the post-therapy SSA PET/CT imaging. EANM (European Association of Nuclear Medicine) recommends SSA PET/CT for monitoring response to therapy, whereas NCCN (National Comprehensive Cancer Network) guidelines recommend SSA PET/CT or PET/MRI in patients with unresectable locally advanced or metastatic disease only as clinically indicated.[93,94] Consequently, integration with monitoring biomarkers, such as NETest,

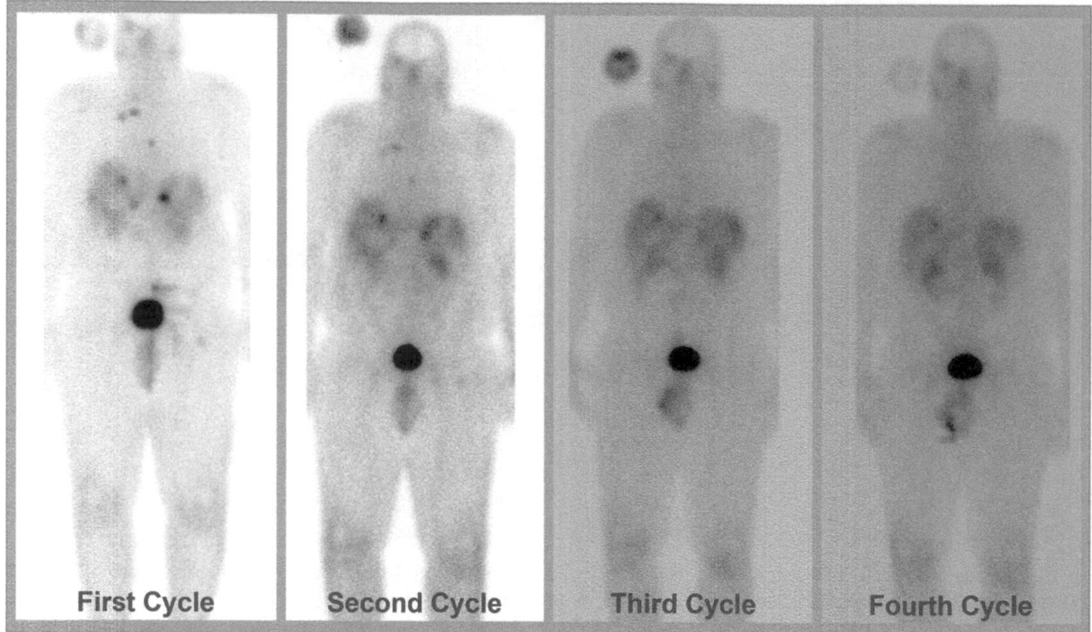

Fig. 10. 73-year-old man with well-differentiated insulin secreting G1 neuroendocrine tumor (Ki-67 2%) metastatic to the liver and bone. Whole-body planar images 3 hours after the completion of each cycle of ^{177}Lu-DOTATATE infusion demonstrating distribution in the blood pool, liver, kidneys, and spleen, as well as decreasing (and resolving) uptake in the pancreatic, liver, and skeletal lesions over the course of treatment.

able to identify treatment response before its completion, have been advocated.[57]

There are a few potential limitations when assessing response with post-therapy PET imaging. Standardized response criteria are yet to be defined. PERCIST use is not validated in the assessment of SSR PET/CT. There is no convincing correlation between changes in post-PRRT SUV changes and patient outcome. Increase in lesion SUVmax values on the post-therapy scan does not necessarily equate to disease progression as it does on FDG PET/CT. Increased SUVmax may imply increased SSR expression and tumor differentiation, whereas decreased uptake may indicate dedifferentiation and loss of SSR. When there is biochemical or

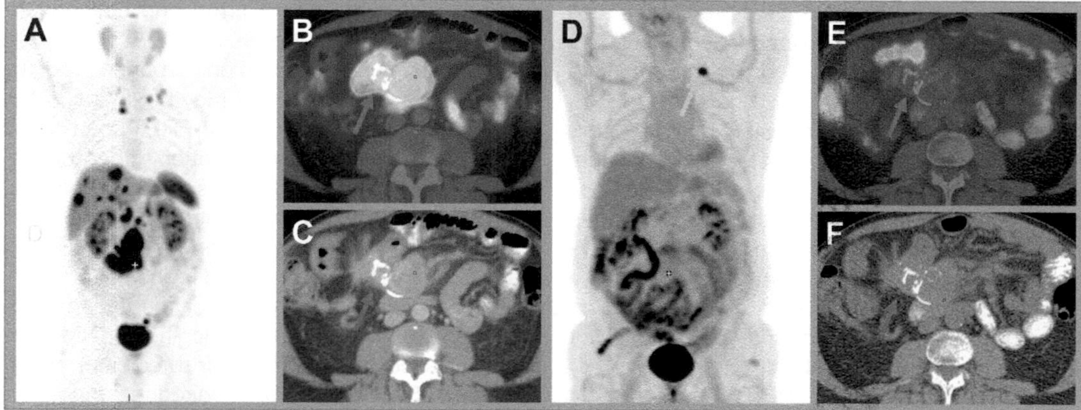

Fig. 11. 70-year-old man with metastatic well-differentiated GI neuroendocrine tumor, low grade, Ki-67 1% and mitotic rate of 1 per 10 HPFs, 6 years after diagnosis. ^{68}Ga-DOTATATE MIP (*A*), fused axial PET/CT (*B*), and contrast-enhanced CT (*C*) show a chronically stable mesenteric mass with partial calcification (*blue arrows*) and intense SSR positivity. ^{18}F-FDG (MIP) (*D*), fused axial PET/CT (*E*) and low-dose companion CT (*F*) show no appreciable FDG avidity within the mesenteric mass, consistent with low-grade disease. Incidental note is made of a synchronous FDG avid primary lung cancer within the left lung apex (*yellow arrow*).

clinical suspicion of disease progression, a new lesion on the SSR PET/CT may be considered unequivocal progression. However, a new lesion seen on the SSA PET/CT on a background of stable clinical and morphologic findings would be indeterminate.

Reporting clinicians must be aware of the pitfalls on the SSA PET/CT scans following ^{177}Lu-DOTATATE therapy. Small liver lesions may be difficult to assess on SSR imaging alone. DOTATATE uptake secondary to physiologic activities, benign pathology such as inflammation or nonneuroendocrine malignancies, may obscure response in NEN lesions.[95] For example, prominent physiologic uptake with the uncinate process can impede the response assessment in pancreatic head lesions. Potential changes in the intensity of uptake may be related to therapy with somatostatin analog.[96] With long-acting SSA, there is nearly 20% to 40% decrease of the DOTATATE SUVmax of the spleen, thyroid, and liver with associated rise in tumor SUVmax over background ratio. This may be misinterpreted as progression of disease. Tumors-sink effect, seen because of sequestration of radio pharmaceutical within intensely avid widespread tumor tissues, can lead to a decrease in healthy tissue uptake, and potentially mask uptake within the smaller metastases.[97,98] In addition, there may be disease differentiation during the course of treatment, which may affect the SSR activity and uptake.

A dual-tracer approach using SSA PET/CT and FDG PET/CT can offer some additional insight into the tumor heterogeneity, selection of biopsy site, prognostication, and response assessment (**Fig. 11**). In a retrospective evaluation of 52 patients with progressive advanced NEN treated with PRRT, a negative FDG PET/CT was associated with improved PFS compared with FDG-positive disease (26% vs 48%).[99] Thapa and colleagues[100] noted that high pretherapy FDG uptake was associated with increased incidences of refractoriness to PRRT. In a meta-analysis of 12 studies, higher percentage of pooled disease control rate (DCR) was seen in patients with negative FDG PET/CT before PRRT compared to those with positive FDG PET CT (91.9% vs 74.2%;

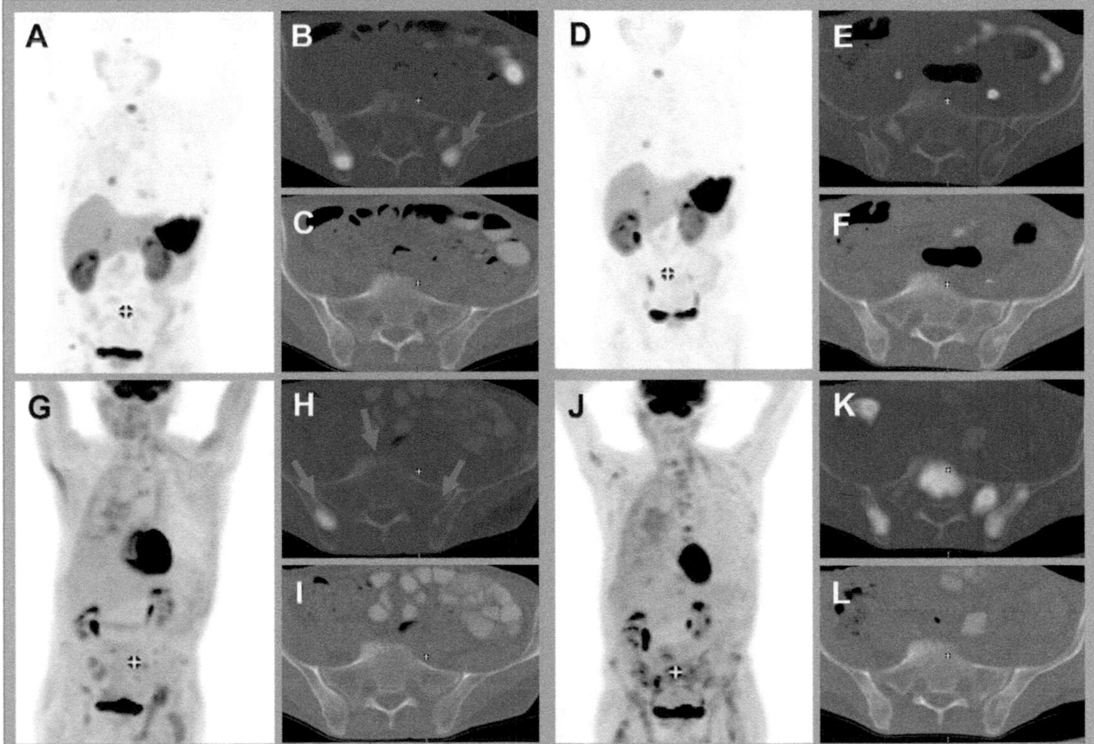

Fig. 12. 76-year-old man with neuroendocrine tumor of the lung 12 years after diagnosis. Baseline ^{68}Ga-DOTATATE MIP (*A*), fused axial PET/CT (*B*), and CT (*C*) images, and ^{18}F-FDG (MIP) (*G*), fused axial PET/CT (*H*) and CT (*I*) prior to 177Lu-DOTATATE therapy show discordant tracer avidity with increased SSR positivity within the pelvic osseus metastases compared with FDG uptake (*blue arrows*). Following 2 cycles of ^{177}Lu-DOTATATE, there is decreased SSR positivity (*D–F*) within the osseous metastases with increased metabolic activity (*J–L*) (*red arrowheads*), suggesting worsening de-differentiation.

random effects OR:4.85; 95% CI: 2.27–10.36).[101] The FDG PET/CT-positive patients also showed decreased OS, with an HR of 2.25 (95% CIs: 1.55–3.28). In patients with mixed differentiation, the NEN can show positivity to both SSR and FDG tracers. Treatment with PRRT is not considered ideal in these patients, as the PRRT may target the SSR-positive disease, leaving the non-SSTR disease to grow unchecked and cause progression (**Fig. 12**).

Response assessment in liver-targeted therapy

The liver is the most common site of metastases in patients with NEN and is associated with poor prognosis.[102,103] In recent years, there has been an increased interest in liver-directed therapy. Liver metastasis resection is performed in patients with completely resectable disease without extrahepatic metastases.[104] In patients with unresectable liver disease or extrahepatic metastases, treatment options include local ablations (radiofrequency, laser, or microwave) and angiographic techniques (transarterial embolization [TAE], transarterial chemoembolization [TACE], and selective internal radiotherapy [TARE]) (**Fig. 13**). Locally ablative therapy is suitable for a small number of lesions less than 5 cm, whereas transarterial therapy is offered for liver dominant large-volume disease. Liver metastases tend to be hypervascular and are best assessed on multiphase contrast-enhanced CT or MRI. Fiore and colleagues[105] reported similar results in patients treated with TAE and TACE with significant reduction in size of the liver lesions when compared with baseline studies (TAE - 2.2 ± 1.4 vs 3.3 ± 1.5; TACE - 2.2 ± 1.5 vs 3.4 ± 1.7 cm). Both TACE and TARE result in significant symptom control, particularly in patients with carcinoid syndrome or insulinoma.[106,107] Response assessment by contrast-enhanced ultrasound in patients after TAE or TACE showed decreased regional blood flow and relative blood volume tumor vitality index (P=.005, P=.04, and P=.03 respectively).[108]

FUTURE DIRECTIONS

In the coming years, SSR PET/MRI imaging is expected to play a bigger role in the evaluation of the patients with NEN. With recent technological advancements in acquisition parameters, PET/MRI is a clinically feasible option that offers a favorable combination of excellent anatomic visualization

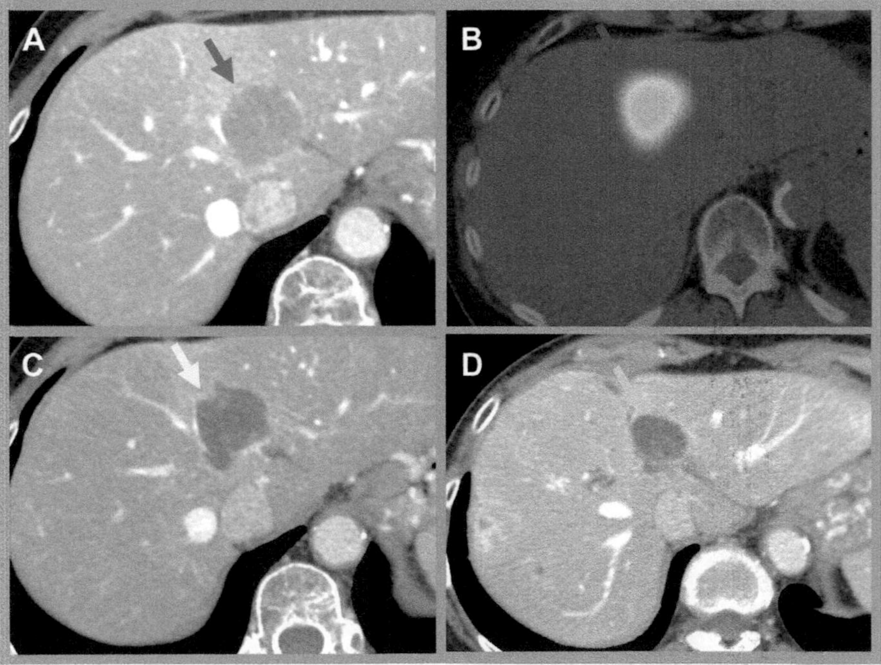

Fig. 13. 71-year-old woman with nonfunctional metastatic pancreatic neuroendocrine tumor 11 years after diagnosis, status after multiple lines of therapy including PRRT with progressive disease in the liver (*A*) (*blue arrow*). Patient underwent Y-90 SIR-Spheres radioembolization with intense bremsstrahlung activity within the metastasis (*B*) (*red arrow*). One month post-treatment CT image shows slightly increased size with decreased attenuation (*C*) (*yellow arrow*). Follow-up CT image 1 year after treatment shows increased contraction of lesion with persistent decreased attenuation (*D*) (*green arrow*).

along with functional and molecular assessment. An additional advantage is the option of addition of a dedicated site-specific (such as liver) protocol if clinically needed. Few studies are available looking at the response assessment on PET/MRI. In small cohort of mixed malignancies, including NEN, PET/MRI following ^{90}Y-microspheres showed significantly higher dose histogram (DVH) in responders compared with nonresponders.[109] Use of artificial intelligence (AI), machine learning, and radiomics has gained interest in the recent years. Radiomics features from CT and MRI have been analyzed to predict tumor grade, aggressiveness, and metastases. However, evidence for use of radiomics to predict response is still sparse.[110] Currently, the NETest offers the best sensitivity and specificity in identifying NEN and monitoring PRRT, whereas PPQ is best for predicting efficacy of the PPRT as well as a marker for radiosensitivity. In the near future, it would be safe to assume that these 2 biomarkers will play a major role in the clinical management of NEN patients.

SUMMARY

Diverse morphologic and functional characteristics of the NENs, along with availability of varied treatment strategies, pose a singular challenge in response assessment of these tumors. Because of these inherent and unavoidable variabilities, there is no standard approach to management of these patients. Treatment strategies and response assessment methodologies also vary in accordance with availability, affordability, and local expertise. In-depth understanding of the tumor biology, understanding the weaknesses and strengths of each investigative modalities, and a combined multidisciplinary personalized treatment strategy are essential in evaluation of patients with NEN.

CLINICS CARE POINTS

- Specific tumor characteristics of NENs and different mechanisms of action of the treating agents present unique challenges in the response assessment which benefits of the synergistic utilization of molecular and morphologic imaging techniques.
- CT or MRI alone may not depict the true extent or nature of response, as response to targeted therapies may occur via decrease in tumor vascularity, increase in tumor necrosis, or cavitation with or without significant change in size.
- ^{68}Ga-DOTA-SSA-peptides plays an integral role in response assessment. While standardized reporting system has been proposed and selection for PRRT is performed through a modified Krenning score, standardized response criteria are yet to be defined.
- Currently, various prognostic and predictive clinical, genomic, morphologic, and functional biomarkers are available in the management of patients with NEN.

ACKNOWLEDGMENT

This work was supported in part by NIH grants P30 CA008748 (S.J., L.B.)

REFERENCES

1. Strosberg J, El-Haddad G, Wolin E, et al. Phase 3 trial of (177)Lu-DOTATATE for midgut neuroendocrine tumors. N Engl J Med 2017;376(2):125–35.
2. Strosberg JR, Caplin ME, Kunz PL, et al. (177)Lu-DOTATATE plus long-acting octreotide versus high-dose long-acting octreotide in patients with midgut neuroendocrine tumours (NETTER-1): final overall survival and long-term safety results from an open-label, randomised, controlled, phase 3 trial. Lancet Oncol 2021;22(12):1752–63.
3. Krenning EP, de Jong M, Kooij PP, et al. Radiolabelled somatostatin analogue(s) for peptide receptor scintigraphy and radionuclide therapy. Ann Oncol 1999;10(Suppl 2):S23–9.
4. Bodei L, Mueller-Brand J, Baum RP, et al. The joint IAEA, EANM, and SNMMI practical guidance on peptide receptor radionuclide therapy (PRRNT) in neuroendocrine tumours. Eur J Nucl Med Mol Imaging 2013;40(5):800–16.
5. Bodei L, Cremonesi M, Grana C, et al. Receptor radionuclide therapy with 90Y-[DOTA]0-Tyr3-octreotide (90Y-DOTATOC) in neuroendocrine tumours. Eur J Nucl Med Mol Imaging 2004;31(7):1038–46.
6. de Jong M, Breeman WA, Bernard BF, et al. [177Lu-DOTA(0),Tyr3] octreotate for somatostatin receptor-targeted radionuclide therapy. Int J Cancer 2001;92(5):628–33.
7. Kwekkeboom DJ, Bakker WH, Kam BL, et al. Treatment of patients with gastro-entero-pancreatic (GEP) tumours with the novel radiolabelled somatostatin analogue [177Lu-DOTA(0),Tyr3]octreotate. Eur J Nucl Med Mol Imaging 2003;30(3):417–22.
8. Strosberg J, Wolin E, Chasen B, et al. Health-related quality of life in patients with progressive midgut neuroendocrine tumors treated with (177) Lu-DOTATATE in the phase III NETTER-1 trial. J Clin Oncol 2018;36(25):2578–84.

9. Strosberg J, Kunz PL, Hendifar A, et al. Impact of liver tumour burden, alkaline phosphatase elevation, and target lesion size on treatment outcomes with (177)Lu-DOTATATE: an analysis of the NETTER-1 study. Eur J Nucl Med Mol Imaging 2020;47(10):2372–82.
10. Mariniello A, Bodei L, Tinelli C, et al. Long-term results of PRRT in advanced bronchopulmonary carcinoid. Eur J Nucl Med Mol Imaging 2016; 43(3):441–52.
11. Pavel ME, Rinke A, Baum RP. 1335TiP - COMPETE trial: peptide receptor radionuclide therapy (PRRT) with 177Lu-edotreotide vs. everolimus in progressive GEP-NET. Ann Oncol 2018;29:viii478.
12. Jungels C, Deleporte A. State of the art and future directions in the systemic treatment of neuroendocrine neoplasms. Curr Opin Oncol 2021;33(4): 378–85.
13. Halfdanarson TR, Reidy DL, Vijayvergia N, et al. Pivotal phase III COMPOSE trial will compare 177Lu-edotreotide with best standard of care for well-differentiated aggressive grade 2 and grade 3 gastroenteropancreatic neuroendocrine tumors. J Clin Oncol 2022;40(4_suppl):TPS514–.
14. Kratochwil C, Apostolidis L, Rathke H, et al. Dosing (225)Ac-DOTATOC in patients with somatostatin-receptor-positive solid tumors: 5-year follow-up of hematological and renal toxicity. Eur J Nucl Med Mol Imaging 2021;49(1):54–63.
15. Bruchertseifer F, Kellerbauer A, Malmbeck R, et al. Targeted alpha therapy with bismuth-213 and actinium-225: meeting future demand. J Labelled Comp Radiopharm 2019;62(11):794–802.
16. Cazzato RL, Hubelé F, De Marini P, et al. Liver-directed therapy for neuroendocrine metastases: from interventional radiology to nuclear medicine procedures. Cancers (Basel) 2021;13(24):6368.
17. Rudisile S, Gosewisch A, Wenter V, et al. Salvage PRRT with (177)Lu-DOTA-octreotate in extensively pretreated patients with metastatic neuroendocrine tumor (NET): dosimetry, toxicity, efficacy, and survival. BMC Cancer 2019;19(1):788.
18. Bodei L, Kidd M, Paganelli G, et al. Long-term tolerability of PRRT in 807 patients with neuroendocrine tumours: the value and limitations of clinical factors. Eur J Nucl Med Mol Imaging 2015;42(1): 5–19.
19. Sabet A, Ezziddin K, Pape UF, et al. Long-term hematotoxicity after peptide receptor radionuclide therapy with 177Lu-octreotate. J Nucl Med 2013; 54(11):1857–61.
20. Kwekkeboom DJ, Kam BL, van Essen M, et al. Somatostatin-receptor-based imaging and therapy of gastroenteropancreatic neuroendocrine tumors. Endocr Relat Cancer 2010;17(1):R53–73.
21. Singh S, Granberg D, Wolin E, et al. Patient-reported burden of a neuroendocrine tumor (NET) diagnosis: results from the first global survey of patients with NETs. J Glob Oncol 2017;3(1):43–53.
22. Halperin DM, Huynh L, Beaumont JL, et al. Assessment of change in quality of life, carcinoid syndrome symptoms and healthcare resource utilization in patients with carcinoid syndrome. BMC Cancer 2019;19(1):274.
23. Warsame R, D'Souza A. Patient reported outcomes have arrived: a practical overview for clinicians in using patient reported outcomes in oncology. Mayo Clin Proc 2019;94(11):2291–301.
24. Barcaccia B, Esposito G, Matarese M, et al. Defining quality of life: a wild-goose chase? Eur J Psychol 2013;9(1):185–203.
25. Basch E, Deal AM, Kris MG, et al. Symptom monitoring with patient-reported outcomes during routine cancer treatment: a randomized controlled trial. J Clin Oncol 2016;34(6):557–65.
26. Chau I, Casciano R, Willet J, et al. Quality of life, resource utilisation and health economics assessment in advanced neuroendocrine tumours: a systematic review. Eur J Cancer Care (Engl) 2013; 22(6):714–25.
27. Oken MM, Creech RH, Tormey DC, et al. Toxicity and response criteria of the Eastern Cooperative Oncology Group. Am J Clin Oncol 1982;5(6): 649–55.
28. Aaronson NK, Ahmedzai S, Bergman B, et al. The European Organization for Research and Treatment of Cancer QLQ-C30: a quality-of-life instrument for use in international clinical trials in oncology. J Natl Cancer Inst 1993;85(5):365–76.
29. Cella DF, Tulsky DS, Gray G, et al. The functional assessment of cancer therapy scale: development and validation of the general measure. J Clin Oncol 1993;11(3):570–9.
30. Yadegarfar G, Friend L, Jones L, et al. Validation of the EORTC QLQ-GINET21 questionnaire for assessing quality of life of patients with gastrointestinal neuroendocrine tumours. Br J Cancer 2013; 108(2):301–10.
31. Vinik E, Carlton CA, Silva MP, et al. Development of the Norfolk quality of life tool for assessing patients with neuroendocrine tumors. Pancreas 2009;38(3): e87–95.
32. Kwekkeboom DJ, de Herder WW, Kam BL, et al. Treatment with the radiolabeled somatostatin analog [177 Lu-DOTA 0,Tyr3]octreotate: toxicity, efficacy, and survival. J Clin Oncol 2008;26(13): 2124–30.
33. Marinova M, Mücke M, Mahlberg L, et al. Improving quality of life in patients with pancreatic neuroendocrine tumor following peptide receptor radionuclide therapy assessed by EORTC QLQ-C30. Eur J Nucl Med Mol Imaging 2018;45(1):38–46.
34. Khan S, Krenning EP, van Essen M, et al. Quality of life in 265 patients with gastroenteropancreatic or

bronchial neuroendocrine tumors treated with [^{177}Lu-DOTA^{0},Tyr^{3}]Octreotate. J Nucl Med 2011; 52(9):1361.
35. Ma ZY, Gong YF, Zhuang HK, et al. Pancreatic neuroendocrine tumors: a review of serum biomarkers, staging, and management. World J Gastroenterol 2020;26(19):2305–22.
36. Oberg K, Modlin IM, De Herder W, et al. Consensus on biomarkers for neuroendocrine tumour disease. Lancet Oncol 2015;16(9): e435–46.
37. Feldman SA, Eiden LE. The chromogranins: their roles in secretion from neuroendocrine cells and as markers for neuroendocrine neoplasia. Endocr Pathol 2003;14(1):3–23.
38. Kidd M, Bodei L, Modlin IM. Chromogranin A: any relevance in neuroendocrine tumors? Curr Opin Endocrinol Diabetes Obes 2016;23(1):28–37.
39. Brabander T, van der Zwan WA, Teunissen JJM, et al. Pitfalls in the response evaluation after peptide receptor radionuclide therapy with [(177)Lu-DOTA(0),Tyr(3)]octreotate. Endocr Relat Cancer 2017;24(5):243–51.
40. Zissimopoulos A, Vradelis S, Konialis M, et al. Chromogranin A as a biomarker of disease activity and biologic therapy in inflammatory bowel disease: a prospective observational study. Scand J Gastroenterol 2014;49(8):942–9.
41. Biondi A, Malaguarnera G, Vacante M, et al. Elevated serum levels of chromogranin A in hepatocellular carcinoma. BMC Surg 2012;12(Suppl 1):S7.
42. Hong P, Guo RQ, Song G, et al. Prognostic role of chromogranin A in castration-resistant prostate cancer: a meta-analysis. Asian J Androl 2018; 20(6):561–6.
43. Hong L, Wang Y, Zhang T, et al. Chromogranin A: a valuable serum diagnostic marker for non-insulinoma neuroendocrine tumors of the pancreas in a Chinese population. Med Sci Monit 2020;26: e926635.
44. Oberg K, Jelic SO. Neuroendocrine gastroenteropancreatic tumors: ESMO clinical recommendation for diagnosis, treatment and follow-up. Ann Oncol 2009;20:iv150–3.
45. Burghuber OC, Worofka B, Schernthaner G, et al. Serum neuron-specific enolase is a useful tumor marker for small cell lung cancer. Cancer 1990; 65(6):1386–90.
46. Gambichler T, Abu Rached N, Susok L, et al. Serum neuron-specific enolase independently predicts outcomes of patients with Merkel cell carcinoma. Br J Dermatol 2022;187(5):806–8.
47. Nobels FR, Kwekkeboom DJ, Coopmans W, et al. Chromogranin A as serum marker for neuroendocrine neoplasia: comparison with neuron-specific enolase and the alpha-subunit of glycoprotein hormones. J Clin Endocrinol Metab 1997;82(8): 2622–8.
48. Tirosh A, Nilubol N, Patel D, et al. Prognostic utility of 24-hour urinary 5-HIAA doubling time in patients with neuroendocrine tumors. Endocr Pract 2018; 24(8):710–7.
49. Feldman JM, O'Dorisio TM. Role of neuropeptides and serotonin in the diagnosis of carcinoid tumors. Am J Med 1986;81(6b):41–8.
50. Adaway JE, Dobson R, Walsh J, et al. Serum and plasma 5-hydroxyindoleacetic acid as an alternative to 24-h urine 5-hydroxyindoleacetic acid measurement. Ann Clin Biochem 2016;53(Pt 5): 554–60.
51. Oberg K, Couvelard A, Delle Fave G, et al. ENETS consensus guidelines for standard of care in neuroendocrine tumours: biochemical markers. Neuroendocrinology 2017;105(3):201–11.
52. Janson ET, Holmberg L, Stridsberg M, et al. Carcinoid tumors: analysis of prognostic factors and survival in 301 patients from a referral center. Ann Oncol 1997;8(7):685–90.
53. Huizing DMV, Aalbersberg EA, Versleijen MWJ, et al. Early response assessment and prediction of overall survival after peptide receptor radionuclide therapy. Cancer Imaging 2020;20(1):57.
54. Kidd M, Drozdov I, Modlin I. Blood and tissue neuroendocrine tumor gene cluster analysis correlate, define hallmarks and predict disease status. Endocr Relat Cancer 2015;22(4):561–75.
55. Sang M, Wu X, Fan X, et al. Multiple MAGE-A genes as surveillance marker for the detection of circulating tumor cells in patients with ovarian cancer. Biomarkers 2014;19(1):34–42.
56. Barrera-Saldaña HA, Fernández-Garza LE, Barrera-Barrera SA. Liquid biopsy in chronic liver disease. Ann Hepatol 2021;20:100197.
57. Bodei L, Kidd MS, Singh A, et al. PRRT neuroendocrine tumor response monitored using circulating transcript analysis: the NETest. Eur J Nucl Med Mol Imaging 2020;47(4):895–906.
58. Modlin IM, Kidd M, Malczewska A, et al. The NETest: the clinical utility of multigene blood analysis in the diagnosis and management of neuroendocrine tumors. Endocrinol Metab Clin North Am 2018; 47(3):485–504.
59. Modlin IM, Drozdov I, Kidd M. The identification of gut neuroendocrine tumor disease by multiple synchronous transcript analysis in blood. PLoS One 2013;8(5):e63364.
60. Liu E, Paulson S, Gulati A, et al. Assessment of NETest clinical utility in a U.S. Registry-based study. Oncologist 2019;24(6):783–90.
61. Malczewska A, Oberg K, Bodei L, et al. NETest liquid biopsy is diagnostic of lung neuroendocrine tumors and Identifies progressive disease. Neuroendocrinology 2019;108(3):219–31.

62. Bodei L, Kidd MS, Singh A, et al. PRRT genomic signature in blood for prediction of (177)Lu-octreotate efficacy. Eur J Nucl Med Mol Imaging 2018; 45(7):1155–69.
63. Schueller G, Schima W, Schueller-Weidekamm C, et al. Multidetector CT of pancreas: effects of contrast material flow rate and individualized scan delay on enhancement of pancreas and tumor contrast. Radiology 2006;241(2):441–8.
64. Eisenhauer EA, Therasse P, Bogaerts J, et al. New response evaluation criteria in solid tumours: revised RECIST guideline (version 1.1). Eur J Cancer 2009;45(2):228–47.
65. de Mestier L, Dromain C, d'Assignies G, et al. Evaluating digestive neuroendocrine tumor progression and therapeutic responses in the era of targeted therapies: state of the art. Endocr Relat Cancer 2014;21(3):R105–20.
66. Luo Y, Chen J, Huang K, et al. Early evaluation of sunitinib for the treatment of advanced gastroenteropancreatic neuroendocrine neoplasms via CT imaging: RECIST 1.1 or Choi Criteria? BMC Cancer 2017;17(1):154.
67. Solis-Hernandez MP, Fernandez Del Valle A, Carmona-Bayonas A, et al. Evaluating radiological response in pancreatic neuroendocrine tumours treated with sunitinib: comparison of Choi versus RECIST criteria (CRIPNET_ GETNE1504 study). Br J Cancer 2019;121(7):537–44.
68. Zwirtz K, Hardt J, Acker G, et al. Comparison of CHOI, RECIST and somatostatin receptor PET/CT based criteria for the evaluation of response and response prediction to PRRT. Pharmaceutics 2022;14(6):1278.
69. Das S, Pineda G, Berlin J, et al. Hidden figures: occult intra-cardiac metastases in asymptomatic neuroendocrine tumor patients. J Oncol Cancer Res 2018;2:23–7.
70. Blažević A, Zandee WT, Franssen GJH, et al. Mesenteric fibrosis and palliative surgery in small intestinal neuroendocrine tumours. Endocr Relat Cancer 2018;25(3):245–54.
71. Blažević A, Brabander T, Zandee WT, et al. Evolution of the mesenteric mass in small intestinal neuroendocrine tumours. Cancers (Basel) 2021; 13(3):443.
72. Choi H, Charnsangavej C, de Castro Faria S, et al. CT evaluation of the response of gastrointestinal stromal tumors after imatinib mesylate treatment: a quantitative analysis correlated with FDG PET findings. AJR Am J Roentgenol 2004;183(6): 1619–28.
73. Chen MY, Bechtold RE, Savage PD. Cystic changes in hepatic metastases from gastrointestinal stromal tumors (GISTs) treated with Gleevec (imatinib mesylate). AJR Am J Roentgenol 2002; 179(4):1059–62.
74. Grimaldi S, Terroir M, Caramella C. Advances in oncological treatment: limitations of RECIST 1.1 criteria. Q J Nucl Med Mol Imaging 2018;62(2): 129–39.
75. Choi H, Charnsangavej C, Faria SC, et al. Correlation of computed tomography and positron emission tomography in patients with metastatic gastrointestinal stromal tumor treated at a single Institution with imatinib mesylate: proposal of new computed tomography response criteria. J Clin Oncol 2007;25(13):1753–9.
76. Oberg K, Krenning E, Sundin A, et al. A delphic consensus assessment: imaging and biomarkers in gastroenteropancreatic neuroendocrine tumor disease management. Endocr Connect 2016;5(5): 174–87.
77. Rodallec M, Vilgrain V, Couvelard A, et al. Endocrine pancreatic tumours and helical ct: contrast enhancement is correlated with microvascular density, histoprognostic factors and survival. Pancreatology 2006;6(1):77–85.
78. Arai T, Kobayashi A, Fujinaga Y, et al. Contrast-enhancement ratio on multiphase enhanced computed tomography predicts recurrence of pancreatic neuroendocrine tumor after curative resection. Pancreatology 2016;16(3):397–402.
79. Pettersson O, Fröss-Baron K, Crona J, et al. Tumor contrast-enhancement for monitoring of PRRT (177)Lu-DOTATATE in pancreatic neuroendocrine tumor patients. Front Oncol 2020;10:193.
80. Yao J, Phan A, Fogleman D, et al. Randomized run-in study of bevacizumab (B) and everolimus (E) in low-to intermediate-grade neuroendocrine tumors (LGNETs) using perfusion CT as functional biomarker. J Clin Oncol 2010;28(15_ suppl):4002.
81. Ng CS, Charnsangavej C, Wei W, et al. Perfusion CT findings in patients with metastatic carcinoid tumors undergoing bevacizumab and interferon therapy. Am J Roentgenol 2011;196:569–76.
82. Weikert T, Maas OC, Haas T, et al. Early prediction of treatment response of neuroendocrine hepatic metastases after peptide receptor radionuclide therapy with (90)Y-DOTATOC using diffusion weighted and dynamic contrast-enhanced MRI. Contrast Media Mol Imaging 2019;2019:1517208.
83. Miyazaki K, Orton MR, Davidson RL, et al. Neuroendocrine tumor liver metastases: use of dynamic contrast-enhanced MR imaging to monitor and predict radiolabeled octreotide therapy response. Radiology 2012;263(1):139–48.
84. Werner RA, Solnes LB, Javadi MS, et al. SSTR-RADS version 1.0 as a reporting system for SSTR PET imaging and selection of potential PRRT candidates: a proposed standardization framework. J Nucl Med 2018;59(7):1085–91.

85. Zidan L, Iravani A, Oleinikov K, et al. Efficacy and safety of (177)Lu-DOTATATE in lung neuroendocrine tumors: a bicenter study. J Nucl Med 2022; 63(2):218–25.
86. Ambrosini V, Campana D, Polverari G, et al. Prognostic value of 68Ga-DOTANOC PET/CT SUVmax in patients with neuroendocrine tumors of the pancreas. J Nucl Med 2015;56(12):1843–8.
87. Kratochwil C, Stefanova M, Mavriopoulou E, et al. SUV of [68Ga]DOTATOC-PET/CT predicts response probability of PRRT in neuroendocrine tumors. Mol Imaging Biol 2015;17(3):313–8.
88. Durmo R, Filice A, Fioroni F, et al. Predictive and prognostic role of pre-therapy and interim 68Ga-DOTATOC PET/CT parameters in metastatic advanced neuroendocrine tumor patients treated with PRRT. Cancers (Basel) 2022;14(3):592.
89. Sharma R, Wang WM, Yusuf S, et al. 68)Ga-DOTATATE PET/CT parameters predict response to peptide receptor radionuclide therapy in neuroendocrine tumours. Radiother Oncol 2019;141: 108–15.
90. Ortega C, Wong RKS, Schaefferkoetter J, et al. Quantitative (68)Ga-DOTATATE PET/CT parameters for the prediction of therapy response in patients with progressive metastatic neuroendocrine tumors treated with (177)Lu-DOTATATE. J Nucl Med 2021;62(10):1406–14.
91. Mahajan S, O'Donoghue J, Weber W, et al. Integrating early rapid post-peptide receptor radionuclide therapy quality assurance scan into the outpatient setting. J Nucl Med Radiat Ther 2019; 10(1):395.
92. Aalbersberg EA, de Vries-Huizing DMV, Tesselaar MET, et al. Post-PRRT scans: which scans to make and what to look for. Cancer Imaging 2022;22(1):29.
93. Bozkurt MF, Virgolini I, Balogova S, et al. Guideline for PET/CT imaging of neuroendocrine neoplasms with (68)Ga-DOTA-conjugated somatostatin receptor targeting peptides and (18) F-DOPA. Eur J Nucl Med Mol Imaging 2017; 44(9):1588–601.
94. Shah MH, Goldner WS, Benson AB, et al. Neuroendocrine and adrenal tumors, version 2.2021, NCCN clinical practice guidelines in oncology. J Natl Compr Canc Netw 2021;19(7):839–68.
95. Hofman MS, Lau WF, Hicks RJ. Somatostatin receptor imaging with 68Ga DOTATATE PET/CT: clinical utility, normal patterns, pearls, and pitfalls in interpretation. Radiographics 2015;35(2):500–16.
96. Cherk MH, Kong G, Hicks RJ, et al. Changes in biodistribution on (68)Ga-DOTA-Octreotate PET/CT after long acting somatostatin analogue therapy in neuroendocrine tumour patients may result in pseudoprogression. Cancer Imaging 2018; 18(1):3.
97. Beauregard JM, Hofman MS, Kong G, et al. The tumour sink effect on the biodistribution of 68Ga-DOTA-octreotate: implications for peptide receptor radionuclide therapy. Eur J Nucl Med Mol Imaging 2012;39(1):50–6.
98. Basu S, Ranade R, Abhyankar A. "Tumour sink effect" on the diagnostic or posttreatment radioiodine scan due to sequestration into large-volume functioning metastasis of differentiated thyroid carcinoma influencing uptake in smaller metastatic sites or remnant thyroid tissue: an uncommon but possible phenomenon in thyroid cancer practice. World J Nucl Med 2020;19(2): 141–3.
99. Severi S, Nanni O, Bodei L, et al. Role of 18FDG PET/CT in patients treated with 177Lu-DOTATATE for advanced differentiated neuroendocrine tumours. Eur J Nucl Med Mol Imaging 2013;40(6): 881–8.
100. Thapa P, Ranade R, Ostwal V, et al. Performance of 177Lu-DOTATATE-based peptide receptor radionuclide therapy in metastatic gastroenteropancreatic neuroendocrine tumor: a multiparametric response evaluation correlating with primary tumor site, tumor proliferation index, and dual tracer imaging characteristics. Nucl Med Commun 2016; 37(10):1030–7.
101. Alevroudis E, Spei ME, Chatziioannou SN, et al. Clinical utility of (18)F-FDG PET in neuroendocrine tumors prior to peptide receptor radionuclide therapy: a systematic review and meta-analysis. Cancers (Basel) 2021;13(8):1813.
102. Pape UF, Berndt U, Müller-Nordhorn J, et al. Prognostic factors of long-term outcome in gastroenteropancreatic neuroendocrine tumours. Endocr Relat Cancer 2008;15(4):1083–97.
103. Rindi G, D'Adda T, Froio E, et al. Prognostic factors in gastrointestinal endocrine tumors. Endocr Pathol 2007;18(3):145–9.
104. Frilling A, Modlin IM, Kidd M, et al. Recommendations for management of patients with neuroendocrine liver metastases. Lancet Oncol 2014;15(1): e8–21.
105. Fiore F, Del Prete M, Franco R, et al. Transarterial embolization (TAE) is equally effective and slightly safer than transarterial chemoembolization (TACE) to manage liver metastases in neuroendocrine tumors. Endocrine 2014;47(1):177–82.
106. Paprottka PM, Hoffmann RT, Haug A, et al. Radioembolization of symptomatic, unresectable neuroendocrine hepatic metastases using yttrium-90 microspheres. Cardiovasc Intervent Radiol 2012; 35(2):334–42.
107. Dermine S, Palmieri LJ, Lavolé J, et al. Non-pharmacological therapeutic options for liver metastases in advanced neuroendocrine tumors. J Clin Med 2019;8(11):1907.

108. Guibal A, Lefort T, Chardon L, et al. Contrast-enhanced ultrasound after devascularisation of neuroendocrine liver metastases: functional and morphological evaluation. Eur Radiol 2013;23:805–15.
109. Fowler KJ, Maughan NM, Laforest R, et al. PET/MRI of hepatic 90Y microsphere Deposition Determines individual tumor response. Cardiovasc Intervent Radiol 2016;39(6):855–64.
110. Staal FCR, Aalbersberg EA, van der Velden D, et al. GEP-NET radiomics: a systematic review and radiomics quality score assessment. Eur Radiol 2022;32(10):7278–94.

9780323938433